Communications
in Computer and Information Science   1993

Rationale

The CCIS series is devoted to the publication of proceedings of computer science conferences. Its aim is to efficiently disseminate original research results in informatics in printed and electronic form. While the focus is on publication of peer-reviewed full papers presenting mature work, inclusion of reviewed short papers reporting on work in progress is welcome, too. Besides globally relevant meetings with internationally representative program committees guaranteeing a strict peer-reviewing and paper selection process, conferences run by societies or of high regional or national relevance are also considered for publication.

Topics

The topical scope of CCIS spans the entire spectrum of informatics ranging from foundational topics in the theory of computing to information and communications science and technology and a broad variety of interdisciplinary application fields.

Information for Volume Editors and Authors

Publication in CCIS is free of charge. No royalties are paid, however, we offer registered conference participants temporary free access to the online version of the conference proceedings on SpringerLink (http://link.springer.com) by means of an http referrer from the conference website and/or a number of complimentary printed copies, as specified in the official acceptance email of the event.

CCIS proceedings can be published in time for distribution at conferences or as post-proceedings, and delivered in the form of printed books and/or electronically as USBs and/or e-content licenses for accessing proceedings at SpringerLink. Furthermore, CCIS proceedings are included in the CCIS electronic book series hosted in the SpringerLink digital library at http://link.springer.com/bookseries/7899. Conferences publishing in CCIS are allowed to use Online Conference Service (OCS) for managing the whole proceedings lifecycle (from submission and reviewing to preparing for publication) free of charge.

Publication process

The language of publication is exclusively English. Authors publishing in CCIS have to sign the Springer CCIS copyright transfer form, however, they are free to use their material published in CCIS for substantially changed, more elaborate subsequent publications elsewhere. For the preparation of the camera-ready papers/files, authors have to strictly adhere to the Springer CCIS Authors' Instructions and are strongly encouraged to use the CCIS LaTeX style files or templates.

Abstracting/Indexing

CCIS is abstracted/indexed in DBLP, Google Scholar, EI-Compendex, Mathematical Reviews, SCImago, Scopus. CCIS volumes are also submitted for the inclusion in ISI Proceedings.

How to start

To start the evaluation of your proposal for inclusion in the CCIS series, please send an e-mail to ccis@springer.com.

Hua Xu · Qingcai Chen · Hongfei Lin · Fei Wu ·
Lei Liu · Buzhou Tang · Tianyong Hao ·
Zhengxing Huang
Editors

Health Information Processing

9th China Health Information Processing Conference, CHIP 2023
Hangzhou, China, October 27–29, 2023
Proceedings

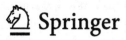 Springer

Editors
Hua Xu
The University of Texas Health Science
Center at Houston
Houston, TX, USA

Hongfei Lin (iD)
Dalian University of Technology
Dalian, China

Lei Liu
Fudan University
Shanghai, China

Tianyong Hao (iD)
South China Normal University
Guangzhou, China

Qingcai Chen
Harbin Institute of Technology
Shenzhen, China

Fei Wu
Zhejiang University
Hangzhou, China

Buzhou Tang (iD)
Harbin Institute of Technology
Shenzhen, China

Zhengxing Huang (iD)
Zhejiang University
Zhejiang, China

ISSN 1865-0929   ISSN 1865-0937 (electronic)
Communications in Computer and Information Science
ISBN 978-981-99-9863-0   ISBN 978-981-99-9864-7 (eBook)
https://doi.org/10.1007/978-981-99-9864-7

This Springer imprint is published by the registered company Springer Nature Singapore Pte Ltd.
The registered company address is: 152 Beach Road, #21-01/04 Gateway East, Singapore 189721, Singapore

Paper in this product is recyclable.

Preface

Health information processing and applications is an essential field in data-driven health and clinical medicine and it has been highly active in recent decades. The China Health Information Processing Conference (CHIP) is an annual conference held by the Medical Health and Biological Information Processing Committee of the Chinese Information Processing Society (CIPS) of China, with the theme of "large models and smart healthcare". CHIP is one of the leading conferences in the field of health information processing in China and turned into an international event in 2022. It is also an important platform for researchers and practitioners from academia, business and government departments around the world to share ideas and further promote research and applications in this field. CHIP 2023 was organized by Zhejiang University and held with a hybrid format both online and offline, whereby people face-to-face or freely connected to live broadcasts of keynote speeches and presentations.

CHIP 2023 received 66 submissions, of which 27 high-quality papers were selected for publication in this volume after double-blind peer review, leading to an acceptance rate of just 40%. These papers have been categorized into 3 main topics: Healthcare Information Extraction, Healthcare Natural Language Processing, and Healthcare Data Mining and Applications.

The authors of each paper in this volume reported their novel results in computing methods or applications. The volume cannot cover all aspects of Medical Health and Biological Information Processing but may still inspire insightful thoughts for the readers. We hope that more secrets of Health Information Processing will be unveiled, and that academics will drive more practical developments and solutions.

November 2023

Hua Xu
Qingcai Chen
Hongfei Lin
Fei Wu
Lei Liu
Buzhou Tang
Tianyong Hao
Zhengxing Huang

Organization

Honorary Chairs

Hua Xu   UTHealth, USA
Qingcai Chen   Harbin Institute of Technology (Shenzhen), China

General Co-chairs

Hongfei Lin   Dalian University of Technology, China
Fei Wu   Zhejiang University, China
Lei Liu   Fudan University, China

Program Co-chairs

Buzhou Tang   Harbin Institute of Technology (Shenzhen) & Pengcheng Laboratory, China
Tianyong Hao   South China Normal University, China
Yanshan Wang   University of Pittsburgh, USA
Maggie Haitian Wang   Chinese University of Hong Kong, China

Young Scientists Forum Co-chairs

Zhengxing Huang   Zhejiang University, China
Yonghui Wu   University of Florida, USA

Publication Co-chairs

Fengfeng Zhou   Jilin University, China
Yongjun Zhu   Yonsei University, South Korea

Evaluation Co-chairs

Jianbo Lei   Medical Informatics Center of Peking University,
                                   China
Zuofeng Li   Takeda Co. Ltd, China

Publicity Co-chairs

Siwei Yu   Guizhou Medical University, China
Lishuang Li   Dalian University of Technology, China

Sponsor Co-chairs

Jun Yan   Yidu Cloud (Beijing) Technology Co., Ltd. China
Buzhou Tang   Harbin Institute of Technology (Shenzhen) &
                                   Pengcheng Laboratory, China

Web Chair

Kunli Zhang   Zhengzhou University, China

Program Committee

Wenping Guo   Taizhou University, China
Hongmin Cai   South China University of Technology, China
Chao Che   Dalian University, China
Mosha Chen   Alibaba, China
Qingcai Chen   Harbin Institute of Technology (Shenzhen), China
Xi Chen   Tencent Technology Co., Ltd, China
Yang Chen   Yidu Cloud (Beijing) Technology Co., Ltd, China
Zhumin Chen   Shandong University, China
Ming Cheng   Zhengzhou University, China
Ruoyao Ding   Guangdong University of Foreign Studies, China
Bin Dong   Ricoh Software Research Center (Beijing) Co.,
                                   Ltd, China
Guohong Fu   Soochow University, China
Yan Gao   Central South University, China
Tianyong Hao   South China Normal University, China

Shizhu He	Institute of Automation, Chinese Academy of Sciences, China
Zengyou He	Dalian University of Technology, China
Na Hong	Digital China Medical Technology Co., Ltd, China
Li Hou	Institute of Medical Information, Chinese Academy of Medical Sciences, China
Yong Hu	Jinan University, China
Baotian Hu	Harbin University of Technology (Shenzhen), China
Guimin Huang	Guilin University of Electronic Science and Technology, China
Zhenghang Huang	Zhejiang University, China
Zhiwei Huang	Southwest Medical University, China
Bo Jin	Dalian University of Technology, China
Xiaoyu Kang	Southwest Medical University, China
Jianbo Lei	Peking University, China
Haomin Li	Children's Hospital of Zhejiang University Medical College, China
Jiao Li	Institute of Medical Information, Chinese Academy of Medical Sciences, China
Jinghua Li	Chinese Academy of Traditional Chinese Medicine, China
Lishuang Li	Dalian University of Technology, China
Linfeng Li	Yidu Cloud (Beijing) Technology Co., Ltd, China
Ru Li	Shanxi University, China
Runzhi Li	Zhengzhou University, China
Shasha Li	National University of Defense Technology, China
Xing Li	Beijing Shenzhengyao Technology Co., Ltd, China
Xin Li	Zhongkang Physical Examination Technology Co., Ltd, China
Yuxi Li	Peking University First Hospital, China
Zuofeng Li	Takeda China, China
Xiangwen Liao	Fuzhou University, China
Hao Lin	University of Electronic Science and Technology, China
Hongfei Lin	Dalian University of Technology, China
Bangtao Liu	Southwest Medical University, China
Song Liu	Qilu University of Technology, China
Lei Liu	Fudan University, China
Shengping Liu	Unisound Co., Ltd, China

Xiaoming Liu	Zhongyuan University of Technology, China
Guan Luo	Institute of Automation, Chinese Academy of Sciences, China
Lingyun Luo	Nanhua University, China
Yamei Luo	Southwest Medical University, China
Hui Lv	Shanghai Jiaotong University, China
Xudong Lv	Zhejiang University, China
Yao Meng	Lenovo Research Institute, China
Qingliang Miao	Suzhou Aispeech Information Technology Co., Ltd, China
Weihua Peng	Baidu Co., Ltd, China
Buyue Qian	Xi'an Jiaotong University, China
Longhua Qian	Suzhou University, China
Tong Ruan	East China University of Technology, China
Ying Shen	South China University of Technology, China
Xiaofeng Song	Nanjing University of Aeronautics and Astronautics, China
Chengjie Sun	Harbin University of Technology, China
Chuanji Tan	Alibaba Dharma Hall, China
Hongye Tan	Shanxi University, China
Jingyu Tan	Shenzhen Xinkaiyuan Information Technology Development Co., Ltd, China
Binhua Tang	Hehai University, China
Buzhou Tang	Harbin Institute of Technology (Shenzhen), China
Jintao Tang	National Defense University of the People's Liberation Army, China
Qian Tao	South China University of Technology, China
Fei Teng	Southwest Jiaotong University, China
Shengwei Tian	Xinjiang University, China
Dong Wang	Southern Medical University, China
Haitian Wang	Chinese University of Hong Kong, China
Haofen Wang	Tongji University, China
Xiaolei Wang	Hong Kong Institute of Sustainable Development Education, China
Haolin Wang	Chongqing Medical University, China
Yehan Wang	Unisound Intelligent Technology, China
Zhenyu Wang	South China Institute of Technology Software, China
Zhongmin Wang	Jiangsu Provincial People's Hospital, China
Leyi Wei	Shandong University, China
Heng Weng	Guangdong Hospital of Traditional Chinese Medicine, China

Gang Wu	Beijing Knowledge Atlas Technology Co., Ltd, China
Xian Wu	Tencent Technology (Beijing) Co., Ltd, China
Jingbo Xia	Huazhong Agricultural University, China
Lu Xiang	Institute of Automation, Chinese Academy of Sciences, China
Yang Xiang	Pengcheng Laboratory, China
Lei Xu	Shenzhen Polytechnic, China
Liang Xu	Ping An Technology (Shenzhen) Co., Ltd, China
Yan Xu	Beihang University, Microsoft Asia Research Institute, China
Jun Yan	Yidu Cloud (Beijing) Technology Co., Ltd, China
Cheng Yang	Institute of Automation, Chinese Academy of Sciences, China
Hai Yang	East China University of Technology, China
Meijie Yang	Chongqing Medical University, China
Muyun Yang	Harbin University of Technology, China
Zhihao Yang	Dalian University of Technology, China
Hui Ye	Guangzhou University of Traditional Chinese Medicine, China
Dehui Yin	Southwest Medical University, China
Qing Yu	Xinjiang University, China
Liang Yu	Xi'an University of Electronic Science and Technology, China
Siwei Yu	Guizhou Provincial People's Hospital, China
Hongying Zan	Zhengzhou University, China
Hao Zhang	Jilin University, China
Kunli Zhang	Zhengzhou University, China
Weide Zhang	Zhongshan Hospital Affiliated to Fudan University, China
Xiaoyan Zhang	Tongji University, China
Yaoyun Zhang	Alibaba, China
Yijia Zhang	Dalian University of Technology, China
Yuanzhe Zhang	Institute of Automation, Chinese Academy of Sciences, China
Zhichang Zhang	Northwest Normal University, China
Qiuye Zhao	Beijing Big Data Research Institute, China
Sendong Zhao	Harbin Institute of Technology, China
Tiejun Zhao	Harbin Institute of Technology, China
Deyu Zhou	Southeast University, China
Fengfeng Zhou	Jilin University, China
Guangyou Zhou	Central China Normal University, China
Yi Zhou	Sun Yat-sen University, China

Conghui Zhu	Harbin Institute of Technology, China
Shanfeng Zhu	Fudan University, China
Yu Zhu	Sunshine Life Insurance Co., Ltd, China
Quan Zou	University of Electronic Science and Technology, China
Xi Chen	University of Electronic Science and Technology, China
Yansheng Li	Mediway Technology Co., Ltd, China
Daojing He	Harbin Institute of Technology (Shenzhen), China
Yupeng Liu	Harbin University of Science and Technology, China
Xinzhi Sun	The First Affiliated Hospital of Zhengzhou University, China
Chuanchao Du	Third People's Hospital of Henan Province, China
Xien Liu	Beijing Huijizhiyi Technology Co., Ltd, China
Shan Nan	Hainan University, China
Xinyu He	Liaoning Normal University, China
Qianqian He	Chongqing Medical University, China
Xing Liu	Third Xiangya Hospital of Central South University, China
Jiayin Wang	Xi'an Jiaotong University, China
Ying Xu	Xi'an Jiaotong University, China
Xin Lai	Xi'an Jiaotong University, China

Contents

Healthcare Information Extraction

Healthcare Natural Language Processing

Healthcare Data Mining and Applications

Healthcare Information Extraction

Cross-Lingual Name Entity Recognition from Clinical Text Using Mixed Language Query

Kunli Shi[1], Gongchi Chen[1], Jinghang Gu[2], Longhua Qian[1(✉)], and Guodong Zhou[1]

[1] School of Computer Science and Technology, Soochow University, Suzhou, China
qianlonghua@suda.edu.cn
[2] Chinese and Bilingual Studies, Hong Kong Polytechnic University, Hong Kong, China

Abstract. Cross-lingual Named Entity Recognition (Cross-Lingual NER) addresses the challenge of NER with limited annotated data in low-resource languages by transferring knowledge from high-resource languages. Particularly, in the clinical domain, the lack of annotated corpora for Cross-Lingual NER hinders the development of cross-lingual clinical text named entity recognition. By leveraging the English clinical text corpus I2B2 2010 and the Chinese clinical text corpus CCKS2019, we construct a cross-lingual clinical text named entity recognition corpus (CLC-NER) via label alignment. Further, we propose a machine reading comprehension framework for Cross-Lingual NER using mixed language queries to enhance model transfer capabilities. We conduct comprehensive experiments on the CLC-NER corpus, and the results demonstrate the superiority of our approach over other systems.

Keywords: Cross-Lingual NER · Clinical Text · Mixed Language Query · Machine Reading Comprehension

1 Introduction

Named Entity Recognition (NER) is a task aimed at accurately locating entities within a given text and categorizing them into predefined entity types. It plays a crucial role in many downstream applications such as relation extraction and question answering. The development of deep learning technology has led to significant breakthroughs in this task. However, supervised learning methods often require a large amount of manually annotated training data, which can be costly and time-consuming, especially for low-resource languages. Therefore, many researchers have focused on zero-shot cross-lingual NER scenarios, which involve using annotated data from a resource-rich source language to perform NER in a target language without labeled data.

Zero-shot cross-lingual NER methods can typically be categorized into two types: annotation projection and direct model transfer. Annotation projection utilize annotated data from a source language to generate pseudo-labeled data in the target language [1–3]. Subsequently, they train NER models on the target language, enabling NER in the target language. One drawback of these methods is that the automatic translation used to generate target language data may introduce translation errors and label alignment errors.

H. Xu et al. (Eds.): CHIP 2023, CCIS 1993, pp. 3–21, 2024.
https://doi.org/10.1007/978-981-99-9864-7_1

On the other hand, direct model transfer learn language-agnostic features through feature space alignment, thereby transferring models trained on the source language to the target language [3–5]. The limitation of these methods is that they require a certain degree of similarity between the source and target languages, making them less applicable to languages with significant differences, such as Chinese and English.

Currently, most research efforts are concentrated on zero-shot cross-lingual NER tasks in general domains, with relatively little exploration in domain-specific cross-lingual NER. For instance, in the field of clinical medicine, the lack of relevant cross-lingual annotated data has hindered the development of cross-lingual clinical name entity recognition tasks. Furthermore, cross-lingual clinical name entity recognition poses more challenges due to variations in data volume, quality, structure, format, as well as differences in the naming conventions, abbreviations, and terminology usage of biomedical entities among different languages.

To facilitate the development of cross-lingual clinical entity recognition, we constructed a corpus for cross-lingual clinical name entity recognition (CLC-NER) using existing monolingual annotated corpora through label alignment. We employed cross-lingual pre-trained models (XLM-R) for knowledge transfer. Additionally, we introduced a machine reading comprehension framework and, based on this, proposed a cross-lingual named entity method using mixed language queries. By integrating prior knowledge from labels in different languages and exploring potential relationships between different annotated corpora in cross-lingual scenarios, we aimed to enhance task transfer performance.

2   Related Work

2.1   Cross-Lingual NER Corpus

Currently, cross-lingual named entity recognition tasks primarily rely on the CoNLL2002/2003 shared task data [6, 7] and the WikiAnn dataset [8]. The CoNLL2002/2003 dataset includes four closely related languages: English, German, Spanish, and Dutch, and focuses on four types of named entities in the news domain: person (PER), location (LOC), organization (ORG), and miscellaneou (MISC). WikiAnn, on the other hand, is a dataset encompassing 282 languages and includes various entity types such as person (PER), location (LOC), and organization (ORG). Previous research mainly employed CoNLL2002/2003 for studying transfer tasks in languages with similar linguistic systems, while WikiAnn was utilized to evaluate NER transfer performance when dealing with languages with more significant linguistic differences.

2.2   Cross-Lingual NER

Based on the shared content between the source language and the target language, cross-lingual named entity recognition methods are typically categorized into two approaches: annotation projection and direct model transfer.

Annotation projection method involves projecting annotated data from the source language to generate pseudo-labeled data in the target language. Previous methods often relied on parallel corpora [9]. Mayhew et al. [1] used a dictionary-based greedy decoding algorithm to establish word-to-word mappings between the source and target languages, reducing the dependency of annotation projection methods on parallel texts. However, word-to-word projection methods cannot consider contextual meaning, which can affect the quality of entity label projection. Jain et al. [10] employed machine translation to translate sentences and entities separately. They used dictionaries to generate candidate matches for translated entities and employed features such as orthography and phonetic recognition to match the translated entities, resulting in high-quality entity annotation projection.

Direct model transfer methods leverage shared representations between two languages, applying a model trained on the source language to the target language. Tsai et al. [4] generated Wikipedia features for cross-lingual transfer by linking the target language to Wikipedia entries. Ni et al. [9] built mapping functions between word vectors in different languages using dictionaries, enabling the mapping of target language vectors into source language vectors. However, direct model transfer cannot utilize lexicalized features when applied to the target language. Therefore, Xie et al. [2] improved upon methods like Ni et al. by incorporating a nearest-neighbor word vector translation approach, effectively leveraging lexicalized features and enhancing model transfer performance.

With the advancement of pre-trained models, models like BERT [11] have made significant progress in natural language understanding tasks by leveraging large-scale unlabeled text corpora for self-supervised learning to acquire latent knowledge in natural language texts. Multilingual models such as mBERT and XLM [9] further propelled the latest developments in cross-lingual understanding tasks. These cross-lingual models are trained on extensive multilingual unlabeled data, obtaining multilingual word embeddings and shared model parameters, thus enabling effective cross-lingual transfer on multilingual corpora. Keung et al. [5] built upon mBERT by using adversarial learning to align word vectors across different languages to enhance task performance. Wu et al. [12] proposed the Teacher-Student Learning (TSL) model for NER task transfer, which involves training a teacher model using source language annotated data and distilling knowledge from the teacher model to a student model using unannotated data in the target language, improving both single-source and multi-source transfer capabilities. Wu et al. [13] introduced the UniTrans framework, employing ensemble learning to fully utilize pseudo-labeled and unlabeled data for knowledge transfer, enhancing data reliability in transfer learning. Li et al. (2022) [14] extended the teacher-student model by proposing a multi-teacher multi-task framework (MTMT). By introducing a similarity task, they trained two teacher models to obtain pseudo-labeled data in the target language, and conducted multi-task learning on the student model, ultimately achieving strong performance on datasets like CoNLL2002/2003.

2.3 Machine Reading Comprehension

Machine Reading Comprehension (MRC) is originally a natural language understanding task used to test a machine's ability to answer questions given context. Levy et al. [15] were among the first to simplify relation extraction as a reading comprehension problem and effectively extended it to Zero-Shot scenarios. With the rise of deep learning and large-scale datasets, especially after the emergence of pre-trained models like BERT, many MRC systems based on pre-trained models have performed well on question-answering datasets such as SQuAD [16] and MS MARCO [17]. Some researchers began to recognize the versatility of the machine reading comprehension framework. Li et al. [18] proposed applying the MRC framework to named entity recognition, designing specific question templates for different entity categories, and providing a unified paradigm for nested and non-nested entities. To enhance information interaction between entity heads and tails, Cao et al. [19] introduced double affine transformations into MRC, achieving an F1 score of 92.8 on the CCKS2017 dataset. Zheng et al. [20] integrated the CRF-MT-Adapt model and MRC model using a voting strategy, achieving superior performance on the CCKS2020 dataset.

3   Dataset Construction

Due to the lack of existing cross-lingual clinical text Named Entity Recognition (NER) task datasets, we developed a dataset for investigating cross-lingual clinical text NER, referred to as CLC-NER, by aligning the labels of the CCKS 2019 dataset, which is designed for Chinese electronic medical records NER, and the 2010 I2B2/VA dataset, intended for English concept extraction. This alignment process enabled us to unify the labels of the two datasets, forming the basis for our research in cross-lingual clinical text NER.

3.1 CCKS 2019

CCKS 2019 (referred to as CCKS) [21] is part of a series of evaluations conducted by CCKS in the context of semantic understanding of Chinese electronic medical records. Building upon the medical named entity recognition evaluation tasks of CCKS2017 and 2018, CCKS2019 extends and expands the scope. It consists of two sub-tasks: medical named entity recognition and medical entity attribute extraction. Our work focuses on the first sub-task, which involves extracting relevant entities from medical clinical texts and identifying them into six predefined categories. These categories include diseases and diagnosis (疾病和诊断), imaging examination (影像检查), laboratory test (实验室检验), surgery (手术), medication (药物), and anatomical site (解剖部位).

3.2 I2B2 2010

The I2B2 2010 dataset [22] (referred to as I2B2)was jointly provided by I2B2 and the VA. This evaluation task consists of three sub-tasks: concept extraction, assertion classification, and relation classification. All three sub-tasks share the same dataset, comprising 349 training documents, 477 test documents, and 877 unlabeled documents. However, only a portion of the data has been publicly released after the evaluation. The publicly available I2B2 dataset includes 170 training documents and 256 test documents. Our focus is on the concept extraction task, which defines three concept entity types: medical problem, medical treatment, and medical test.

3.3 Correlation

The above subsection provide descriptions of the concepts or entity types in the two datasets. We can observe that while their annotation schemes differ somewhat, there are certain corresponding relationships between some types. One notable difference is that CCKS includes the "anatomical site" class of entities, used to specify the anatomical site in the human body where diseases or symptoms occur, whereas I2B2 does not annotate such entities.

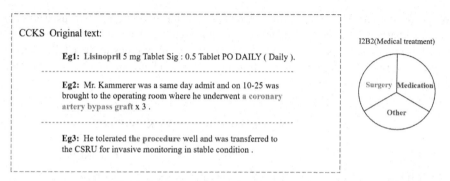

Fig. 1. Differences in entity annotation scope.

On the other hand, the concepts annotated in the I2B2 dataset are broader in scope than the entities in the CCKS dataset. As shown in Fig. 1, the "Medical Treatment" type in I2B2 encompasses not only explicit treatment methods, such as "Surgery" and "Medication", as seen in the first two examples, but also includes some general treatment concepts, as in the third example where "the procedure" refers to a certain treatment process. As illustrated in Fig. 2, although both "Medical problem" in I2B2 and "Disease and Diagnosis" in CCKS annotate disease names, their scope and granularity differ. "Medical Problem" covers a wider range, including some clinical symptoms, such as infection, redness, and drainage. In contrast, "Disease and Diagnosis" entities strictly adhere to the medical definition of diseases and include fine-grained annotations such as "Hepatoblastoma, hypodermic type (fetal and embryonic) " within the broader category.

I2B2(Medical problem):

Original text: Coronary artery disease s/p Coronary Artery Bypass Graft x3

Original text: Monitor wounds for infection- redness, drainage, or increased pain

---

CCKS(Disease and Diagnosis):

Original text: 肝母细胞瘤可能（侵犯肝右、左叶），术后病理：肝母细胞瘤，下皮型（胎儿及胚胎型）。

Translation: Possible hepatoblastoma (invasion of right and left lobes of the liver), postoperative pathology:hepatoblastoma, hypodermic type (fetal and embryonic).

Fig. 2. Differences in annotation scope between "Disease and Diagnosis" and "Medical Problem".

3.4 Label Alignment

Based on the similarities and differences between the two corpora, we used a label alignment approach to unify similar concept entity types and discarded entity types that couldn't be aligned. Specifically, we mapped the six entity types in the CCKS dataset to three entity types, aligning them with the annotation scheme of the I2B2dataset. This alignment is shown in Table 1:

Table 1. Label alignment rules between CCKS and I2B2.

CCKS	I2B2	CLC-NER
疾病和诊断 (diseases and diagnosis)	Medical problem	Medical problem
影像检查 (imaging examination)	Medical test	Medical test
实验室检验 (laboratory test)		
手术 (surgery)	Medical treatment	Medical treatment
药物 (medication)		
解剖部位 (anatomical site)	–	–

From the table, it can be seen that the "Imaging Examination" and "Laboratory Test" entity types in CCKS are similar in meaning to the "Medical Test" concept type in the 2010 I2B2 corpus. Therefore, we grouped "Imaging Examination" and "Laboratory Test" into one category. Similarly, we mapped the "Surgery" and "Medication" entity types in CCKS to the "Medical Treatment" concept type in I2B2. Since there is no corresponding concept type for "Anatomical Site" in the 2010 I2B2 corpus, we removed it.

4   Framework

4.1   Machine Reading Comprehension

Figure 3 depicts a cross-lingual named entity recognition framework based on the MRC architecture, consisting of three main components: the input layer, encoding layer, and classification layer. Due to the pointer-labeling scheme used for output, multiple questions are posed to the context to extract entities of different types. First, we convert the token sequence generated by concatenating the query and context into vectors through embedding. Next, they are encoded into hidden representations using the XLM-R model. Finally, a classifier determines whether each token marks the beginning or end of entity.

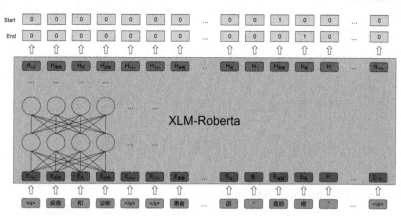

Fig. 3. NER framework based on machine reading comprehension.

Input Layer
Its role is to segment the text composed of queries and context into token sequences and then transform them into vector sequences through token embedding. Specifically, given an input sequence $X = \{x_i\}_{i=1}^{N}$ with N tokens, it produces a sequence of vectors $V = \{v_i\}_{i=1}^{N}$. v_i is the vector corresponding to the i-th token.

Encoding Layer
The encoder maps the sequence of lexical element vectors from the input layer to a sequence of hidden vectors $H = \{h_i\}_{i=1}^{N}$:

$$H = \text{Encoder}(V) \tag{1}$$

The Encoder model can be any encoder model that uses cross-lingual, in this paper we have chosen the XLM-roberta_base model. h_i is the hidden vector corresponding to the i-th token.

Classification Layer
After obtaining the hidden vectors for each token, they are fed into the two linear classification layers and the probability distributions for each token as the start and end of

the entity are computed using the softmax function, respectively:

$$p^{s/e}(x_i) = \text{softmax}\left(W^{s/e}h_i + b^{s/e}\right) \tag{2}$$

$$\hat{y}^{s/e} = \text{argmax}\left(p^{s/e}(x_i)\right) \tag{3}$$

Here $p^s(x_i)$ and $p^e(x_i)$ denote the probability that the ith token starts and ends as an entity, respectively, and $\hat{y}_i^{s/e}$ denotes the final classification result that the i-th token starts and ends as an entity.

Loss Function
We use the cross-entropy loss function to compute the loss for the training task, which consists of two components:

$$L = L_{START} + L_{END} \tag{4}$$

$$L_{START} = \frac{1}{N} \sum_{i=1}^{N} -[y_i^s \log p_i^s + (1 - y_i^s) \log(1 - p_i^s)] \tag{5}$$

$$L_{END} = \frac{1}{N} \sum_{i=1}^{N} -[y_i^e \log p_i^e + (1 - y_i^e) \log(1 - p_i^e)] \tag{6}$$

where L_{START} and L_{END} are computed as follows, and $y_i^{s/e}$ denotes the i-th token's as the real label of the start and end of the entity.

Finally, we use a proximity matching strategy on the final classification result to determine the boundary of an entity.

4.2 Construction of Mixed Language Query

In the context of named entity recognition (NER) based on the machine reading comprehension (MRC) framework, the choice of queries has a notable impact on recognition performance. Similarly, constructing rational and effective queries is highly significant for knowledge transfer in cross-lingual NER.

In monolingual NER, incorporating prior knowledge containing entity type information can induce the model to enhance task performance. However, in the context of cross-lingual NER, which involves multiple languages, using a single query clearly cannot effectively guide the model to learn the prior knowledge across different languages, thus limiting the performance of model transfer. Therefore, this paper proposes a mixed language query construction method, wherein by integrating prior knowledge from multiple languages into the queries, the model can learn the corresponding relationships between different languages, thereby improving the transfer performance of cross-lingual tasks.

Specifically, given a two-language query set $Q = \{Q_{zh}, Q_{en}\}$, where each language query set contains a priori knowledge of m entity types, i.e.:

$$Q_{zh} = \left\{E_{zh}^1, E_{zh}^2...E_{zh}^m\right\} \tag{7}$$

$$Q_{en} = \left\{ E_{en}^1, E_{en}^2 ... E_{en}^m \right\} \tag{8}$$

where E^i denotes the label of the i-th entity type, and E_{zh}^i and E_{en}^i are translations of each other.

We use the separator "/" to splice the type information of Chinese and English, so as to merge the a priori knowledge of the two languages. As an example, we show the concatenation method with English followed by Chinese, i.e.,:

$$Q_{mix} = \left\{ E_{en}^1/E_{zh}^1, E_{en}^2/E_{zh}^2 ... E_{en}^m/E_{zh}^m \right\} \tag{9}$$

4.3 Query Template Set

In order to investigate the impact of different query templates on model transfer performance, we defined various query templates by combining language and task aspects. This task comprises two language types, Zh (Chinese) and En (English), and two tasks, Src (source task) and Tgt (target task). Taking CCKS as the source task and I2B2 as the target task, we provide an example of the templates combined from the "Medical treatment" entity type in the CLC-NER corpus, as shown in Table 2.

Table 2. Combination of query templates.

Query Type	Query Templates
Src_Zh	<s> 药物, 手术 </s>
Src_En	<s> medication, surgery </s>
Src_ZhEn	<s> 药物/medication, 手术/surgery </s>
Src_EnZh	<s> medication/药物, surgery/手术 </s>
Tgt_Zh	<s> 医疗治疗 </s>
Tgt_En	<s> Medical treatment </s>
Tgt_ZhEn	<s> 药物/medication, 手术/surgery </s>
Tgt_EnZh	<s> medication/药物, surgery/手术 </s>

For example, Src_Zh denotes the use of Chinese labels (i.e., "药物" and "手术") from the source language task to generate query templates as prior knowledge. Src_ZhEn represents the generation of mixed language query templates using labels from the source language task, with Chinese first and English second. Similarly, Tgt_ZhEn uses labels from the target language task to create mixed language query templates.

5 Experiments

5.1 Experiment Settings

Datasets

The experiments use the CLC-NER introduced in Sect. 3, and the dataset sizes are shown in Table 3. Both datasets are divided into two subsets for training and testing. "Abstract/Note" and "Entity" denote the number of abstracts and entities in the subset, respectively. It should be noted that the number of entities in the CCKS dataset is the number after excluding the "anatomical site" entities. From the table, we can see that the entity size of I2B2 is larger than that of CCKS, and the entity size of its test set is larger than training set.

Table 3. CLC-NER dataset statistics.

Dataset	Subset	Abstract/Note	Entity
I2B2 2010(En)	Train	170	16,525
	Test	256	31,161
CCKS 2019(Zh)	Train	1,001	9,257
	Test	379	2,908

The number of CLC-NER entities is shown in Table 4, from which it can be seen that the number of entities for "medical problem" is the highest in both corpora. In the I2B2 dataset, there is not much difference between the number of "Medical treatment" entities and the number of "Medical test" entities. In the CCKS dataset, the training set exhibits the lowest count of "Medical treatment" entities, while the test set displays the lowest count of "Medical test" entities.

Table 4. Statistics on the number of entities in the CLC-NER dataset.

Entity Type	I2B2 2010 (En)				CCKS 2019 (Zh)			
	Training		Test		Training		Test	
	Entity	%	Entity	%	Entity	%	Entity	%
Medical problem	7,073	43	12,592	40	4,242	46	1,323	45
Medical treatment	4,844	29	9,344	30	2,164	23	938	32
Medical test	4,608	28	9,225	30	2,851	31	647	23
Sum	11,917	7200	21,936	100	9,257	100	2,908	100

Implementation Details

The XLM-R-base trained by Conneau et al. [23] is used as Encoding model. The hyperparameters used for training are listed in Table 5. Throughout this study, all experiments are conducted on a 2080Ti. The standard P/R/F1 metrics are adopted to evaluate the performance.

Table 5. Hyper-Parameter Settings

Hyper Parameter	Value
Batch size	64
Maximum sequence length	128
Learning rate	2e−5
Epoch	10
Dropout	0.1
Optimizer	AdamW

5.2   Experimental Results

The Impact of Different Query Templates on Cross-Language Transfer Performance

Tables 6 and 7 compare the effects of different query templates on the transfer performance in two transfer directions, where the transfer direction in Table 6 is from CCKS source task to I2B2 target task and vice versa in Table 7. Tables (a) and (b) indicate the performance of using the source and target task labels as the query templates. For example, the cell value in the "Src_Zh" row and "Src_En" column indicate the performance when predicting with the Chinese label of the source task on the training set and the English label of the source task on the test set of the target task. Since preliminary experiments show poor performance when different task labels are used for training and testing, this paper only considers the transfer performance between source task labels (four templates) and target task labels (four templates). The experiments take the average of five runs as the final performance value, and the values in the right bracket are the standard variance of the five runs. The same query template was used for training, and the highest performance values for the test templates are shown in bold.

Table 6. The impact of different query templates on cross-language transfer performance (CCKS to I2B2).

(a) the source task (CCKS) labels as query templates

Train\Test	Src_Zh	Src_En	Src_ZhEn	Src_EnZh
Src_Zh	36.5(±3.1)	26.7(±4.2)	35.6(±2.2)	**37.0**(±2.6)
Src_En	22.9(±4.7)	**38.1**(±1.5)	34.7(±2.2)	37.7(±1.6)
Src_ZhEn	30.0(±1.7)	31.9(±2.3)	**38.7**(±1.0)	37.2(±1.2)
Src_EnZh	31.1(±3.0)	33.8(±3.0)	38.1(±0.9)	**38.7**(±0.6)

(b) the target task (I2B2) labels as query templates

Train\Test	Tgt_Zh	Tgt_En	Tgt_ZhEn	Tgt_EnZh
Tgt_Zh	38.7(±1.6)	35.1(±5.2)	**38.8**(±1.4)	38.7(±1.5)
Tgt_En	30.6(±5.2)	**39.7**(±1.7)	37.9(±2.6)	39.7(±1.9)
Tgt_ZhEn	35.1(±2.3)	35.3(±2.9)	**40.8**(±1.6)	39.9(±1.6)
Tgt_EnZh	37.0(±1.8)	38.9(±1.1)	39.1(±1.8)	**39.7**(±1.3)

Table 7. The impact of different query templates on cross-language transfer performance (I2B2 to CCKS).

(a) the source task (I2B2) labels as query templates

Train\Test	Src_Zh	Src_En	Src_ZhEn	Src_EnZh
Src_Zh	**25.5**(±1.5)	22.6(±1.5)	24.4(±1.0)	22.6(±1.4)
Src_En	22.9(±2.4)	23.1(±1.6)	**23.6**(±2.3)	23.1(±1.6)
Src_ZhEn	**26.5**(±4.3)	25.3(±3.1)	23.8(±1.0)	24.2(±1.2)
Src_EnZh	**25.8**(±1.9)	24.4(±0.9)	24.3(±1.1)	23.8(±0.8)

(b) the target task (CCKS) labels as query templates

Train\Test	Tgt_Zh	Tgt_En	Tgt_ZhEn	Tgt_EnZh
Tgt_Zh	**23.8**(±1.1)	18.2(±7.6)	18.9(±1.5)	21.8(±4.3)
Tgt_En	21.7(±4.7)	**24.9**(±1.0)	22.0(±6.5)	21.3(±2.8)
Tgt_ZhEn	25.2(±4.6)	25.3(±3.9)	25.6(±1.2)	**26.9**(±1.2)
Tgt_EnZh	22.8(±2.1)	24.0(±1.2)	**24.3**(±2.7)	23.0(±1.1)

As can be seen in Table 6:

- The highest performance was achieved when using a mixture of English and Chinese labels of the target task as the query template(F1 value of nearly 41). This indicates that using labels that are semantically similar to the target task entities can better induce cross-lingual prior knowledge in the model.
- Whether using source task labels or target task labels as query templates, when both training and prediction utilize the same queries, the F1 performance metric generally outperforms other scenarios. This suggests that employing identical query templates

for both training and prediction is advantageous for the model's induction of prior knowledge.

- When training and prediction are conducted using mixed-language queries, regardless of the order of Chinese and English, the transfer performance generally surpasses other scenarios. This indicates that the position of labels within the template has a relatively minor impact on the induction of prior knowledge.

The differences between the scenarios presented in Table 7 and those in Table 6 are shown as follows:

- In Table 7(a), during training, using source task labels that include Chinese as query templates, and during testing, employing the "Src_Zh" query template containing only Chinese, achieved relatively better performance. This might be attributed to the fact that the target task's text is in Chinese, and the labels from the source task (I2B2) are relatively broad and general.
- As observed in Table 6, the absence of achieve the optimum values, when training and prediction use the same query templates in Table 6. It may be attributed to the fact that the entities annotated in the I2B2 dataset are more generic compared to the CCKS dataset. Furthermore, mixed language queries induce more information in the model, allowing models trained on the I2B2 corpus to recognize a broader range of entities. This results in more generic false positives when predicting the CCKS dataset, thereby having an impact on the model's performance.

Comparison of Performance for Different Entity Types

To explore performance differences between different entity types in different transfer directions, we selected the highest performance values in two transfer directions for analysis. Table 8 compares the performance of different entity types under mixed-language query templates, with the highest values among the three entity types indicated in bold.

Table 8. Comparison of performance for different entity types.

Entity Type	Tgt_ZhEn (CCKS to I2B2)			Tgt_ZhEn (I2B2 to CCKS)		
	P (%)	R (%)	F1 (%)	P (%)	R (%)	F1 (%)
Medical problem	**75.7**	21.2	33.1	15.6	44.0	23.1
Medical treatment	72.9	**38.5**	**50.4**	29.2	34.6	31.7
Medical test	59.5	30.3	40.1	**34.8**	**45.0**	**39.3**
Micro Avg	68.3	29.1	40.8	19.3	44.3	26.9

As shown in Table 8:

- Although the "Medical problem" type has the largest proportion in both datasets, it has the lowest F1 score in both transfer directions, and it is lower than the overall F1 score. This is due to the semantic differences between the annotated entities in the two corpora, and the more entities there are, the greater the impact of noise on the transfer.

- The "Medical treatment" entity achieved the highest performance in the transfer direction from CCKS to I2B2, but it performed poorly in the reverse direction. This is because the I2B2 training set contains too many broad concept entities, which have a negative impact on the model's transfer effectiveness.
- The performance of "Medical test" did not vary significantly in both transfer directions, mainly due to the relatively small semantic differences in the annotation of "Medical test" entities between the two corpora. Additionally, "Medical test" entities appear in a relatively fixed format, and a considerable portion of entities in the Chinese dataset are represented using English abbreviations, such as "CT".

Performance Comparison with Baseline Systems

In Table 9, we compare our method with several commonly used methods in Cross-lingual NER. BDS_BERT (Bio_Discharge_Summary_BERT) [19] and Chinese_BERT_wwm [24] represent the best monolingual encoder models in Chinese and English, respectively. We employ cross-lingual word alignment information to project the source language into the target language and treat the task as monolingual NER. For a fair comparison, we also introduce the MRC framework into their methods. The XLM-R model refers to the direct model transfer using sequence labeling on a cross-lingual pretrained model.

Our proposed method is divided into two categories: "Sgl", where query templates contain only one language, and "Mix", where query templates contain both languages. The performance in the table corresponds to the highest values for these two approaches. Similarly, the highest Precision/Recall/F1 scores among these methods are represented in bold.

Table 9. Performance comparison with baseline systems.

(a) CCKS to I2B2

Model	P(%)	R(%)	F1(%)
BDS_BERT+MRC	64.7	**29.7**	40.7(±0.8)
XLM-R	54.7	27.7	36.8(±2.2)
XLM-R+MRC(Sgl)	65.5	28.5	39.7(±1.7)
XLM-R+MRC(Mix)	**68.3**	29.1	**40.8(±1.6)**

(b) I2B2 to CCKS

Model	P(%)	R(%)	F1(%)
Chinese-BERT-wwm+MRC	15.2	**58.8**	24.1(±0.7)
XLM-R	13.2	56.8	21.4(±0.6)
XLM-R+MRC(Sgl)	17.7	45.4	25.5(±1.5)
XLM-R+MRC(Mix)	**19.3**	44.3	**26.9(±1.2)**

- After adopting the MRC framework, the model's transfer performance in both transfer directions significantly outperformed the sequence labeling approach, demonstrating the advantages of MRC in cross-lingual named entity recognition tasks.
- In both transfer directions, XLM-R +MRC with mixed language query templates achieved the highest F1 values among all baseline systems. Compared to using single-language templates, it obtained a positive improvement of 1.05 and 1.46, demonstrating the effectiveness of the mixed-query approach in cross-lingual pretrained models.
- Our proposed XLM-R+MRC(Mix) approach showed comparable performance to BDS_BERT+MRC and a significant improvement over the Chinese-BERT-wwm+MRC method. This is because BDS_BERT was pretrained on clinical domain text, endowing the model with domain-specific knowledge. When combined with MRC, it can better utilize prior knowledge to induce domain-specific knowledge into the model, thereby enhancing task performance.

6 Discussion and Case Study

6.1 Mixed Language Query and Single Language Query

To investigate the reasons behind the improved model transfer performance of mixed language query templates, we selected the settings with the highest values achieved using mixed language queries and single-language queries in both transfer directions for comparison. The highest values in the comparison results are indicated in bold, as shown in Table 10.

Table 10. Comparison of single and mixed templates.

(a) CCKS to I2B2

Entity Type	Tgt_En			Tgt_ZhEn		
	P(%)	R(%)	F1(%)	P(%)	R(%)	F1(%)
Medical problem	**76.3**	19.6	31.2	75.7	**21.2**	**33.1**
Medical treatment	70.5	36.8	48.3	**72.9**	**38.5**	**50.4**
Medical test	55.3	**32.3**	40.8	**59.5**	30.3	40.1
Micro Avg	65.5	28.5	39.7	**68.3**	**29.1**	**40.8**

(b) I2B2 to CCKS

Entity Type	Tgt_En			Tgt_ZhEn		
	P(%)	R(%)	F1(%)	P(%)	R(%)	F1(%)
Medical problem	11.1	59.1	18.7	**15.6**	44.0	**23.1**
Medical treatment	**30.6**	**42.2**	**35.5**	29.2	34.6	31.7
Medical test	34.8	**48.0**	**40.4**	34.8	45.0	39.3
Micro Avg	16.4	**51.7**	24.9	**19.3**	44.3	**26.9**

From Table 10, we can observe the following:

• The use of mixed language query templates results in a more noticeable improvement in precision, particularly for the "Medical problem" and "Medical treatment" entity types. This suggests that mixed language query templates, compared to single-language templates, enable the model to acquire more prior knowledge to enhance the accuracy of predicting entities.

• In the CCKS to I2B2 direction, the results generally exhibit a "high precision, low recall" pattern, whereas in the I2B2 to CCKS direction, a "high recall, low precision" scenario is observed. This is due to the semantic differences in entities and concepts annotated in the two monolingual datasets. The broad concepts annotated in I2B2 lead to more false positives when transferred to CCKS, while the fine-grained entities annotated in CCKS result in the recognition of some fine-grained entities within the broad concepts when transferred to I2B2, leading to the opposite pattern.

6.2 Source Task Labels and Target Task Labels

To investigate the reasons behind the improved model transfer performance using source task label templates, we selected the settings with the highest values achieved using source task labels and target task labels in both transfer directions for comparison. The highest values in the comparison results are indicated in bold, as shown in Table 11.

Table 11. Comparison of source and target task labels.

(a) CCKS to I2B2

Entity Type	Src_ZhEn			Tgt_ZhEn		
	P(%)	R(%)	F1(%)	P(%)	R(%)	F1(%)
Medical problem	72.0	17.3	27.9	**75.7**	**21.2**	**33.1**
Medical treatment	71.6	36.3	48.2	**72.9**	**38.5**	**50.4**
Medical test	51.5	**32.9**	**40.2**	**59.5**	30.3	40.1
Micro Avg	63.0	27.6	38.7	**68.3**	**29.1**	**40.8**

(b) I2B2 to CCKS

Entity Type	Src_ZhEn			Tgt_ZhEn		
	P(%)	R(%)	F1(%)	P(%)	R(%)	F1(%)
Medical problem	14.3	**52.5**	22.4	**15.6**	44.0	**23.1**
Medical treatment	23.8	**37.2**	29.1	**29.2**	34.6	**31.7**
Medical test	**35.4**	43.3	39.0	34.8	**45.0**	**39.3**
Micro Avg	**20.1**	39.0	26.5	19.3	**44.3**	**26.9**

In both transfer directions, using target task labels contributes to an improvement in recall and enhances transfer performance. Employing labels that are similar to the target corpus as queries aids the model in capturing the relationship between prior knowledge and context entities. For example, in the I2B2 dataset sentence, "She also received Cisplatin 35 per meter squared on 06/19 and Ifex and Mesna on 06/18", using "Src_ZhEn" did not identify "Ifex" and "Mesna" entities, while "Tgt_ZhEn" recognized all of them. The machine reading comprehension framework assists the model in capturing the relationship between the prior knowledge "Medical treatment" and the context word "received", thereby inducing the model to recognize more correct entities and enhancing transfer performance.

7 Conclusion

In this paper, we constructed a corpus for cross-lingual clinical named entity recognition (CLC-NER) using label alignment on existing monolingual datasets, demonstrating the effectiveness of the mixed-language query approach. Given that the semantic differences in annotated entities in the corpus limit the model's transfer performance, manual annotation of cross-lingual NER data in the clinical domain is necessary in future research.

Funding. This research is supported by the National Natural Science Foundation of China [61976147] and the research grant of The Hong Kong Polytechnic University Projects [#1-W182].

References

1. Mayhew, S., Tsai, C.-T., Roth, D.: Cheap translation for cross-lingual named entity recognition. In: Proceedings of the 2017 Conference on Empirical Methods in Natural Language Processing, pp. 2536–2545. Association for Computational Linguistics, Copenhagen (2017). https://doi.org/10.18653/v1/D17-1269
2. Xie, J., Yang, Z., Neubig, G., Smith, N.A., Carbonell, J.: Neural cross-lingual named entity recognition with minimal resources (2018). http://arxiv.org/abs/1808.09861
3. Wu, S., Dredze, M.: Beto, bentz, becas: the surprising cross-lingual effectiveness of BERT. In: Proceedings of the 2019 Conference on Empirical Methods in Natural Language Processing and the 9th International Joint Conference on Natural Language Processing (EMNLP-IJCNLP), pp. 833–844. Association for Computational Linguistics, Hong Kong (2019). https://doi.org/10.18653/v1/D19-1077
4. Tsai, C.-T., Mayhew, S., Roth, D.: Cross-lingual named entity recognition via wikification. In: Proceedings of the 20th SIGNLL Conference on Computational Natural Language Learning, pp. 219–228. Association for Computational Linguistics, Berlin (2016). https://doi.org/10. 18653/v1/K16-1022
5. Keung, P., Lu, Y., Bhardwaj, V.: Adversarial learning with contextual embeddings for zero-resource cross-lingual classification and NER. In: Proceedings of the 2019 Conference on Empirical Methods in Natural Language Processing and the 9th International Joint Conference on Natural Language Processing (EMNLP-IJCNLP), pp. 1355–1360. Association for Computational Linguistics, Hong Kong (2019). https://doi.org/10.18653/v1/D19-1138
6. Sang, T.K., Erik, F.: Introduction to the CoNLL-2002 shared task: language-independent named entity recognition. In: Proceedings of CoNLL-2002/Roth, Dan [edit], pp. 155–158 (2002)
7. Sang, E.T.K., De Meulder, F.: Introduction to the CoNLL-2003 shared task: language-independent named entity recognition. In: Proceedings of the Seventh Conference on Natural Language Learning at HLT-NAACL 2003, pp. 142–147 (2003)

8. Pan, X., Zhang, B., May, J., Nothman, J., Knight, K., Ji, H.: Cross-lingual name tagging and linking for 282 languages. In: Proceedings of the 55th Annual Meeting of the Association for Computational Linguistics (Volume 1: Long Papers), pp. 1946–1958. Association for Computational Linguistics, Vancouver (2017). https://doi.org/10.18653/v1/P17-1178

9. Ni, J., Dinu, G., Florian, R.: Weakly supervised cross-lingual named entity recognition via effective annotation and representation projection. In: Proceedings of the 55th Annual Meeting of the Association for Computational Linguistics (Volume 1: Long Papers), pp. 1470–1480. Association for Computational Linguistics, Vancouver (2017). https://doi.org/10.18653/v1/P17-1135

10. Jain, A., Paranjape, B., Lipton, Z.C.: Entity projection via machine translation for cross-lingual NER. In: Proceedings of the 2019 Conference on Empirical Methods in Natural Language Processing and the 9th International Joint Conference on Natural Language Processing (EMNLP-IJCNLP), pp. 1083–1092. Association for Computational Linguistics, Hong Kong (2019). https://doi.org/10.18653/v1/D19-1100

11. Devlin, J., Chang, M.-W., Lee, K., Toutanova, K.: BERT: pre-training of deep bidirectional transformers for language understanding. In: Proceedings of NAACL-HLT, vol. 1, p. 2 (2019)

12. Wu, Q., Lin, Z., Karlsson, B., Lou, J.-G., Huang, B.: Single-/multi-source cross-lingual NER via teacher-student learning on unlabeled data in target language. In: Proceedings of the 58th Annual Meeting of the Association for Computational Linguistics, pp. 6505–6514. Association for Computational Linguistics (2020). https://doi.org/10.18653/v1/2020.acl-main.581

13. Wu, Q., Lin, Z., Karlsson, B.F., Huang, B., Lou, J.-G.: UniTrans: unifying model transfer and data transfer for cross-lingual named entity recognition with unlabeled data. Presented at the Twenty-Ninth International Joint Conference on Artificial Intelligence (2020). https://doi.org/10.24963/ijcai.2020/543

14. Li, Z., Hu, C., Guo, X., Chen, J., Qin, W., Zhang, R.: An unsupervised multiple-task and multiple-teacher model for cross-lingual named entity recognition. In: Proceedings of the 60th Annual Meeting of the Association for Computational Linguistics (Volume 1: Long Papers), pp. 170–179 (2022)

15. Levy, O., Seo, M., Choi, E., Zettlemoyer, L.: Zero-shot relation extraction via reading comprehension. In: Proceedings of the 21st Conference on Computational Natural Language Learning (CoNLL 2017), pp. 333–342. Association for Computational Linguistics, Vancouver (2017). https://doi.org/10.18653/v1/K17-1034

16. Rajpurkar, P., Jia, R., Liang, P.: Know what you don't know: unanswerable questions for SQuAD. In: Proceedings of the 56th Annual Meeting of the Association for Computational Linguistics (Volume 2: Short Papers), pp. 784–789. Association for Computational Linguistics, Melbourne (2018). https://doi.org/10.18653/v1/P18-2124

17. Nguyen, T., et al.: MS MARCO: a human generated machine reading comprehension dataset (2017)

18. Li, X., Feng, J., Meng, Y., Han, Q., Wu, F., Li, J.: A unified MRC framework for named entity recognition. In: Proceedings of the 58th Annual Meeting of the Association for Computational Linguistics, pp. 5849–5859. Association for Computational Linguistics (2020). https://doi.org/10.18653/v1/2020.acl-main.519

19. Cao, J., et al.: Electronic medical record entity recognition via machine reading comprehension and biaffine. Discrete Dyn. Nat. Soc. **2021**, 1–8 (2021)

20. Zheng, H., Qin, B., Xu, M.: Chinese medical named entity recognition using CRF-MT-adapt and NER-MRC. Presented at the 2021 2nd International Conference on Computing and Data Science (CDS) (2021). https://doi.org/10.1109/CDS52072.2021.00068

21. Han, X., et al.: Overview of the CCKS 2019 knowledge graph evaluation track: entity, relation, event and QA. arXiv preprint arXiv:2003.03875 (2020)

22. Uzuner, Ö., South, B.R., Shen, S., DuVall, S.L.: 2010 i2b2/VA challenge on concepts, assertions, and relations in clinical text. J. Am. Med. Inform. Assoc. **18**, 552–556 (2011). https://doi.org/10.1136/amiajnl-2011-000203

23. Conneau, A., Lample, G.: Cross-lingual language model pretraining. In: Advances in Neural Information Processing Systems, vol. 32 (2019)

24. Cui, Y., Che, W., Liu, T., Qin, B., Yang, Z.: Pre-training with whole word masking for Chinese BERT. IEEE/ACM Trans. Audio Speech Lang. Process. **29**, 3504–3514 (2021). https://doi.org/10.1109/TASLP.2021.3124365

PEMRC: A Positive Enhanced Machine Reading Comprehension Method for Few-Shot Named Entity Recognition in Biomedical Domain

Yuehu Dong[1], Dongmei Li[1], Jinghang Gu[2], Longhua Qian[1(✉)], and Guodong Zhou[1]

[1] Natural Language Processing Lab, School of Computer Science and Technology, Soochow University, Suzhou, China
{20215227045,20224027005}@stu.suda.edu.cn,
{qianglonghua,gzzhou}@suda.edu.cn
[2] Chinese and Bilingual Studies, The Hong Kong Polytechnic University, Hung Hom, Hong Kong

Abstract. In this paper, we propose a simple and effective few-shot named entity recognition (NER) method for biomedical domain, called PEMRC (**P**ositive **E**nhanced **M**achine **R**eading **C**omprehension). PEMRC is based on the idea of using machine reading comprehension reading comprehension (MRC) framework to perfome few-shot NER and fully exploit the prior knowledge implied in the label information. On one hand, we design three different query templates to better induce knowledge from pre-trained language models (PLMs). On the other hand, we design a positive enhanced loss function to improve the model's accuracy in identifying the start and end positions of entities under low-resources scenarios. Extensive experimental results on eight benchmark datasets in biomedical domain show that PEMRC significantly improves the performance of few-shot NER.

Keywords: Few-shot Named Entity Recognition · Machine Reading Comprehension · Biomedical Domain

1 Introduction

NER is a fundamental task in information extraction, which aims to identify text segments according to predefined entity categories. Current methods use neural network approaches [3,14,25] to solve the NER task. However, neural-based methods require a large amount of annotated data to achieve good performance, and data annotation requires rich domain expertise. Due to the high complexity in the biomedical expertise, which poses challenges for biomedical NER in low-resource scenarios. Recently, few-shot NER [4,5,7,17,26] has received wide attention.

The current mainstream method for few-shot named entity recognition is metric learning based on Similarity Learning. Similarity-based metric learning methods [5, 24, 26] make the distance between entities of the same class smaller and the distance between entities of different types larger by learning a metric space. However, the entity and non-entity clustering information learned by this similarity metric function in the source domain cannot be well transferred to the task in the target domain. At the same time, the tokens of other entity types in the source domain is uniformly encoded as non-entities, reducing the expressiveness of the model.

Prompt Learning method can achieve the consistency of upstream and downstream tasks by designing prompt templates and label words. The method proposed by [4] solves this problem by scoring. By incorporating distinct label words in both the source and target domains, the prompt-based approach effectively mitigates discrepancies arising from inconsistent training objectives during pretraining and fine-tuning. Moreover, its well-crafted template design facilitates information induction within the pre-trained language model. However, prompt learning cannot design templates for token-level tasks, and the high complexity caused by enumerating all spans is unacceptable.

In order to deal with the above problems, this paper introduces the method of Machine Reading Comprehension (MRC) [16]. We adopt a span extraction machine reading comprehension method, which can unify upstream and downstream tasks by designing task-specific queries on upstream and downstream tasks. Compared with prompt learning, machine reading comprehension can effectively reduce the complexity of training and inference. In order to further utilize the knowledge in the pre-trained language model, we design three different types of query templates and conduct extensive experiments. To our knowledge, we are the first to introduce the machine reading comprehension method into the few shot named entity recognition in the biomedical domain.

2 Related Work

2.1 Few-Shot NER

In this section, we review two types of methods for few-shot NER: similarity-based metric learning and prompt learning.

Similarity-Based Metric Learning. Similarity based approach is a common solution in few-shot named entity recognition. The tokens are classified by assessing the similarity between the entity type representation in the support set and tokens in the test set. The few shot named entity recognition primarily relies on metric learning. Currently, there are two main approaches to metric learning: the prototype network [7, 10, 23] and contrastive learning [5, 11].

The method based on the prototype network learns a metric space that encompasses a class of data around a single type prototype representation, enabling classification into the nearest class by calculating the distance between instance representation and class prototype during inference.

[26] proposed a Nearest Neighbor (NN) classification method which divides the test set token into categories based on comparing distances with support set tokens. Contrastive learning employs distance metric function (such as Euclidean distance) and relative entropy (Kullback-Leibler Divergence, KLD) to design various contrastive methods aiming to narrow distances between tokens of the same category while pushing away tokens from different categories for improved token representation.

Prompt Learning. Prompt learning originates from GPT [1,19] (Generative Pre-training Transformer) models and has been widely used in few-shot learning. Prompt learning organizes the downstream task into a cloze task, and with excellent template and label word design, prompt learning effectively bridges the gap between pre-training and fine-tuning. [20,21] used prompt learning in sentence-level tasks and achieved good results.

The performance of the model can be effectively enhanced by designing prompt templates. [20,21] employ human-crafted templates for text classification tasks. [22] utilize a gradient-based method to search for discrete templates. [8,22,27] generate discrete prompt templates using pre-trained generative models. Meanwhile, [15] adopt continuous prompt templates for classification and generation tasks, thereby avoiding the necessity for intricate template design. Additionally, [9] propose P-Tuning, which involves incorporating learnable continuous prompt into discrete prompt templates.

[4] employed a template-based approach in few-shot Named Entity Recognition. In this methodology, the original sentence is fed into the encoder, while the prompt template and all text spans within the sentence are combined in the decoder. The amalgamated templates are evaluated based on loss. However, this exhaustive enumeration of all spans introduces significant complexity to the method. To address these limitations, [17] proposed an innovative template-free approach that eliminates intricate template design altogether. This alternative method restructures the task as an entity-oriented language model task by predicting label words corresponding to tokens at respective positions.

2.2   Few-Shot NER in Biomedical Domain

The study conducted by [18] introduced task hardness information based on [13] to enhance transfer learning in biomedical domain for few-shot named entity recognition tasks. MetaNER [13], which adopts a multi-task learning framework, employs an adversarial training strategy to obtain a more robust, generalizable, and transferable representation method for named entity recognition. Additionally, [13] utilizes a meta-learning training approach that enables it to perform effectively in low resources scenarios.

3   Problem Definition

We adopt the task setup from [5] (as depicted in Fig. 1 below). Amongst the four named entity recognition tasks (Disease, Chem/Drug, Gene/Protein, Species), we select three tasks (e.g., Disease, Chem/Drug, Gene/Protein) as source tasks with rich resources. The remaining task served as a low-resource target task (e.g., Species). For this target task, we employ a model pre-trained on the standard training set X_{tr} lines of the source tasks and fine-tune it using the support set X_{supp} of the target task. The support set is generated by sampling instances from the training set in the target task. Finally, evaluation was conducted on the standard test set X_{test} of that particular target task.

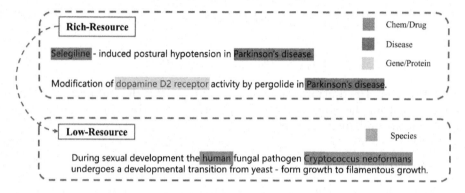

Fig. 1. Task Description.

4 Methodology

The proposed method utilizes a span-extraction approach for machine reading comprehension and incorporates a loss function that focuses on positive tokens. The methodology outlined in this section comprises four components: model architecture, query template design, loss function formulation, and training process implementation. We will present our approach sequentially in the subsequent sections.

4.1 Model Framework

Given the input $X = \{x_1, x_2, x_3, ..., x_n\}$, we concatenate it with the query $Q = \{q_1, q_2, q_3, ..., q_m\}$ to obtain the model input. Then we feed it into the pre-trained model [12] to encode it and obtain the representation $\mathbf{H}$, as shown in Eq. 1.

$$H(e_{cls}, e_1, e_2, ..., e_{m+n}, e_{sep}) = PLM([CLS], q_1, q_2, ..., q_m, x_1, x_2, ..., x_n, [SEP]) \tag{1}$$

We apply a dropout layer to randomly drop the representation $\mathbf{H}$ twice, obtaining the representation H_{start} for predicting the start position and the representation H_{end} for predicting the end position, as shown in Eq. 2.

$$H_{start} = Dropout(H), H_{end} = Dropout(H) \tag{2}$$

Start Position Prediction. For the obtained representation H_{start}, we feed it into a classifier FFN to get a score matrix $S \in R^{(m+n)\times 2}$, and then apply softmax to get a probability matrix $P \in R^{(m+n)\times 2}$. Finally, we select the index with the highest probability as its prediction label $\hat{Y}_{start}$. Regarding the obtained labels, '1' signifies that the current token marks the start of an entity, and '0' indicates that the current token does not mark the start of an entity, as shown in Eq. 3 and Eq. 4.

$$P_{start} = Softmax(FFN(H_{start})) \in R^{(m+n)\times 2} \tag{3}$$

$$\hat{Y}_{start} = Argmax(P_{start}) \in (0,1) \tag{4}$$

End Position Prediction. The prediction process for the end position is the same as that for the start position, except that we use the representation H_{end} to obtain the probability matrix P_{end}.

4.2   Construction of Queries

In prompt learning, designing prompt template can effectively induce prior knowledge in pre-trained language models. Taking inspiration from prompt learning's template design [15, 16, 20, 21], we construct discrete, continuous, and hybrid query templates respectively.

The discrete query template is manually crafted while learnable vectors of varying lengths are employed as continuous query templates without any prior knowledge. In hybrid queries, entity type identifiers, such as disease, are substituted with continuous learnable vectors. The hybrid template incorporates some prior knowledge (discrete query) but excludes entity label information. Examples of these three types of query templates are provided in Table 1.

Table 1. An examples of three query templates.

Query Type	Query Example
Discrete Query	Find disease entities in the next sentence
Continuous Query	v1 v2 v3 v4 v5 v6 v7
Hybrid Query	Find v1 entities in the next sentence

The expression "v1-v7" denotes a learnable vector, akin to the continuous prompt template employed in prompt learning. The "[unused]" symbols are utilized as learnable vectors to seamlessly integrate into the input during the implementation.

4.3   Loss Function Formulation

In the context of machine reading comprehension models, it is a common practice to compute the sequence loss ζ_{seq} by applying cross-entropy between the probability matrix P representing start and end positions, and the label Y. The formula is shown in Eq. 5 below.

$$\zeta_{seq} = CrossEntropy(P_{start}, Y_{start}) + CrossEntropy(P_{end}, Y_{end}) \quad (5)$$

To improve the accuracy of the model in identifying the start and end positions of entities, we augment the loss of gold labeled tokens, namely positive enhanced loss. The objective is for the model to acquire more information about entity head and tail tokens. The loss function can be defined as Eq. 6: where Y_{start_p} represents a positive token with its starting position, P_{start_p} corresponds to the token probability matrix of that positive token; likewise for P_{end_p} and Y_{end_p}.

$$\zeta_{pos} = CrossEntropy(P_{start\_p}, Y_{start\_p}) + CrossEntropy(P_{end\_p}, Y_{end\_p}) \quad (6)$$

We combine these two functions into ultimate loss function as Eq. 7:

$$\zeta_{final} = \zeta + \zeta_{pos} \quad (7)$$

4.4   Training Process

The BioBERT model serves as the base model F and is trained on a rich resources training set X_{tr}. At this stage, we do not incorporate a positive enhanced loss L_{tr}. Subsequently, We then fine-tune model with positive enhanced loss $L_s upp$ on a few-shot support set X_{supp}. Training on a support set may lead to severe overfitting, we maintain a fixed number of training epochs on the support set throughout the process. The algorithmic details regarding the model's training procedure are elucidated in Algorithm 1.

Algorithm 1: Training and Fine Tuning

Require: Training Data X_{tr}, Support Data X_{supp},
Train loss function L_{tr}, Finetune loss function L_{supp}, Model F

1   epoch = num_epoches //initialize fixed nums epoch
2   // training in source domain
3   for sampled(w/o replacement) minibatch X in X_{tr} do
4       $L_{tr} = F(X)$ // L_{tr} without ζ_{pos}
5   update F by backpropagation to reduce L_{tr}
6   end for
7   $F_{source} \leftarrow F$
8   // finetuning to target domain
9   While epoch >0 do
10   for sampled(w/o replacement) minibatch x in X_{supp} do
11          $L_{supp} = F_{source}(x)$ // L_{supp} with ζ_{pos}
12   update F_{source} by backpropagation to reduce L_{supp}
13   end for
14   epoch $\leftarrow$ epoch-1
15   end while
16   $F_{target} \leftarrow F_{source}$
17   return F_{target}

---

5   Experiment

5.1   Datasets

The benchmark NER corpora preprocessed by BioBERT [12] are utilized in this study. We have conducted an analysis of entity counts in both the training and test sets within the corpus, with the statistical findings presented in Table 2 below.

Table 2. Corpus Statistic

Task	Corpus	Num of Entities	
		Train	Test
Disease	NCBI	5,145	960
	BC5CDR	9,385	9,809
Drug/Chem	BC5CDR	9,385	9,593
	BC4CHEMD	29,478	25,346
Gene/Protein	JNLPBA	32,178	6,241
	BC2GM	15,197	6,325
Species	LINNAEUS	2,119	1,433
	S800	2,557	767

5.2   Sampling Strategy

The previous sampling has primarily employed two predominant methods, namely the N-way K-shot [6] sampling method and the precision sampling [2,4,17] method. Both of these methods are instance-oriented samplings that select a specific number of entities randomly using different strategies. However, in real-world scenarios, inputs do not exist solely as instances. To address this limitation, HGDA [18] proposed a sentence-level oriented sampling method. In the few-shot setting, K sentences containing entities are sampled as the support set. In this paper, we also adopt HGDA's [18] sampling strategy to obtain the support set by performing sampling within the standard train set.

5.3   Experimental Settings

The BioBERT model is used as the base encoder, while the span extraction network is employed for extracting entity spans. The loss calculation involves the utilization of the positive enhanced loss function, and Adam serves as the optimizer. Throughout this study, all experiments are conducted on a 3090Ti, and after employing 5 different seeds for experimentation purposes, an average F1 value is obtained. To provide a clearer details, Table 3 presents all training-related hyperparameters.

Table 3. Hyper-Parameter Settings

Hyper Parameter	Value
Max input length	256
Source batch size	8
Target batch size	2
Source task encoder lr	1e−5
Target task encoder lr	1e−4
Source task classifier lr	1e−4
Target task classifier lr	1e−4
Dropout rate	0.1
Number of epochs	10
Number of learnable vectors in continuous query	7
Number of learnable vectors in hybrid query	3

5.4   Experimental Results

In this section, we present the results of performance differences among different query templates, loss function and finally the comparison with SOTA systems.

Impact of Query Template. The impact of query templates on performance is investigated in this section, aiming to explore how the form of label information as prior knowledge in the machine reading comprehension framework affects recognition performance. Table 4 compares the F1 values of different query templates on the NCBI corpus under various few-shot settings (K = 5, 10, 20, 50), with the highest value for each quantity highlighted in bold.

Table 4. Performance of three different query templates on NCBI dataset.

Query Type	5	10	20	50
Continuous	50.83	58.30	65.58	**69.86**
Hybrid	49.81	54.11	66.94	69.39
Discrete	**57.84**	**61.06**	**67.40**	69.03

The table above clearly demonstrates that the discrete query template outperforms the continuous and hybrid query templates, particularly when K = 5, 10, and 20. However, at K = 50, all three templates show comparable performance. Notably, the discrete query template exhibits a larger performance gain when the support set is small; however, as the size of the support set increases, this advantage gradually diminishes. Further detailed analysis can be found in Subsect. 5.5 of this paper. Consequently, in all subsequent experiments conducted in this study, discrete templates are exclusively employed as query templates for MRC baseline and PEMRC.

The Influence of Positive Enhanced Loss. The effectiveness of the positive enhanced loss function is examined by comparing the disparities between two methods, MRC and PEMRC, with F1 value results presented in Table 5. Here, MRC denotes the machine reading comprehension model employing solely the cross-entropy loss function, and PEMRC incorporates the positive enhanced loss. The maximum value for each setting is highlighted in bold.

Table 5. MRC and PEMRC performance comparison

K	Method	Disease		Drug/Chem		Gene/Protein		Species	
		NCBI	BC5	BC5	BC4	JNL	BC2	LINN	S800
5	MRC	**57.84**	64.85	74.78	52.52	46.73	47.20	52.27	52.56
	PEMRC	55.77	**64.87**	**79.07**	**53.71**	**46.87**	**48.75**	**52.89**	**53.26**
10	MRC	61.06	65.50	76.93	53.26	52.63	52.00	60.64	**55.89**
	PEMRC	**62.37**	**66.27**	**79.57**	**55.56**	**52.79**	**52.67**	**62.55**	55.74
20	MRC	67.40	**67.96**	78.93	59.46	**57.33**	54.02	63.10	57.00
	PEMRC	**69.87**	**67.96**	**82.64**	**60.58**	56.61	**55.33**	**67.82**	**57.88**
50	MRC	69.03	**71.61**	81.16	59.78	59.39	56.10	68.28	59.79
	PEMRC	**72.48**	69.36	**84.08**	**61.29**	**60.53**	**57.42**	**71.79**	**59.82**

Table 5 demonstrates that PEMRC outperforms the MRC baseline model on most of the eight datasets. When averaging performance across all datasets, PEMRC achieves a 2.1% improvement over the MRC baseline system, highlighting the effectiveness of the positive enhanced loss function.

Comparison with Other SOTA Systems. In this section, we use PEMRC as a baseline for the methodology. We conduct extensive experiments on 8 datasets and compare them with similar systems. The SOTA systems used for comparison, the experimental results, and the analysis of the results are described below.

SOTA systems

(i) MetaNER [13] is a multi-task learning method for domain adaptation, which combines supervised meta-learning and adversarial training strategies. It can obtain more robust, general and transferable representation methods in named entity recognition tasks.

(ii) HGDA [18] introduces hardness information based on MetaNER and applies it to biomedical domains.

Table 6. Compared with the performance of SOTA systems, some dataset names are replaced by abbreviations.

K	Method	Disease		Drug/Chem		Gene/Protein		Species		AVG
		NCBI	BC5	BC5	BC4	JNL	BC2	LINN	S800	
5	MetaNER	27.29	21.71	57.84	22.12	21.75	24.43	12.14	15.16	23.87
	HGDA	31.25	26.98	61.02	25.71	37.76	35.73	17.53	28.80	33.10
	PEMRC	**55.77**	**64.87**	**79.07**	**53.71**	**46.86**	**48.75**	**52.89**	**53.26**	**56.90**
10	MetaNER	33.30	36.88	66.59	33.60	33.74	32.65	30.38	31.64	37.35
	HGDA	43.86	42.44	70.97	42.47	47.90	44.89	32.01	37.03	45.14
	PEMRC	**62.37**	**66.27**	**79.57**	**55.56**	**52.79**	**52.67**	**62.55**	**55.74**	**60.94**
20	MetaNER	46.12	47.22	73.01	43.83	41.67	39.26	49.52	29.77	46.30
	HGDA	56.31	55.29	74.72	49.44	54.66	51.24	48.43	52.05	55.26
	PEMRC	**69.87**	**67.96**	**82.64**	**60.58**	**56.61**	**55.33**	**67.82**	**57.88**	**64.84**
50	MetaNER	57.31	61.06	74.78	50.82	53.37	50.58	61.25	36.07	55.65
	HGDA	62.08	61.90	80.23	**62.73**	**61.46**	**60.16**	63.73	58.55	63.90
	PEMRC	**72.48**	**69.36**	**84.08**	61.29	60.53	57.42	**71.79**	**59.82**	**67.10**

As shown in Table 6, our performance is better than other systems in most cases, and our method achieves significant performance in low-resource situations. This may be due to the fact that our designed query templates can use the information in the pre-trained language model more directly, just like prompt learning. The less annotated data, the more obvious the effect of using the information in the PLM. In addition, the machine reading comprehension method has only one classifier for all tasks, while HGDA and MetaNER have multiple classifiers for multi-task learning. We believe that this unified classifier can learn the knowledge transfer between different tasks, while the task-specific classifier will lose some of the knowledge learned on the source tasks to some extent.

5.5   Discussion and Analysis

We offer insightful explanations to analyze the performance disparities resulting from different query template types. There are two potential reasons for this phenomenon:

Firstly, in the low-resource scenario (K = 5), natural language text can effectively leverage the knowledge within the pretrained language model, whereas continuous and hybrid query templates constructed from random vectors fail to align with the model's input during pretraining and thus cannot directly harness the knowledge embedded in the pretrained language model.

Secondly, the structure of learnable vectors present in continuous and hybrid templates remains fixed, necessitating more training data to discover an optimal vector. Consequently, they achieve comparable performance to discrete query templates only when greater resources are available (K = 50).

To further demonstrate how prior knowledge and label information impact experimental performance in low-resource scenarios, we analyzed error cases generated on the NCBI (disease) test set with K = 5.

Table 7. The following table shows two cases. Gold represents the sentence and the entity that should be predicted, where the entity is marked in red font.

Case 1	The predicted entities
Gold	The risk of cancer, especially lymphoid neoplasias, is substantially elevated in A - T patients and has long been associated with chromosomal instability.
Discrete	cancer — lymphoid neoplasias — A-T
Continuous	lymphoid neoplasias
Hybrid	None
Case 2	The predicted entities
Gold	These clustered in the region corresponding to the kinase domain, which is highly conserved in ATM - related proteins in mouse, yeast and Drosophila.
Discrete	None
Continuous	Drosophila
Hybrid	proteins — mouse — yeast — Drosophila

From Table 7, it is evident that in Case 1, only the discrete query accurately identifies all entities, while the continuous query successfully identifies one entity and the hybrid query fails to identify any entity. In Case 2, sentences without entities are correctly predicted solely by discrete queries, whereas both continuous and hybrid queries incorrectly detect false positives. Upon analysis, it becomes apparent that the continuous query possesses limited prior knowledge, resulting in its failure to correctly identify or recognize entities. The hybrid query incorporates some prior knowledge but lacks explicit label information, leading to identification of other types of entities in Case 2 such as proteins/genes (ATM-related proteins) and species (mouse, yeast, Drosophila).

6   Conclusion and Future Work

In this paper, we present a simple yet effective approach to machine reading comprehension. Our query template is designed to better leverage the knowledge in pre-trained language model and facilitate knowledge transfer between source and target tasks. Additionally, our positive enhanced loss function further boosts model performance. This method yields significant improvements in low-resource settings and even outperforms state-of-the-art methods in challenging biomedical domains. Moving forward, we plan to explore machine reading comprehension techniques across various domains with limited resources while also refining our query design.

Funding. This research is supported by the National Natural Science Foundation of China [61976147] and the research grant of The Hong Kong Polytechnical University Projects [# 1-W182].

References

1. Brown, T.B., et al.: Language models are few-shot learners. In: Proceedings of the 34th International Conference on Neural Information Processing Systems. NIPS'20, Curran Associates Inc., Red Hook, NY, USA (2020)
2. Chen, X., et al.: LightNER: A lightweight tuning paradigm for low-resource NER via pluggable prompting. In: Proceedings of the 29th International Conference on Computational Linguistics, pp. 2374–2387. Gyeongju, Republic of Korea (2022)
3. Chiu, J.P., Nichols, E.: Named entity recognition with bidirectional LSTM-CNNs. Trans. Assoc. Comput. linguist. **4**, 357–370 (2016)
4. Cui, L., Wu, Y., Liu, J., Yang, S., Zhang, Y.: Template-based named entity recognition using BART. In: Findings of the Association for Computational Linguistics: ACL-IJCNLP 2021, pp. 1835–1845. Association for Computational Linguistics (2021)
5. Das, S.S.S., Katiyar, A., Passonneau, R., Zhang, R.: CONTaiNER: few-shot named entity recognition via contrastive learning. In: Proceedings of the 60th Annual Meeting of the Association for Computational Linguistics (Volume 1: Long Papers), pp. 6338–6353. Association for Computational Linguistics, Dublin, Ireland (2022)
6. Ding, N., et al.: Few-NERD: a few-shot named entity recognition dataset. In: Proceedings of the 59th Annual Meeting of the Association for Computational Linguistics and the 11th International Joint Conference on Natural Language Processing (Volume 1: Long Papers), pp. 3198–3213. Association for Computational Linguistics (2021)
7. Fritzler, A., Logacheva, V., Kretov, M.: Few-shot classification in named entity recognition task. In: Proceedings of the 34th ACM/SIGAPP Symposium on Applied Computing, pp. 993–1000 (2019)
8. Gao, T., Fisch, A., Chen, D.: Making pre-trained language models better few-shot learners. In: Proceedings of the 59th Annual Meeting of the Association for Computational Linguistics and the 11th International Joint Conference on Natural Language Processing (Volume 1: Long Papers), pp. 3816–3830. Association for Computational Linguistics (2021). https://doi.org/10.18653/v1/2021.acl-long.295. https://aclanthology.org/2021.acl-long.295
9. Han, X., Zhao, W., Ding, N., Liu, Z., Sun, M.: PTR: prompt tuning with rules for text classification. ArXiv abs/2105.11259 (2021). https://api.semanticscholar.org/CorpusID:235166723
10. Hou, Y., et al.: Few-shot slot tagging with collapsed dependency transfer and label-enhanced task-adaptive projection network. In: Proceedings of the 58th Annual Meeting of the Association for Computational Linguistics, pp. 1381–1393. Association for Computational Linguistics (2020)

11. Huang, Y., et al.: COPNER: contrastive learning with prompt guiding for few-shot named entity recognition. In: Proceedings of the 29th International Conference on Computational Linguistics, pp. 2515–2527. International Committee on Computational Linguistics, Gyeongju, Republic of Korea (2022)
12. Lee, J., et al: BioBERT: a pre-trained biomedical language representation model for biomedical text mining. Bioinformatics **36**(4), 1234–1240 (2019)
13. Li, J., Shang, S., Shao, L.: MetaNER: named entity recognition with meta-learning. In: Proceedings of The Web Conference 2020, pp. 429–440. WWW '20, Association for Computing Machinery, New York, NY, USA (2020)
14. Li, J., Sun, A., Han, J., Li, C.: A survey on deep learning for named entity recognition. IEEE Trans. Knowl. Data Eng. **34**(1), 50–70 (2020)
15. Li, X.L., Liang, P.: Prefix-tuning: optimizing continuous prompts for generation. In: Proceedings of the 59th Annual Meeting of the Association for Computational Linguistics and the 11th International Joint Conference on Natural Language Processing (Volume 1: Long Papers), pp. 4582–4597. Association for Computational Linguistics (2021)
16. Liu, S., Zhang, X., Zhang, S., Wang, H., Zhang, W.: Neural machine reading comprehension: methods and trends. ArXiv abs/1907.01118 (2019)
17. Ma, R., et al.: Template-free prompt tuning for few-shot NER. In: Proceedings of the 2022 Conference of the North American Chapter of the Association for Computational Linguistics: Human Language Technologies, pp. 5721–5732. Association for Computational Linguistics, Seattle, United States (2022)
18. Nguyen, N.D., Du, L., Buntine, W., Chen, C., Beare, R.: Hardness-guided domain adaptation to recognise biomedical named entities under low-resource scenarios. In: Proceedings of the 2022 Conference on Empirical Methods in Natural Language Processing, pp. 4063–4071. Abu Dhabi, United Arab Emirates (2022)
19. Radford, A., Wu, J., Child, R., Luan, D., Amodei, D., Sutskever, I.: Language models are unsupervised multitask learners (2019)
20. Schick, T., Schütze, H.: Exploiting cloze-questions for few-shot text classification and natural language inference. In: Proceedings of the 16th Conference of the European Chapter of the Association for Computational Linguistics: Main Volume, pp. 255–269. Association for Computational Linguistics (2021)
21. Schick, T., Schütze, H.: It's not just size that matters: small language models are also few-shot learners. In: Proceedings of the 2021 Conference of the North American Chapter of the Association for Computational Linguistics: Human Language Technologies, pp. 2339–2352. Association for Computational Linguistics (2021). https://doi.org/10.18653/v1/2021.naacl-main.185. https://aclanthology.org/2021.naacl-main.185
22. Shin, T., Razeghi, Y., Logan IV, R.L., Wallace, E., Singh, S.: AutoPrompt: eliciting knowledge from language models with automatically generated prompts. In: Proceedings of the 2020 Conference on Empirical Methods in Natural Language Processing (EMNLP), pp. 4222–4235. Association for Computational Linguistics (2020). https://doi.org/10.18653/v1/2020.emnlp-main.346. https://aclanthology.org/2020.emnlp-main.346
23. Snell, J., Swersky, K., Zemel, R.: Prototypical networks for few-shot learning, pp. 4080–4090. NIPS'17, Curran Associates Inc., Red Hook, NY, USA (2017)
24. Wiseman, S., Stratos, K.: Label-agnostic sequence labeling by copying nearest neighbors. In: Proceedings of the 57th Annual Meeting of the Association for Computational Linguistics, pp. 5363–5369. Association for Computational Linguistics, Florence, Italy (2019)

25. Yadav, V., Bethard, S.: A survey on recent advances in named entity recognition from deep learning models. In: Proceedings of the 27th International Conference on Computational Linguistics, pp. 2145–2158. Association for Computational Linguistics, Santa Fe, New Mexico, USA (2018)
26. Yang, Y., Katiyar, A.: Simple and effective few-shot named entity recognition with structured nearest neighbor learning. In: Proceedings of the 2020 Conference on Empirical Methods in Natural Language Processing (EMNLP), pp. 6365–6375. Association for Computational Linguistics (2020)
27. Zhang, Y., Fei, H., Li, D., Li, P.: PromptGen: automatically generate prompts using generative models. In: Findings of the Association for Computational Linguistics: NAACL 2022, pp. 30–37. Association for Computational Linguistics, Seattle, United States (2022). https://doi.org/10.18653/v1/2022.findings-naacl.3. https://aclanthology.org/2022.findings-naacl.3

Medical Entity Recognition with Few-Shot Based on Chinese Character Radicals

Jiangfeng Xu, Yuting Li, Kunli Zhang[✉], Wenxuan Zhang, Chenghao Zhang, Yuxiang Zhang, and Yunlong Li

School of Computer and Artificial Intelligence, Zhengzhou University, Zhengzhou, China
{iejfxu,ieklzhang}@zzu.edu.cn

Abstract. In medical text entity recognition tasks, Chinese character radicals are often closely related to the semantics of the characters. Based on this insight, we proposed the CSR-ProtoLERT model to integrate Chinese character radical information into few-shot entity recognition to enhance the contextual representation of the text. We optimized the pre-training embeddings, extracted radicals corresponding to Chinese characters from an online Chinese dictionary for the extensive collection of medical texts we acquired, and stored these radicals as key-value pairs. Concurrently, we employed CNN to optimize the radical embedding representation. We input the static embedding vectors of multiple Chinese characters sharing the same radical into the CNN network, extracting common feature representations for Chinese characters, ultimately obtaining the embedding representation of the Chinese character radicals. The Cross Star-Transformer model we proposed employs two Star-Transformers to model the embeddings of the input medical text character sequence and the corresponding radical sequence embedding. It fuses the Chinese character radical features with the character features, enabling the few-shot entity recognition model to learn more about medical Chinese character entity features. In the CMF 5-way 1-shot and 5-way 5-shot scenarios of the Chinese medical text few-shot entity recognition dataset we constructed, we achieved F1 values of 54.07% and 57.01%, respectively.

Keywords: Medical Text · Entity Recognition · Few-shot Learning · Fusion of Chinese Radicals

1 Introduction

Medical informatization involves a large number of medical terms and entities, which are important for knowledge graph construction. Named Entity Recognition (NER) can identify and extract entities with specific meanings from text and determine their categories or attributes. In applications in the medical field, NER can extract entities such as diseases, symptoms, and parts in medical texts, and organize them into structured data according to certain rules and formats, thereby building a medical knowledge graph [1] and medical intelligent question answering [2], clinical decision support [3] and other tasks to provide data support.

© The Author(s), under exclusive license to Springer Nature Singapore Pte Ltd. 2024
H. Xu et al. (Eds.): CHIP 2023, CCIS 1993, pp. 36–50, 2024.
https://doi.org/10.1007/978-981-99-9864-7_3

In the medical field, annotated data is relatively scarce for two main reasons: On the one hand, clinical data such as electronic medical records involve patients' personal privacy and sensitive information, such as name, age, gender, medical history, and these data cannot be disclosed or shared at will, restricting the circulation and utilization of data. On the other hand, texts in the medical field involve a large number of professional terms and abbreviations. At the same time, the professional level of annotators is required to be high, which also increases the difficulty of data annotation. For example, the evaluation dataset of the CCKS2019 named entity recognition task for Chinese electronic medical records only has 1,379 annotated data, and the CHIP2020 traditional Chinese medicine instructions entity recognition evaluation task contains a total of 1,997 drug instructions after deduplication. In the medical field, the accuracy of entity recognition tasks is required to be high, and the scarcity of annotated data is often insufficient to establish an accurate deep learning model. In this case, few-shot entity recognition [4] (Few-Shot NER) can reduce the model's dependence on data annotation, using only a small amount of annotated data for training, and improving the performance and efficiency of the entity recognition model. In 2021, Tsinghua University and Alibaba collaborated to complete the first small few-shot entity recognition dataset Few-NERD [5]. Apart from this, there are few public benchmark datasets. Existing research on few-shot entity recognition is mainly focused on general fields, and there is a lack of research on few-shot entity recognition of medical texts.

In this paper, we proposed a few-shot entity recognition model (ProtoLERT based on Cross-Star transformer with Chinese Radicals, CSR-ProtoLERT) that fuses Chinese radical information. The model includes a text embedding module and a Chinese radical fusion module. The text embedding module employs the pre-trained language model LERT to map input character sequences of medical texts into vector space. Then, the embedding representation of Chinese character radicals in Tencent Chinese pre-trained word embedding [6] (Tencent AI Lab Embedding Corpus for Chinese Words and Phrases) is analyzed and optimized to bring the radical and its corresponding Chinese character embedding representation closer, making the semantic information contained closer. The Chinese radical fusion module employs a transformer structure to deeply encode text sequences. It utilizes the simplified Star-Transformer structure to reduce the model's reliance on extensive annotated data, thereby enhancing the model's computational efficiency. We proposed an improved Cross Star-Transformer model for the integration of Chinese character radical information into the input text sequence through shared central nodes. Finally, prototype learning is employed to conduct entity classification on the fused span representations. All span representations in the query set are classified based on the prototypes derived from the category span representations learned from the support set.

We took medical text as the research object, analyzed and sampled multiple medical text entity recognition datasets, and constructed a Chinese medical text few-shot entity recognition dataset (CMF). It can not only reduce the cost of annotating medical texts, but also improve the model's ability to automatically obtain medical entities, providing a data basis for medical informatization. Finally, the main contributions of this article include three aspects as follows:

1) We proposed a few-shot entity recognition model, CSR-ProtoLERT, based on the Cross-Star transformer with Chinese Radicals, which fuses Chinese character radical information to learn the radical structure of Chinese characters within entities.

2) A strategy based on weighted random sampling was proposed to balance the entity distribution of the data set in the process of constructing the data set, and a Chinese medical text few-shot entity recognition (CMF) data set was constructed. Experiments were conducted using a few-shot named entity recognition model based on meta-learning, and the F1 value was used to conduct experiments and analysis on the CMF data set.

3) We Conducted comparative experiments on the CMF dataset, and proved the effectiveness of the Chinese character radical fusion module through different model experimental comparisons.

2   Related Work

Traditional machine learning methods design feature extraction and learning algorithms based on target tasks, which usually require a large amount of labeled data for training. Few-shot learning means that when faced with new tasks, there are only a few samples available for learning. In this case, traditional machine learning algorithms may overfit and fail to generalize well to new tasks. The few-shot learning algorithm aims to solve this problem by learning reusable knowledge from other tasks to assist the learning of new tasks. Different from few-shot learning, meta-learning pays more attention to how to design a learning algorithm so that the algorithm can quickly adapt to new tasks.

2.1   Task Definition

Given a sentence sequence, the named entity recognition task is dedicated to identifying the labels of pre-categorized numbers in the sentence. The purpose is to identify entities with specific meanings or categories from the text, such as person names, place names, organization names, time, numbers, and percentages, etc. Named entity recognition can be used in information extraction, question answering systems, text summarization, machine translation and other application scenarios.

2.2   Few-Shot Learning

Few-shot learning is a subcategory of machine learning that deals with a limited number of examples with supervised information. Specifically, few-shot classification learns classifiers given only a few labeled examples of each class. Formally, few-shot classification learns a classifier h which predicts label y_i for each input x_i. Typically, we consider the N-way-K-shot classification [7, 8], in which D_{train} contains S $=$ KN examples from N classes each with K examples.

Pre-Trained Language Models (PLM) are trained on large-scale corpora using unsupervised or weakly supervised learning methods, expecting the model to acquire a large amount of language knowledge and then fine-tune it for use. Early explorations focused on pre-training shallow networks to capture the semantics of words such as Word2Vec

[9] and GloVe [10], which play an important role in various NLP tasks. Since each word is represented by only one vector, but the same word may have different meanings in different contexts, until the introduction of Transformer, it became possible to train deep neural models for NLP tasks. In 2018, Transformer proposed deep PLMs for NLP tasks, such as Generative Pre-Training Transformer (GPT) [11] and Bidirectional Encoder Representation from Transformers (BERT) [12]. As the scale of PLMs increases, large-scale PLMs with hundreds of millions of parameters can capture word sense disambiguation, lexical and syntactic structure, and factual knowledge from text.

BERT [13] uses a bidirectional Transformer as the main structure and adopts Masked Language Model (MLM) for unsupervised training. Similar to cloze completion, it randomly masks characters in the input sequence with a special token [MASK] and predicts the hidden position words through context. The BERT model obtains a richer vector representation, which can extract complex relationship features of characters, words, sentences and text segments at multiple levels and more finely, greatly promoting the research and development of NLP tasks.

3 Research on Few-Shot Entity Recognition Integrating Chinese Character Radical Information

In few-shot entity recognition of Chinese medical texts, the Chinese radical structure of the Chinese medical entity itself also implies the semantic information of the entity. In this section, the CSR-ProtoLERT model is introduced, which leverages the Cross Star-Transformer model to integrate Chinese character and radical structural information, aiming to enhance the accuracy of named entity recognition in Chinese medical text under the few-shot scenario.

3.1 CSR-ProtoLERT Model

There are a large number of entities in medical texts, and the same entity may have different entity types in the context of different medical texts. Due to the inconsistent classification of entity categories in different datasets, it is difficult for the model to learn good entity feature representation. In the Chinese context, the radicals of Chinese characters are often closely related to their meanings. Integrating Chinese character radical information into few-shot entity recognition can enhance the context representation of the text, classify entities with the help of radical features, and improve the accuracy of few-shot entity recognition. The CSR-ProtoLERT model architecture proposed in this article is shown in Fig. 1, and mainly includes the following two modules:

1) Text embedding module: First, the pre-trained language model LERT is used to map the input character sequence of medical text to vector space. Then, the embedding representation of Chinese character radicals in Tencent Chinese pre-trained word embedding [6] (Tencent AI Lab Embedding Corpus for Chinese Words and Phrases) is analyzed and optimized to make the radical and its corresponding Chinese character embedding representation closer, that is the semantic information contained is closer.

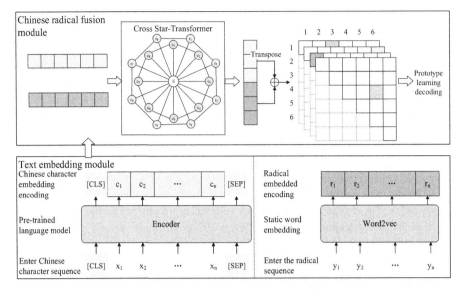

Fig. 1. CSR-ProtoLERT Model structure diagram

2) Chinese radical fusion module: Deep encoding of text sequences is achieved using the Transformer architecture. To reduce the model's dependency on a large amount of labeled data and improve computational efficiency, a simplified Star-Transformer structure is employed. An enhanced model, the Cross Star-Transformer, incorporates Chinese character radical information into the input text sequences through a shared central node. Finally, prototype learning is used to classify the fused span representations, based on prototypes learned from the support set, and to classify all span representations in the query set, resulting in the final entity classification.

3.2 Text Embedding Module

For the input character sequence $X = x_1, x_2, \cdots, x_n$ of medical text, use the LERT pre-trained language model to encode it to obtain the character embedding representation of the medical text $C = c_1, c_2, \cdots, c_n$. The Chinese characters radicals are often related to their structural form. In most Chinese dictionaries, the radicals are typically components or parts within the characters that convey the approximate meaning of the characters. When people encounter unknown Chinese characters in their daily lives, they often judge the general semantics of the Chinese characters through structures such as radicals. As shown in Table 1, in medical texts "艹" (grass) and "木" (tree) usually represent plants and traditional Chinese medicine. "月" (moon) represents human body parts or organs, and "疒" (radical of illness) represents disease. "艾, 芷, 芝, 莲, 蔻, 芪" (ai, zhi, zhi, lotus, kou, qi) usually appear in Chinese characters for herbal plants. "肝, 肺, 胆, 胃, 肘, 脖" (liver, lungs, gallbladder, stomach, elbows, neck) are commonly found in body parts. "疟, 痢, 疝, 疮, 癌, 疽" (malaria, dysentery, hernia, sore, cancer, and subcutaneous ulcer) are often associated with diseases.

Table 1. Examples of Chinese Radicals in Medical Texts

Radical	Meaning	Example
艹	Herb	艾, 芷, 芝, 莲, 蔻, 芪
月	Body parts	肝, 肺, 胆, 胃, 肘, 脖
疒	Disease	疟, 痢, 疝, 疮, 癌, 疽

The semantics of Chinese characters with the same radicals are relatively similar, and there is little difference in different semantic scenarios. Therefore, for the radical $Y = y_1, y_2, \cdots, y_n$ corresponding to the Chinese character in the input medical text sequence, the static embedding based on context training is used to represent the radical embedding representation $R = r_1, r_2, \cdots, r_n$ of the medical text entity.

The pre-trained embedding representation is generated by large-scale high quality text training in multiple fields. In order to make it more suitable for named entity recognition of medical text, certain fine-tuning is performed on the pre-trained embedding. Principal Component Analysis (PCA) [14] can reduce high-dimensional data to low-dimensional data without losing too much information in the process. The new data is mapped to a new coordinate system, which is helpful for data analysis and visualization. First, perform PCA processing on the pre-trained embedding representation, reduce the 200-dimensional pre-trained embedding vector to 3 dimensions, and use some Chinese characters and radicals in the medical text to perform visual analysis on the reduced dimension feature vector, as shown in Fig. 2.

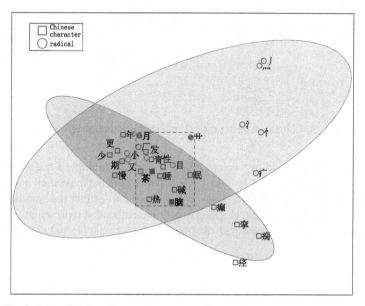

Fig. 2. Visualization of pre-training embedding of Chinese character radicals

The embedded representation of Chinese radicals in medical entities varies greatly. The whole can be divided into two categories: radicals (i.e., "疒" (sickness), "氵" (water), "忄" (heart)) and character radicals (i.e., "月" (moon), "又" (again), "目" (eye)).Compared with radicals, the embedded representation distance of character radicals and Chinese characters is closer, that is, the semantics in the text are closer, such as "月" (moon) and "脑" (brain) and "艹" (grass) and "茶" (tea) in Fig. 2. The radicals are relatively compact, far away from the representation space of Chinese characters, and the semantic representation is inaccurate. Therefore, this section optimizes the pre-training embedding. First, obtain a large number of medical texts related to the content of the original dataset, and count and sort the frequency of Chinese characters in these medical texts. Then, the obtained Chinese characters are deduplicated, the radicals corresponding to the Chinese characters are crawled online from the online Chinese dictionary, and the radicals and their corresponding Chinese characters are stored in the form of key-value pairs. Load the pre-trained embedding and use CNN to optimize the radical embedding representation. The specific process is shown in Fig. 3.

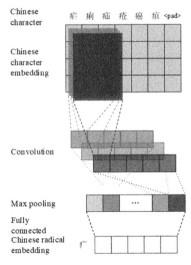

Fig. 3. Chinese character radical embedding optimization process

First, the static embedding vectors $c_1^i, c_2^i, \cdots, c_m^i$ of multiple Chinese characters with the same radical are input into the CNN network, and the maximum pooling layer MaxPooling and the fully connected layer FC are used to extract the common feature representation of Chinese characters, and finally the embedded representation r_i of the Chinese character radical is obtained, as shown in the formula (1) and (2) are shown.

$$t_i = CNN\left(c_1^i, c_2^i, \cdots, c_m^i\right) \tag{1}$$

$$r_i = FC(MaxPooling(t_i)) \tag{2}$$

The optimized pre-training embedding is visually displayed, as shown in Fig. 4. It can be seen that the optimized radical and character radical embedding representation is more

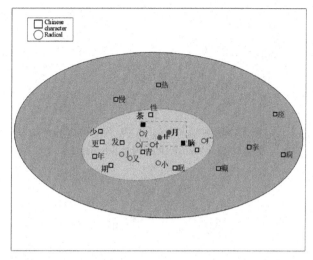

Fig. 4. Optimized visualization of Chinese character radical embedding

reasonable, and the distance between Chinese characters and their corresponding radicals is closer and the semantic representation is closer, such as "月" (moon) and "脑" (brain), "艹" (grass) and "茶" (tea). Reasonable Chinese character radical embedding can help the model better identify entities in medical texts, provide richer feature representation, and help distinguish similarities between entities of different categories.

3.3 Chinese Radical Fusion Module

The parallel capability of the transformer-based method is far better than that of LSTM, but it has many model parameters and requires a large amount of computing resources and memory in training long texts. In the Transformer model, the self-attention mechanism is applied. Each position must establish a direct connection with other positions and obtain contextual information from other positions. The overall structure has many complex parameters and is prone to overfitting when there are few training samples. The Star-Transformer [15] model enables each position to establish direct connections with adjacent positions and indirect connections with other non-adjacent positions through the central node. Star-Transformer has fewer parameters, less dependence on sample size, and is more suitable for few-shot scenarios. As shown in Fig. 5, if the beginning and end of the medical text sequence are connected into a ring, then the connection of transformer is a fully connected graph. The simplified Star-Transformer obtains knowledge for each medical text character h_i from the adjacent characters h_{i-1}, h_{i+1} and the virtual central node S. The central node S obtains the context information of the medical text sequence from all characters h.

We proposed a Cross Star-Transformer to fuse Chinese character radical information, as shown in Fig. 6, where the inner ring is the sequence of Chinese character notes g_i, and the outer ring is the sequence of radical nodes h_i, S is the context center node.

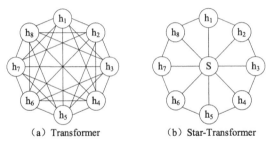

Fig. 5. Star-Transformer structure diagram

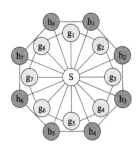

Fig. 6. Cross Star-Transformer structure diagram

Two Star-Transformers are used to model the embedding $C = c_1, c_2, \ldots, c_n$ of the input medical text character sequence and the corresponding radical sequence embedding $R = r_1, r_2, \ldots, r_n$ respectively. The two models are updated using the same central node S, thus making the medical interaction occurs between Chinese characters and radicals in the text. The update process of Cross Star-Transformer is shown in Algorithm 1.

Algorithm 1: The Update of Cross Star-Transformer

Input: Chinese Character Embedding C, Chinese Radical Embedding R

1   $g_1^0, g_2^0, \cdots; g_n^0 \leftarrow c_1, c_2, \cdots; c_n$ // Initialize peripheral nodes

2   $h_1^0, h_2^0, \cdots; h_n^0 \leftarrow r_1, r_2, \cdots; r_n$

3   $S_0 = average(c_1, c_2, \cdots; c_n; r_1, r_2, \cdots; r_n)$ // Initialize central node

4   for t from 1 to T do

5   for i from 1 to n do // Update peripheral nodes

6         $C_i^t = [g_{i-1}^{t-1}; g_i^{t-1}; g_{i+1}^{t-1}; c_i; S^{t-1}]$

7         $R_i^t = [h_{i-1}^{t-1}; h_i^{t-1}; h_{i+1}^{t-1}; r_i; S^{t-1}]$

8         $g_i^t = MultiAtt(g_i^{t-1}, C_i^t)$ $h_i^t = MultiAtt(h_i^{t-1}, R_i^t)$

9         $g_i^t = LayerNorm\left(ReLU(g_i^t)\right)$ $h_i^t = LayerNorm\left(ReLU(h_i^t)\right)$

10      $S^t = MultiAtt(S^{t-1}, [S^{t-1}; G^t; H^t])$ // Update central node

11      $S^t = LayerNorm\left(ReLU(S^t)\right)$

The input is the sequence embedding representation of Chinese characters and radicals C and R. Steps 1–3 initialization stage: first map it to Cross Star-Transformer and initialize surrounding nodes g_i and h_i, and then use the mean value of all surrounding node vectors as the initialization representation S_0 of the central node. Steps 5–9 external node update stage: Chinese character point g_i and radical node h_i are updated in the same way. Taking the Chinese character node g_i^t as an example, the current g_i^t needs to be updated by concatenating the initial embedding c_i, the central node S of the previous moment, the current and adjacent nodes g_i^{t-1}, g_{i-1}^{t-1}, and g_{i+1}^{t-1} of the previous moment with the previous g_i^{t-1}, and then performing multi-head attention calculation and normalization operation. Steps 10–11 central node update stage: The update method is similar to that of surrounding nodes. The central node S^t at the current moment needs to be updated through the central node S^{t-1} at the previous moment and all Chinese character points G^t and radical nodes H^t at the current moment.

First update the peripheral medical text character embedding c_i and radical embedding r_i, and then update the central node S. The visual update process of Cross Star-Transformer is shown in Fig. 7.

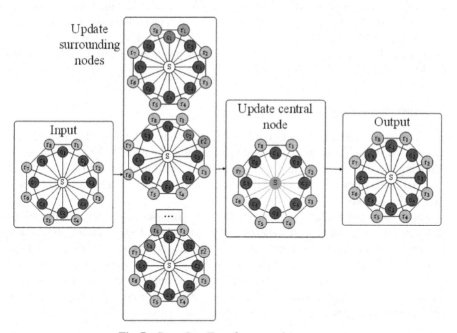

Fig. 7. Cross Star-Transformer update process

4 Experimental Results and Analysis

4.1 Dataset Introduction

The datasets used in the experiment are sourced from various departments and include the following: the public dataset Chinese Medical Named Entity Extraction dataset [16] (CMeEE), the Critical Illness Knowledge Graph dataset (CIKG), the Chinese Pediatric Epilepsy Knowledge Graph (CpeKG), the Cardiovascular Diseases Knowledge Graph dataset (CvdKG) [17], and the Diabetes Electronic Medical Record Entity and Relation Corpus (DEMRC). These datasets constitute the Chinese Medical Text Few-Shot Entity Recognition (CMF) dataset. It encompasses a total of 20 categories and 132,426 medical entities.

Based on the consistency of entity descriptions for each type across different datasets, they are categorized into three groups: identical entities, similar entities, and unique entities. Entities like "disease," "symptom," and "body part" have consistent descriptions across all datasets. In the CMeEE dataset, "examination" is also subdivided into "examination items" and "examination indicators". Some datasets constructed based on medical textbooks, such as CIKG, CPeKG, and CvdkG, also include long entities like "sociology" and "epidemiology". Additionally, some datasets have their unique entity types, such as the "EEG performance" entity in the childhood epilepsy dataset CPeKG and entities like time and modifiers in the diabetes electronic medical record dataset DEMRC.

4.2 Experimental Setup

The experimental settings include the CNN filters, convolution kernels, environment settings used in the experiment and hyperparameter settings of the model used when optimizing the radical embedding representation. The dropout is set to 0.2, a 6-layer Cross Star-Transformer is used, and the internal attention layer is 6 attention heads, each with 256 dimensions.

When constructing a data sample in the few-shot scenario, firstly, N types of medical entities are randomly drawn from the medical entity label set. Then, sentences containing these entities are extracted to form a collection in the N-way K-shot format, and the support set and query set are constructed in turn. Weighted random sampling is a method of random sampling based on sample weights. Each sample is assigned a weight, and then random sampling is carried out with the weight as the probability, thus making the probability of more important samples being selected larger.

Dataset Statistics. The CMF dataset constructed in this chapter is designed for small-sample scenarios with 5-way 1-shot and 5-way 5-shot settings. Specifically, 700 samples and 350 samples are sampled from each original dataset for training, validation, and test data partitions, with a split ratio of 4:2:1. To ensure distinct training and testing tasks, the training set is reorganized. The statistics of the number of 5-way 1-shot and 5-way 5-shot entities in the CMF data set are shown in Table 2.

4.3 Experimental Results and Analysis

We compare the CSR-ProtoLERT model with ProtoBERT [18], NNShot [19], StructShot [18] few-shot entity recognition models on the self-built medical text few-shot entity recognition dataset CMF dataset, in order to verify the effectiveness of the proposed Chinese character radical fusion module. The experimental results are shown in Table 3 and Table 4.

Table 2. Statistics of CMF dataset

Source	Num of sentences (5w1s/5w5s)			Types	Description
	Train	Dev	Test		
CMeEE	400/200	200/100	100/50	9	Clinical Pediatrics
CIKG	400/200	200/100	100/50	11	Lung, liver and breast cancer
CPeKG	400/200	200/100	100/50	19	Pediatric epilepsy
CVdKG	400/200	200/100	100/50	15	Cardiovascular diseases
DEMRC	400/200	200/100	100/50	9	Diabetes

Table 3. Results of CSR-ProtoLERT Model 5-way 1-shot on the CMF Dataset

Model	CMeEE	CIKG	CPeKG	CvdKG	DEMRC	Average
ProtoBERT	26.71 ± 1.11	31.69 ± 0.25	27.48 ± 1.02	29.47 ± 1.31	29.99 ± 0.48	29.07
NNShot	17.25 ± 14.83	26.29 ± 1.47	25.67 ± 1.19	25.21 ± 0.84	43.16 ± 1.55	27.52
StructShot	21.26 ± 18.42	30.07 ± 1.17	30.59 ± 0.74	30.91 ± 0.68	47.13 ± 1.96	31.99
CSR-ProtoBERT	57.82 ± 1.23	50.02 ± 0.93	50.19 ± 0.63	49.11 ± 1.34	51.21 ± 0.59	51.67
CSR-ProtoLERT	$\mathbf{59.25 \pm 1.60}$	$\mathbf{51.34 \pm 0.61}$	$\mathbf{51.83 \pm 1.08}$	$\mathbf{51.85 \pm 1.39}$	$\mathbf{56.08 \pm 0.30}$	**54.07**

Table 4. Results of CSR-ProtoLERT Model 5-way 5-shot on the CMF Dataset

Model	CMeEE	CIKG	CPeKG	CvdKG	DEMRC	Average
ProtoBERT	42.15 ± 1.60	39.92 ± 0.44	39.22 ± 0.28	42.25 ± 0.22	34.34 ± 1.76	39.58
NNShot	24.58 ± 21.27	31.97 ± 1.02	30.89 ± 1.38	22.32 ± 19.34	32.89 ± 28.36	28.53
StructShot	28.88 ± 25.02	38.84 ± 1.64	39.03 ± 0.45	28.22 ± 24.46	30.09 ± 28.63	33.61
CSR-ProtoBERT	61.36 ± 0.62	55.12 ± 0.57	52.12 ± 1.22	56.22 ± 0.61	54.82 ± 0.51	55.93
CSR-ProtoLERT	$\mathbf{61.89 \pm 0.98}$	$\mathbf{56.16 \pm 0.49}$	$\mathbf{53.38 \pm 0.20}$	$\mathbf{57.31 \pm 0.37}$	$\mathbf{56.30 \pm 1.04}$	**57.01**

This section compares the experimental results of each entity category of CPeKG in the CMF dataset, as shown in Fig. 8. Among them, the identification effect of epidemiological entities is poor, because epidemiology is the study of the distribution and determinants of diseases and health conditions in specific populations, and the coverage of entities is wide, and using Chinese character radical features for entity identification is prone to noise. In addition, the improvement of parts in the same medical entities in each task in the CMF dataset is more obvious, and it may be analyzed that diseases and symptoms have entity overlap phenomena, and symptom descriptions may be disease entities in some medical contexts. Among them, the recognition accuracy of surgical entities compared with the experimental results of the MBE-ProtoLERT model has increased by 2.83% on the basis of an F1 value of 37.29%, indicating that the method of fusing Chinese character radicals is effective.

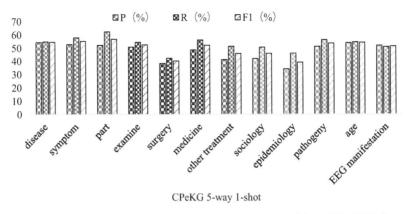

CPeKG 5-way 1-shot

Fig. 8. F1 value of CSR-ProtoLERT model in each category of CPeKG in CMF dataset

In order to analyze the model more intuitively, based on the results of entity recognition, four samples of different tasks were selected to compare the model prediction results, as shown in Table 5.

It can be seen from the four examples that the CSR-ProtoLERT model can accurately identify medical entities in the text, such as "disease", "drug", "symptoms", and "EEG performance", among others. This indicates that the incorporation of knowledge related to Chinese radicals can enhance the accuracy of entity recognition in few-shot medical texts.

Table 5. CSR-ProtoLERT Model Entity Recognition Example Analysis

Example 1	No history of hypertension or heart disease
Real label	"Decorate": (0, 0) "Disease": (1, 3), (5, 8)
Predicted label	"Decorate": (0, 0) √ "Disease": (1, 3), (5, 8) √
Example 2	Epileptic EEG shows alternating sharp and slow waves
Real label	"Disease": (0, 1) "EEG performance": (8, 17)
Predicted label	"Disease": (0, 1) √ "EEG performance": (8, 17) √
Example 3	Fever and pain in the liver area are common
Real label	"Symptom": (2, 3), (5, 8)
Predicted label	"Symptom": (2, 3), (5, 8) √
Example 4	Drugs used to treat lung cancer include paclitaxel, gefitinib, pemetrexed, etc.
Real label	"Disease": (2, 3) "Drug": (9, 11), (13, 16), (18, 21)
Predicted label	"Disease": (2, 3) √ "Drug": (9, 11), (13, 16), (18, 21) √

5 Conclusion

This paper proposed the CSR-ProtoLERT model to conduct research on few-shot medical text entity recognition, and uses a method of integrating Chinese character radical information to improve the accuracy of Chinese medical entities. First, the pre-trained radical embeddings are optimized using a CNN model in the representation learning stage. In the feature fusion stage, considering that medical text sentences are usually long and contain many long entities, and long-distance modeling is easy to lose information, a Cross Star-Transformer structure based on the Transformer structure is proposed to fuse Chinese radicals and character embedding representations. Experiments on the medical text few-shot entity recognition dataset CMF show that some medical entities can be categorized using Chinese character radicals, in these cases, the CSR-ProtoLERT model achieves very high recognition accuracy.

Acknowledgments. Here, we would like to express our gratitude for the valuable suggestions provided by all reviewers. This work was supported in part by the Science and Technology Innovation 2030-"New Generation of Artificial Intelligence" Major Project under Grant No. 2021ZD0111000.

References

1. Fan, Y., Li, Z.: Research and application progress of Chinese medical knowledge graph. Comput. Sci. Explor. **16**(10), 2219–2233 (2022)
2. He, J., Du, J., Nie, B., et al.: Research on the application of intelligent question answering system in the medical field. Med. Inf. **31**(14), 16–19 (2018)

3. Shah, S., Coughlan, J.: How prescribers can use technology to improve patient care. J. Prescribing Pract. **1**(4), 198–203 (2019)
4. Luong, T., Sutskever, I., Le, Q.V., et al.: Addressing the rare word problem in neural machine translation. CoRR (2014)
5. Ding, N., Xu, G., Chen, Y., et al.: Few-NERD: a few-shot named entity recognition dataset. In: Proceedings of the 59th Annual Meeting of the Association for Computational Linguistics and the 11th International Joint Conference on Natural Language Processing (Volume 1: Long Papers), pp. 3198–3213 (2021)
6. Song, Y., Shi, S., Li, J., et al.: Directional skip-gram: explicitly distinguishing left and right context for word embeddings. In: Proceedings of the 2018 Conference of the North American Chapter of the Association for Computational Linguistics: Human Language Technologies, Volume 2 (Short Papers), pp. 175–180 (2018)
7. Finn, C., Abbeel, P., Levine, S.: Model-agnostic meta-learning for fast adaptation of deep networks. In: International Conference on Machine Learning. PMLR, pp. 1126–1135 (2017)
8. Vinyals, O., Blundell, C., Lillicrap, T., et al.: Matching networks for one shot learning. In: Advances in Neural Information Processing Systems, vol. 29 (2016)
9. Mikolov, T., Chen, K., Corrado, G., et al.: Efficient estimation of word representations in vector space. In: Proceedings of the International Conference on Learning Representations (ICLR 2013) (2013)
10. Pennington, J., Socher, R., Manning, C.D.: GloVe: global vectors for word representation. In: Proceedings of the 2014 Conference on Empirical Methods in Natural Language Processing (EMNLP), pp. 1532–1543 (2014)
11. Radford, A., Narasimhan, K., Salimans, T., et al.: Improving language understanding by generative pre-training. Preprint (2018)
12. Devlin, J., Chang, M.-W., Lee, K., Toutanova, K.: BERT: pre-training of deep bidirectional transformers for language understanding. In: Proceedings of NAACL-HLT, pp. 4171–4186 (2019)
13. Devlin, J., Chang, M.W., Lee, K., et al.: BERT: pre-training of deep bidirectional transformers for language understanding. arXiv preprint arXiv:1810.04805 (2018)
14. Pearson, K.: LIII. On lines and planes of closest fit to systems of points in space. Lond. Edinb. Dublin Philos. Mag. J. Sci. **2**(11), 559–572 (1901)
15. Guo, Q., Qiu, X., Liu, P., et al.: Star-transformer. In: Proceedings of the 2019 Conference of the North American Chapter of the Association for Computational Linguistics: Human Language Technologies, Volume 1 (Long and Short Papers), pp. 1315–1325 (2019)
16. Zhang, N., Chen, M., Bi, Z., et al.: CBLUE: a Chinese biomedical language understanding evaluation benchmark. In: Proceedings of the 60th Annual Meeting of the Association for Computational Linguistics (Volume 1: Long Papers), pp. 7888–7915 (2022)
17. Zhang, S., Song, Y., Zhang, K.: Research on knowledge reasoning technology for cardiovascular disease knowledge graph question and answer. Zhengzhou University (2023)
18. Snell, J., Swersky, K., Zemel, R.: Prototypical networks for few-shot learning. In: Advances in Neural Information Processing Systems, vol. 30 (2017)
19. Yang, Y., Katiyar, A.: Simple and effective few-shot named entity recognition with structured nearest neighbor learning. In: Proceedings of the 2020 Conference on Empirical Methods in Natural Language Processing (EMNLP), pp. 6365–6375 (2020)

Biomedical Named Entity Recognition Based on Multi-task Learning

Hui Zhao, Di Zhao[✉], Jiana Meng, Wen Su, and Wenxuan Mu

School of Computer Science and Engineering, Dalian Minzu University,
Dalian 116000, Liaoning, China
{zhaodi,mengjn}@dlnu.edu.cn

Abstract. Under the background of big data era, the literature in the field of biomedicine has increased explosively. Named Entity Recognition (NER) is able to extract key information from large amounts of text quickly and accurately. But the problem of unclear boundary recognition and underutilization of hierarchical information has always existed in the task of entity recognition in the biomedical domain. Based on this, the paper proposes a novel Biomedical Named Entity Recognition (BioNER) model based on multi-task learning that incorporates syntactic dependency information. Syntactic dependency information is extracted through Graph Convolutional Network (GCN) and incorporated into the input sentences. Using a co-attentive mechanism, the input information and the label information encoded by BERT are fused to obtain the interaction matrix. Then, entity recognition is performed through the boundary detection and span classification tasks. The model was experimented on two English datasets, JNLPBA and BC5CDR, as well as a Chinese dataset, CCKS2017. The experimental results reflected the effectiveness of the entity recognition model proposed in this paper.

Keywords: Biomedical Named Entity Recognition · Syntactic Dependency Tree · Graph Convolutional Network · Co-attention Mechanism · Multi-task Learning

1 Introduction

Named Entity Recognition (NER) [1] as an important cornerstone of Natural Language Processing (NLP) tasks. It refers to the recognition of specific meaningful entities in semi-structured or unstructured texts and classifying them into predefined entity types, such as name of people, place, organization, etc. Whereas in the biomedical domain, it is essential to recognize entity types such as chemical, disease, gene, protein. Biomedical Named Entity Recognition (BioNER) accurately recognizes biomedical entity information from texts, providing valuable data resources for researchers. Moreover, it offers vital support for scientific research in fields such as medicine, drug development, and disease diagnosis. BioNER is not only a component of information extraction but also an indispensable part of biomedical research.

© The Author(s), under exclusive license to Springer Nature Singapore Pte Ltd. 2024
H. Xu et al. (Eds.): CHIP 2023, CCIS 1993, pp. 51–65, 2024.
https://doi.org/10.1007/978-981-99-9864-7_4

With the exponential increase in the volume of biomedical texts, accurate and automatic extraction of entity information from large amounts of medical texts has become a key focus of research. BioNER provides the basis for other downstream tasks, such as relation extraction [2], knowledge base construction [3], information retrieval [4] and question answering systems [5].

Early BioNER relied primarily on expert rules and machine learning, requiring domain experts to extract features directly in deep networks, leading to poor generalization and wasteful use of manual effort. Later, deep learning methods reduced labor and training costs, becoming the mainstream research methods.

Compared with NER in general domains, BioNER is more challenging and involves greater difficulties. Biomedical entities are more complex in form, often consisting of multiple words with many acronyms. These acronyms often exist in different forms without clear definitions and descriptions for reference, which makes the entity boundaries difficult to distinguish and increases the difficulty of recognition. In entity recognition, there are also phenomena of nested and overlapping entities, which increase difficulty of recognition. In addition, the limited utilization of syntactic information in the corpus in the medical entity recognition method leads to poor results. Based on this, this paper proposes a BioNER model based on multi-task learning, and the main contributions are as follows:

(1) The BioNER task is transformed from a sequence labeling task to a multi-task, specifically as a joint task of boundary detection and span classification, addressing issues related to ambiguous boundary recognition and nested entity problems.
(2) The dataset undergoes syntactic dependency analysis, and the resulting syntactic parsing graphs are encoded using Graph Convolutional Network (GCN) and integrated into the multi-task. This integration allows the model to comprehensively learn the syntactic elements within the text as well as the relationships between these elements, thereby enhancing the performance of NER.
(3) Multiple sets of comparative experiments were conducted on datasets, and the results demonstrate the effectiveness of the model proposed in this paper.

2   Related Work

NER has been regarded as a crucial metric in evaluating the effectiveness of information extraction [6]. Based on its historical development process, research progress in NER can be divided into three stages: from rule-based and dictionary-based methods to machine learning-based methods, and later to deep learning-based methods. The following will introduce the development process of BioNER from these three aspects.

2.1   Rule-Based and Dictionary-Based Methods

In the early stages, NER based on rules and dictionaries. Rule-based methods typically use fixed rule templates and rely on pattern matching and string matching techniques to filter and process the text. Hanisc et al. [7] proposed a rule-based method for recognizing gene and protein entities. However, these rules are often overfit to specific entity recognition tasks, and their design process is complex, time-consuming and prone to errors.

Later, in the biomedical domain, dictionary-based methods were introduced. Common terminology vocabularies, such as ICD-10, UMLS and RxNorm, were widely utilized in early BioNER. This process primarily relies on matching the text with dictionaries to recognize specific entities. In the biomedical domain, three typical tools have emerged: MedLEE, MedKAT and cTAKES [8]. They represent the applied aspects of this method. However, the effectiveness of this method is largely contingent upon the quality of the dictionaries and algorithmic matching techniques. Xia [9] constructed a gene entity vocabulary based on UMLS and utilized machine learning methods such as Conditional Random Fields (CRF) to recognize gene named entities in GENIA 3.02 dataset. Krauthammer et al. [10] proposed a dictionary-based method to recognize gene and protein entities.

In summary, rule-based and dictionary-based methods have limitations inBioNER. With the growth of data and the emergence of new specialized terms, these methods often require constant maintenance and adjustments. Moreover, they are challenging to generalize across different domains.

2.2 Machine Learning-Based Methods

Machine learning methods plays an important role in entity recognition, which include the Hidden Markov Model (HMM) [11], the Maximum Entropy (ME) [12] model and the CRF [13]. These methods usually have high requirements on feature selection and need to consider features such as prefixes, suffixes, letter cases, special characters, morphemes and roots to train the models. In particular, CRF is widely used in NER tasks and has shown good performance.

Leaman et al. [14] researchers proposed the tmChem model, which integrates two CRF models and combines a variety of manually designed features. Li et al. [15] researchers introduced word frequency and co-occurrence information into the CRF model to improve the performance of recognizing gene entities.

In summary, machine learning-based methods bring significant performance improvements in entity recognition but still suffers from poor generalization and insufficient interpretability capabilities.

2.3 Deep Learning-Based Methods

In recent years, deep learning methods have been widely used in many research domains because they can automatically and efficiently discover hidden features, not only avoiding the complicated process of manually constructing features, but also discovering more nonlinear relationships and obtaining stronger representative information.

Zhu et al. [16] applied the CNN model to NER in the biomedical domain and proposed a new model, GRAM-CNN. Korvigo et al. [17] proposed an end-to-end BioNER model that combines CNN and LSTM to recognize chemical entities and does not require the manual creation of rules. Dang et al. [18] adapted the BiLSTM-CRF model and then proposed the D3NER model. This model can be fine-tuned to recognize a variety of named entities, such as diseases, genes, proteins, etc. SC-LSTM-CRF [19] utilized the method of embedding two channels and sentence levels into the LSTM-CRF. The two channels solve the problem of hidden feature loss in the model, and the sentence-level embedding enables the model to utilize contextual information and improve its performance. Zhao et al. [20] proposed a novel disease NER method based on multi-labeled convolutional neural networks that concatenate character-level embedding, word-level embedding and lexical feature embedding. Then several convolutional layers are stacked on top of the cascade embeddings, and local features are obtained by combining different sizes of convolutional kernels. Yan et al. [21] proposed a span-based NER model that uses a convolutional neural network to model the interactions between segments, which helps the model find more nested entities.

In summary, deep learning-based methods can utilize textual contextual information, including long-distance dependencies, improving the understanding of entity context and recognition accuracy.

3   The Method

In this paper, we propose a BioNER model based on multi-task learning. Firstly, the input sentences $X = \{x_1, x_2, \cdots, x_n\}$ and the labels of entities $L = \{l_1, l_2, \cdots, l_n\}$ in the dataset are encoded by BERT pre-training. The sentences undergo encoding using a syntactic dependency tree through a GCN. Subsequently, the outcomes of the convolution and label encoding processes are computed utilizing a similarity matrix through the co-attentive mechanism. The rows and columns are computed separately by the element-by-element multiplication method, then the boundary detection and span classification tasks are carried out. The overall architecture of the model is shown in Fig. 1.

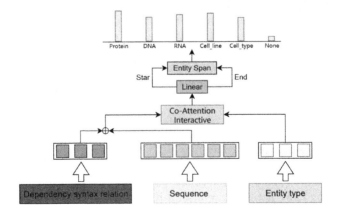

Fig. 1. The overall architecture of the model.

3.1   Feature Extraction Layer

Syntactic Dependency Tree. Syntactic dependency information can extract relationships between words in a text, provide abundant structural information, and have a significant advantage in representing distant lexical relationships. In this paper, we used Standford CoreNLP to obtain medical texts for segmentation and their syntactic dependency trees. The visualization of the result is shown in Fig. 2.

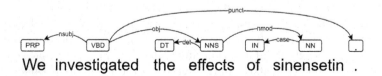

Fig. 2. Example of an English syntactic analysis.

GCN. GCN is a deep learning model for processing graphical data. In NLP, textual data is modeled as a graph. Each word is represented as node information in the graph, and the relationship between words (dependency or co-occurrence) is represented as edges in the graph. GCN has distinct advantages in NER. Firstly, it excels in modeling the context of each node by leveraging information from neighboring nodes. This aspect is particularly valuable in NER, as the context surrounding a named entity often holds pivotal information. Secondly, GCN can capture word-to-word dependencies by examining connections between nodes in the graph. This capability is crucial for NER, enabling the system to handle syntactic dependency information effectively.

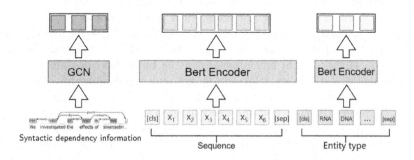

Fig. 3. The architecture of feature representation layer.

Representation of Features. The feature representation part is shown in Fig. 3, where the model first encodes the input sequence and entity type labels using BERT. Syntactic dependency analysis is a method of syntactic analysis that reveals the structure of a sentence and the relationships between its components by analyzing the dependencies between words in the sentence. This method of analysis focuses on the dependencies between words. This helps us to understand the structure and grammatical relationships of the sentence and thus better understand the meaning of the text. Dependency relations are represented by dependency links with the direction pointing from the dependent word to the dominant word, and the markers on the dependency links represent different dependency relations. The dependency syntax tree is represented as the adjacency matrix A and the degree matrix D. GCN is a type of convolutional network that can be used to encode data structures related to graphs.

The GCN makes the input information interact with its syntactic dependency tree, so that the model fully learns the dependency relations present in the sentence. h_1 is the input information after BERT coding, A is the adjacency matrix, D is the degree matrix, and w and b are the learnable parameters and the specific formula for GCN to extract the syntactic features in the sentence is shown as:

$$G_x = RELU(DAh_1w + b) \tag{1}$$

In addition to the syntactic information contained in sentences, we consider that entity types also contain entity-specific information. In order to better represent entity type labeling information, the BERT-encoded entity type labels are mean-pooled to obtain a abundant entity type labeling representation.

3.2   Feature Fusion Layer

Co-attention Mechanism. The co-attention mechanism is an attentional method for processing sequence data and establishing associations between sequences. The co-attention mechanism allows the model to process sequential data without being limited by the length of the sequences. This is different from traditional Recurrent Neural Network (RNN), which suffer from the problem of vanishing or exploding gradients when processing long sequences. The co-attention mechanism makes information transfer in long sequences more efficient by calculating the weighted attention of each element. It can be highly parallelized, which is more advantageous in the biomedical domain where the sentences in the dataset are relatively longer and more numerous. And it can also allow the model to consider all the elements in the input sequences at the same time during the encoding and decoding process and therefore capture the global dependency relations, which allows the model to better understand long-distance dependencies between sequences. By utilizing this mechanism in this paper, the syntactic information in a sentence can be better learned for better feature fusion.

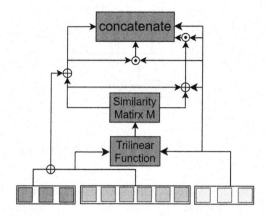

Fig. 4. The architecture of co-attention mechanism.

For better feature fusion, this paper used the co-attention mechanism to fuse features. As shown in Fig. 4, after obtaining the output of the GCN and the output of the label after mean pooling, the co-attentive interaction network is used so that the input sentence and the syntactic information contained in the sentence as well as the specific information contained in the entity label are fully interacted with each other. So the model can better learn the potential interaction information as well as the specific information so that the entity span boundaries can be better represented. The boundary information formula is shown as:

$$M = w^T[h_x, G_x, h_e] \tag{2}$$

W is the trainable weights and M is the final attention weight matrix, the interaction matrices M_r and M_c at the entity boundaries are obtained by row-by-row and column-by-column operations respectively. Label-to-token and token-to-label interactions formulas are obtained as:

$$H_l^t = M_r \bullet h_e \tag{3}$$

$$H_t^l = M_r \bullet M_c^T \bullet h_x \tag{4}$$

3.3 Label Classification Layer

Multi-task Method. NER based on multi-task is a method that integrates multiple related tasks into a single model in order to learn together, and this method has a number of advantages. The model allows data to be shared and utilized across multiple tasks, which improves data utilization. With the multi-task learning, the complexity of maintaining and debugging separate models can be reduced, which helps to reduce computational resource requirements and improve system efficiency. The multi-task learning is flexible enough to allow tasks to be easily incorporated or deleted to accommodate different needs.

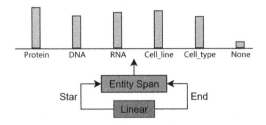

Fig. 5. The architecture of multi-task learning.

Boundary Detection and Span Classification Method. The multi-task method in this paper is shown in Fig. 5, where the head position and tail position of an entity are first recognized, followed by the task of labeling and classifying the entity type. The head entity and tail entity recognition tasks require the model to perform finer-grained recognition near the boundaries of the entity, which provides more contextual information and is more helpful in accurately determining the entity boundaries. The span classification task recognizes the entity type, which provides additional information about the content of the entity, and this multi-task method allows the model to understand the entity from different perspectives, which improves the accuracy of the entity recognition.

Specifically, the start or end position of the entity span is computed as a pre-task of the multi-task method to compute the correct entity boundaries to lay the foundation for the next entity type classification task. During the training process, the cross-entropy loss is used to optimize the boundaries of entity spans. The formulas are shown as:

$$B = [h_x; H_l^t; h_x \bullet H_l^t; h_x \bullet H_t^l] \tag{5}$$

$$p(\theta)_i = \frac{exp(w_1^T B_i)}{\sum_j exp(w_1^T B_j)} \tag{6}$$

$$L_{ht}(\theta) = -\sum_{i=1}^{N} \hat{y}_i log P(\theta)_i \tag{7}$$

The span classification task is based on matching the header and tail labels of each boundary label to classify entity spans into the corresponding semantic labels, or the "None" category if the candidate entity span is not an entity. The entity span V_{span} is defined as:

$$V_{span} = [B_i + B_j; B_i - B_j] \tag{8}$$

Finally, the entity span representation is sent to the Softmax layer to predict the probability of entity labeling P_{span}, which minimizes the entity labeling prediction loss L_{span} formulas as:

$$P_{span}(\theta) = softmax(MLP(w^T V_{span} + b)) \tag{9}$$

$$L_{span}(\theta) = -\sum_{i=1}^{c}(y_{span}^{\Delta i})log(P_{span}^{i}(\theta)) \tag{10}$$

The multi-task method is used to minimize the loss of entity type labels and boundaries during the training phase as:

$$L(\theta) = L_{ht}(\theta) + L_{span}(\theta) \tag{11}$$

4 Experiments and Results

4.1 Datasets

In this paper, experiments were carried out on two English datasets, JNLPBA and BC5CDR, as well as a Chinese dataset, CCKS2017. NER is considered accurate if both entity boundaries and entity types are predicted accurately. The dataset statistics are shown in Table 1:

Table 1. Dataset statistics

	JNLPBA	BC5CDR	CCKS2017
Train	14,690	15,935	1,561
Dev	3,856	4,012	334
Test	3,856	4,012	334

4.2 Results and Analysis

In this paper, to validate the model's effectiveness, three sets of baseline experiments were conducted separately on BC5CDR, JNLPBA and CCKS2017 datasets. Additionally, comparative experiments were conducted with other models. The results of the experiments are shown in Tables 2, 3 and 4.

Table 2. Results of comparison experiments on BC5CDR

Model	P (%)	R (%)	F1 (%)
BERT+CRF	87.0	81.5	84.2
BERT+BiLSTM+CRF	87.7	82.0	84.8
BERT+CNN+CRF	88.7	82.6	85.5
Habibi et al. (2017) [22]	87.6	86.2	86.9
Sachan et al. (2018) [23]	88.1	90.4	89.2
Wang et al. (2019) [24]	89.1	88.4	88.7
BioBERT (2020) [25]	88.1	88.7	88.4
CASN (2021) [26]	89.5	90.9	90.2
BioLinkBERT (2022) [27]	–	–	90.3
BERTForTC (2022) [28]	–	–	90.8
Ours	**90.2**	**92.4**	**91.3**

Table 3. Results of comparison experiments on JNLPBA

Model	P (%)	R (%)	F1 (%)
BERT+CRF	71.8	77.3	74.5
BERT+BiLSTM+CRF	71.0	79.6	75.0
BERT+CNN+CRF	71.2	80.2	75.4
Habibi et al. (2017) [22]	71.3	75.7	73.4
Sachan et al. (2018) [23]	71.3	79.0	75.0
Wang et al. (2019) [24]	70.9	76.3	73.5
BioBERT (2020) [25]	72.2	83.5	77.4
CASN (2021) [26]	75.8	80.0	78.0
MINER (2022) [29]	–	–	77.0
BioDistilBERT (2023) [30]	73.5	**85.5**	79.1
Ours	**78.0**	81.7	**79.8**

Table 4. Results of comparison experiments on CCKS2017

Model	P (%)	R (%)	F1 (%)
BiLSTM+CRF	84.5	87.5	85.9
BiLSTM+CNN+CRF	85.2	88.2	86.8
Bert+CRF	88.7	93.0	90.9
BERT+BiLSTM+CRF	90.9	91.6	91.2
BERT+CNN+CRF	91.3	92.2	91.7
Lattice-LSTM (2018) [31]	91.4	92.3	91.8
IDDNN (2019) [32]	92.0	93.7	92.8
SETL (2019) [33]	92.5	94.8	93.6
Yu et al. (2022) [34]	–	–	93.8
Ours	**93.9**	**95.6**	**94.7**

As shown in Tables 2, 3 and 4, the experimental results of the multi-task learning-based entity recognition method proposed in this paper, with the addition of syntactic dependency parsing, are significantly better than the baseline experiments. The experimental results on the BC5CDR and the JNLPBA datasets show that the multi-task method is better compared to the sequence labeling method. There is an increase of 5.8% and 4.4% in the BC5CDR dataset and the JNLPBA dataset, compared with the baseline experiments with the best results for sequence labeling, and an increase of 3.0% over the sequence labeling method on the CCKS2017 dataset.

The boundary detection and span classification tasks can recognize all entities and effectively solve the unregistered word problem relative to sequence labeling method. After the comparison experiments with other models, the proposed model in this paper also outperforms other methods. Compared with the best experimental results, the proposed model improved by 0.5% on the BC5CDR dataset, 0.7% on the JNLPBA dataset and 0.9% on the CCKS2017 dataset, achieving the optimal F1 score on all three datasets. This proves the effectiveness of incorporating syntactic dependency trees and extracting features with GCN. The model fully learns the syntactic dependency present in the sentences and performs well on the multi-task afterward, which proves the effectiveness and superiority of the model both on the Chinese and English datasets.

4.3 Ablation Experiments

In order to verify the contribution of syntactic dependency information to the model and the validity of multi-task, we conducted the following ablation experiments on BC5CDR, JBNLPBA, and CCKS2017 datasets:

Table 5. Ablation experiments

	BC5CDR			JNLPBA			CCKS2017		
	P (%)	R (%)	F1 (%)	P (%)	R (%)	F1 (%)	P (%)	R (%)	F1 (%)
ALL	**90.2**	**92.4**	**91.3**	**78.0**	81.7	**79.8**	**93.9**	**95.6**	**94.7**
W/O SYN	89.5	90.9	90.2	75.8	80.3	78.0	91.1	94.5	92.7
W/O MT	86.8	89.8	88.3	70.2	**85.0**	76.9	91.3	93.7	92.5
W/O SYN&MT	87.0	81.5	84.2	71.8	77.3	74.5	88.7	93.0	90.9

As shown in Tables 5, when the model removed the syntactic dependency parsing and multi-task modules, the performance decreased in each case. Especially after removing the multi-task module, the performance dropped significantly, highlighting the importance of using the boundary detection and span classification tasks. The multi-task method can recognize all candidate entities, proving that the method is effective for complex biomedical texts. When the syntactic dependency parsing module was removed, the model's performance also decreased, proving the importance of syntactic dependency information in NER.

4.4 Error Analysis

On the BC5CDR and JNLPBA datasets, Habibi et al. [22] utilized a sequence labeling method incorporating BiLSTM and CRF. And Sachan et al. [23] utilized a special weight transfer method for improving parameter initialization. BioBERT [25] is specifically designed for the biomedical domain, providing better contextual understanding and generalization capabilities. CASN [26] is a multi-task model for BioNER. BERTForTC [28] is a BERT-based model specially designed for text classification tasks. The BioDistilBERT [30] is a DistilBERT-based model that had achieved excellent results in fine-tuning biomedical text.

On the CCKS2017 dataset, Lattice-LSTM [31] improved the Chinese NER by increasing the external knowledge base. IDDNN [32] is a neural network model used for incremental learning. SETL [33] is a model that utilized semi-supervised and unsupervised learning techniques. Yu et al. [34] utilized multi-task method for NER. The method overlook the implicit syntactic dependency information within Chinese sentences. In this paper, we propose the boundary detection and span classification tasks related to NER, and the experimental results have demonstrated the superiority.

Compared with the BC5CDR and the JNLPBA datasets, the improvement on the Chinese dataset CCKS2017 is more significant. However, syntactic dependency information has a more significant impact on improvement in Chinese NER compared with English datasets. After removing syntactic dependency information, the experimental results on the BC5CDR, JNLPBA and CCKS2017 datasets decreased by 1.1%, 1.8% and 2.0% respectively. This is because there are great differences between Chinese and English in terms of grammatical structure. In Chinese, the relationship between vocabulary words is usually expressed by the position and the order of words, and Chinese does not have the variation (singular, plural and tense and so on). Chinese relies more on the order between words, modifier relations, word order, etc. The experiments strongly demonstrate the effectiveness of incorporating syntactic dependency information.

4.5   Visualization

In order to show the effect of incorporating syntactic dependency information to the model more intuitively, we have done the visualization of labels in the baseline model on the CCKS2017 dataset to reflect it, as shown in Fig. 6(a) and Fig. 6(b).

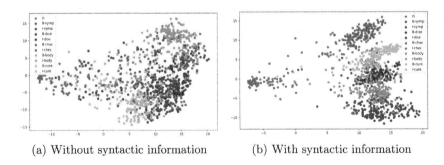

(a) Without syntactic information   (b) With syntactic information

Fig. 6. Visualization of labels on CCKS2017 dataset (Color figure online)

The visualization of labels on the CCKS2017 dataset showed that the various types of labels shown in Fig. 6(a) are almost disordered, and the chaotic distribution between each color. This is not conducive to recognizing entity boundaries and types. But after incorporating syntactic dependency information and using

GCN to extract feature information for the model to learn, the effect of clustering the different colors together as shown in Fig. 6(b) is much more pronounced, and there is almost a clear boundary between each type of color that allows the model to recognize entities better. The two types of entities, non-physical (O) and chemical (chec), are almost all clustered together and have clear boundaries with other entity types. It can also be noticed that the green (symp) and dark blue (dise) are well differentiated, and the symptom entities and disease entities are very similar, as in the case of "骨: B-symp 折: I-symp" 以及 "左: B-dise 侧: I-dise 粗: I-dise 隆: I-dise 间: I-dise 骨: I-dise 折: I-dise" , which are similar to both types of entities, proving that the model has learned the features of the two after incorporating syntactic information.

5 Conclusion

In this paper, we propose a BioNER model based on multi-task learning, which utilizes GCN to extract syntactic dependency information features in sentences. The model incorporates syntactic dependency information into the sentences and integrates it with label encoding through the co-attention mechanism. Then, it combines the boundary detection and span classification tasks for NER.

Acknowledgements. This research was funded by the National Natural Science Foundation of China (No. 61876031), the Natural Science Foundation of Liaoning Province, China (20180550921), the Scientific Research Fund Project of the Education Department of Liaoning Province, China (LJYT201906), and the Natural Science Foundation of Liaoning Province (2022-BS-104).

References

1. Grishman, R., Sundheim, B.: Message understanding conference 6: a brief history. In: Proceedings of the 16th Conference on Computational Linguistics, vol. 1. Association for Computational Linguistics (1996)
2. Bunescu, R., Mooney, R.: A shortest path dependency kernel for relation extraction. In: Proceedings of Human Language Technology Conference and Conference on Empirical Methods in Natural Language Processing, pp. 724–731 (2005)
3. Riedel, S., Yao, L., McCallum, A., et al.: Relation extraction with matrix factorization and universal schemas. In: Proceedings of the Association for Computational Linguistics: Human Language Technologies, pp. 74–84 (2013)
4. Chen, Y., Xu, L., Liu, K., et al.: Event extraction via dynamic multi-polling convolutional neural networks. In: Proceedings of the 53rd Annual Meeting of the Association for Computational Linguistics and the 7th International Joint Conference on Natural Language Processing, pp. 167–176 (2015)
5. Diefenbach, D., Lopez, V., Singh, K., et al.: Core techniques of question answering systems over knowledge bases: a survey. Knowl. Inf. Syst. **55**(3), 529–569 (2018). https://doi.org/10.1007/s10115-017-1100-y
6. United States. Defense Advanced Research Projects Agency. Information Technology Office. Sixth Message Understanding Conference (MUC-6): Proceedings of a Conference Held in Columbia, Maryland, 6–8 November 1995. Morgan Kaufmann Publishers (1995)

7. Hanisch, D., Fundel, K., Mevissen, H.T., et al.: ProMiner: rule-based protein and gene entity recognition. BMC Bioinform. **6**(Suppl 1), 1–9 (2005). Article Number: S14

8. Savova, G.K., Masanz, J.J., Orgen, P.V., et al.: Mayo clinical Text Analysis and Knowledge Extraction System (cTAKES): architecture component evaluation and applications. J. Am. Med. Inform. Assoc. (JAMIA) **17**(5), 507 (2010)

9. Xia, G.: Research on Gene Named Entity Recognition Mechanism Based on Dictionary and Machine Learning. Peking Union Medical College Hospital, Beijing (2013)

10. Krauthammer, M., Rzhetsky, A., Morozov, P., et al.: Using BLAST for identifying gene and protein names in journal articles. Gene **259**(1–2), 245–252 (2001)

11. Todorovic, B.T., Rancic, S.R., Markovic, I.M., et al.: Named entity recognition and classification using context Hidden Markov Model. In: Proceedings of 2008 9th Symposium on Neural Network Applications in Electrical Engineering, pp. 43–46 (2008)

12. Berger, A.L.: A maximum entropy approach to natural language processing. Comput. Linguist. **22**(1), 39–71 (1996)

13. Lafferty, J., McCallum, A., Pereira, F.C.N.: Conditional random fields: probabilistic models for segmenting and labeling sequence data. In: Proceedings of the 18th International Conference on Machine Learning, pp. 282–289 (2001)

14. Leaman, R., Wei, C.H., Lu, Z.Y.: tmChem: a high performance approach for chemical named entity recognition and normalization. J. Cheminformatics **7**(Supplement 1), 1–10 (2015). Article Number: S3

15. Li, Y.P., Lin, H.F., Yang, Z.Z.: Incorporating rich background knowledge for gene named entity classification and recognition. BMC Bioinform. **10**, 1–15 (2009). Article Number: 233

16. Zhu, Q., Li, X., Conesa, A., et al.: GRAM-CNN: a deep learning approach with local context for named entity recognition in biomedical text. Bioinformatics **34**(9), 1547–1554 (2018)

17. Korvigo, I., Holmatov, M., Zaikovskii, A., et al.: Putting hands to rest: efficient deep CNN-RNN architecture for chemical named entity recognition with no handcrafted rules. J. Cheminformatics **10**(1), 1–10 (2018)

18. Dang, T.H., Le, H.Q., Nguyen, T.M., et al.: D3NER: biomedical named entity recognition using CRF-BiLSTM improved with fine-tuned embeddings of various linguistic information. Bioinformatics **34**(20), 3539–3546 (2018)

19. Li, L., Jiang, Y.: Biomedical named entity recognition based on the two channels and sentence level reading control conditioned LSTM-CRF. In: IEEE International Conference on Bioinformatics and Biomedicine, pp. 380–385 (2017)

20. Zhao, Z., Yang, Z., Luo, L., et al.: Disease named entity recognition from biomedical literature using a novel convolutional neural network. BMC Med. Genomics **10**, 75–83 (2017). https://doi.org/10.1186/s12920-017-0316-8

21. Yan, H., Sun, Y., Li, X., Qiu, X.: An embarrassingly easy but strong baseline for nested named entity recognition. In: Proceedings of the 61st Annual Meeting of the Association for Computational Linguistics, vol. 2, pp. 1442–1452 (2023). https://doi.org/10.18653/v1/2023.acl-short.123

22. Habibi, M., Weber, L., Neves, M.L., Wiegandt, D.L., Leser, U.: Deep learning with word embeddings improves biomedical named entity recognition. Bioinformatics **33**(14), i37–i48 (2017)

23. Sachan, D.S., Xie, P., Sachan, M., Xing, E.P.: Effective use of bidirectional language modeling for transfer learning in biomedical named entity recognition. In:

Proceedings of the Machine Learning for Healthcare Conference, MLHC, vol. 85, pp. 383–402. PMLR (2018)

24. Wang, X., et al.: Cross-type biomedical named entity recognition with deep multi-task learning. Bioinformatics **35**(10), 1745–1752 (2019)
25. Lee, J., et al.: BioBERT: a pre-trained biomedical language representation model for biomedical text mining. Bioinformatics **36**(4), 1234–1240 (2020)
26. Chen, P., et al.: Co-attentive span network with multi-task learning for biomedical named entity recognition. In: 2021 IEEE International Conference on Bioinformatics and Biomedicine (BIBM), pp. 649–652. IEEE (2021)
27. Yasunaga, M., Leskovec, J., Liang, P.: LinkBERT: pretraining language models with document links. In: Proceedings of the 60th Annual Meeting of the Association for Computational Linguistics, vol. 1, pp. 8003–8016 (2022). https://doi.org/10.18653/v1/2022.acl-long.551
28. Kocaman, V., Talby, D.: Accurate clinical and biomedical named entity recognition at scale. Softw. Impacts **13**, 100373 (2022)
29. Wang, X., et al.: MINER: improving out-of-vocabulary named entity recognition from an information theoretic perspective. In: Proceedings of the 60th Annual Meeting of the Association for Computational Linguistics, vol. 1, pp. 5590–5600 (2022). https://doi.org/10.18653/v1/2022.acl-long.383
30. Rohanian, O., Nouriborji, M., Kouchaki, S., et al.: On the effectiveness of compact biomedical transformers. Bioinformatics **39**(3), btad103 (2023)
31. Zhang, Y., Yang, J.: Chinese NER using lattice LSTM. In: Proceedings of the 56th Annual Meeting of the Association for Computational Linguistics, pp. 1554–1564 (2018)
32. Wang, Q., Zhou, Y.M., Ruan, T., et al.: Incorporating dictionaries into deep neural networks for the Chinese clinical named entity recognition. J. Biomed. Inform. **92**, 103–133 (2019)
33. Li, N., Luo, L., Ding, Z.Y., et al.: Improving Chinese clinical named entity recognition using stroke ELMo and transfer learning. In: Proceedings of the Evaluation Tasks at the China Conference on Knowledge Graph and Semantic Computing (CCKSTasks 2019) (2019)
34. Yu, P., Chen, Y., Xu, J., et al.: Entity recognition method for electronic medical records based on multi-task learning. In: Computer and Modernization, no. 09, pp. 40–50 (2022)

A Simple but Useful Multi-corpus Transferring Method for Biomedical Named Entity Recognition

Jiqiao Li[1], Chi Yuan[1(✉)], Zirui Li[1], Huaiyu Wang[2], and Feifei Tao[1]

[1] School of Computer and Information, Hohai University, Nanjing, China
{jiqiao,chiyuan,lzr_autumnRay,tff}@hhu.edu.cn
[2] Beijing University of Chinese Medicine, Beijing, China

Abstract. In the biomedical field, understanding biomedical texts requires domain-specific knowledge, and the annotation of biomedical texts often requires a lot of human involvement, which makes annotation costly and time-consuming. Therefore, how to effectively use the existing public-available corpus resources is meaningful for performance improvement in biomedical NLP. In this paper, we present a multi-corpus transferring method for biomedical named entity recognition task. We clearly define the target criteria by adding two artificial tokens at the beginning and end of each input sentence. A comprehensive evaluation was conducted to prove the efficiency of our method. The results illustrate that the multi-corpus transferring method could benefit the current methods and improve its performance. Our method provides a potential solution for biomedical NER enhancement from data perspective, and it could further improve biomedical information extraction with the help of increasingly public available corpus.

Keywords: Multi-corpus transferring · biomedical named entity recognition · Information extraction

1 Introduction

In biomedical texts, there is a wealth of data and knowledge that can be reused. To fully harness such unstructured medical data, it is essential to utilize appropriate biomedical natural language processing techniques and methods, particularly information extraction methods tailored to biomedical texts [1]. Most existing biomedical information extraction systems are still designed based on methods that rely on annotated corpora provided by domain experts. However, such corpus-based approaches often depend on a substantial amount of manually annotated data, and the annotation process consumes significant human and financial resources.

In biomedical domain, understanding biomedical texts requires domain-specific knowledge, and annotated corpora typically rely on the expertise of domain experts for annotation [2]. Compared to corpora in general domains, obtaining relevant corpora in the biomedical field is more challenging and incurs higher annotation costs. This complexity leads to the labor-intensive and intricate task of corpus annotation for efficient information extraction for each scientific question.

In entity recognition tasks, superior results often rely on supervised methods because they can provide high-quality labeled data to the model, resulting in high performance and generalization [3]. However, for entity recognition tasks in the biomedical field, there are challenges of expensive labeling costs and large human input, which makes the application of supervised methods in this field more difficult.

In the face of these challenges, how to effectively use the limited corpus resources has become a crucial issue. In the biomedical field, we need to find innovative ways to overcome the problem of data scarcity. One such approach is to employ few-shot learning methods, which focus on extracting maximum information value from limited labeled data for efficient model training [4]. In addition, we can also consider using corpus augmentation techniques to increase the amount of data available for training in different ways, such as data synthesis, transfer learning or data enhancement.

In this study, we propose a multi-corpus transferring method to solve the problem in the case of labor saving, to obtain better results. Specifically, we adopted a multi-corpus transferring training method with artificial tokens. This involves adding two artificial tokens at the beginning and end of input sentences to specify the target standards, along with proposing a joint multi-standard learning scheme. We conducted various experiments on eight standard corpora, including the comparison experiment of single corpus training, the comparison experiment of increasing the number of aggregate corpora, and the aggregate experiment without tokens and the aggregate experiment with tokens, and obtained satisfactory results.

2   Related Work

2.1   Biomedical Entity Recognition

In recent years, the development of deep learning methods has made rapid progress in the field of biomedical entity recognition. These methods do not need to manually design features but use neural networks to automatically learn text representations. Here are some representative deep learning approaches:

Recurrent Neural Networks were among the early deep learning models used for biomedical entity recognition. They are capable of capturing sequence information in text. However, RNNs suffer from the vanishing gradient problem when handling long-distance dependencies, limiting their performance.

The introduction of transformer models has had a significant impact on biomedical entity recognition. This architecture employs self-attention mechanisms to process text sequences, offering parallelism and improved modeling capabilities. Devlin et al. introduced the BERT (Bidirectional Encoder Representations from Transformers) model, which achieved significant performance improvements in multiple NLP tasks [5].

In addition, some other Transformer models have emerged in recent years. The Text-to-text Transfer Transformer (T5) model proposed by Raffel et al., adopts the text-to-text task approach and regards both input and output as text sequences. This versatility makes it suitable for a variety of NLP tasks, including entity recognition [6]. The GPT-3 (Generative Pre-trained Transformer 3) proposed by Brown et al. is a huge autoregressive language model with 175 billion parameters. GPT-3 emphasizes generative tasks, and its pre-trained model can be used for fine-tuning various NLP tasks [7]. At present, GPT-4 [8] have been successively released, becoming one of the most concerned large models at present.

2.2 Corpus Reuse in Biomedical NER

Biomedical corpus reuse for named entity recognition could be mainly divided into three categories. Transfer learning, Domain adaptation, and Semi-Supervised learning.

Transfer Learning. Transfer learning uses existing knowledge in the source domain to enhance the performance of the model in the target domain. In the context of the biomedical NER, this approach involves adapting a model originally trained on a general corpus to domain-specific biomedical data.

The process of transfer learning begins with the selection of pre-trained models, typically language models such as BERT or BioBERT [9], which are initially trained on large amounts of text from different domains. The pre-trained model is then fine-tuned using a domain-specific biomedical corpus, which typically includes annotated NER datasets. During the fine-tuning process, the model learns to adjust its representation to better capture biomedical entities such as diseases, genes, and proteins.

Domain Adaptation. Domain adaptation is a crucial subfield of transfer learning, particularly applicable for transferring models from one domain (source domain) to another (target domain). Ganin et al. introduced Domain-Adversarial Neural Networks (DANN) to reduce distributional differences between the source and target domains through adversarial training [10]. This approach has shown significant performance improvements in tasks like text classification. Additionally, Lee et al. conducted experiments by transferring LSTM-CRF-based NER models from a large labeled dataset to a smaller one for identifying Protected Health Information (PHI) in Electronic Health Records (EHR) [11]. The study demonstrated that transfer learning improved performance, particularly beneficial for target datasets with limited labels.

Semi-supervised Learning. In semi-supervised learning, building a silver standard corpus is a key approach to fill the gap between the scarcity of gold standard data in biomedical named entity recognition (NER) tasks and the need for large-scale training of models.

John et al. took an innovative approach to melding the Gold Standard and Silver Standard corpora to achieve synergistic advantages. Gold standard data provides high accuracy but is limited in scale, while silver standard data, although larger in scale, is accompanied by greater noise. By combining the two, transfer learning is realized, and the error rate of NER model is significantly reduced, especially on small-scale labeled data sets. This approach highlights the potential to integrate diverse data sources to improve BNER and opens up the prospect of wider applications [12].

3 Materials and Methods

3.1 Overall Workflow

The main idea of our work is to aggregate more other annotated data to enhance named entity recognition performance. Hence, the first priority is to collect a large amount of textual data in relevant fields. These data contain different entities, different types. The construction of this dataset is a key step in ensuring that the NER system can cover diversity and breadth. Secondly, in order to ensure the quality and consistency of the data, we carried out a series of pre-processing steps. This includes text cleaning, removal of unnecessary punctuation, HTML tags and special characters, conversion of data formats and other text standardization operations to ensure the consistency and availability of input data. Then the corpus is fused with our multi-corpus transferring method, and finally it is put into the BERT-BiLSTM-CRF model for training, and the results are output. The whole process is shown as (Fig. 1).

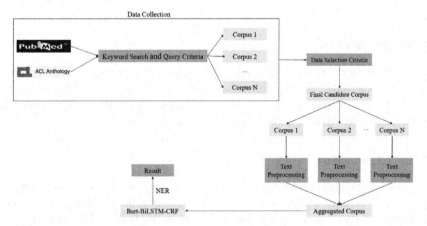

Fig. 1. Overall workflow of our method.

3.2 Data Collection

In order to implement the multi-corpus transferring method in named entity recognition (NER), we design a systematic method to collect corpus for transferring. In this section, we describe our collection process in detail, including search keywords, query criteria, filtering strategies, and the resulting candidate corpus.

Keyword Search and Query Criteria. Our data collection process primarily relied on scientific literature databases, including PubMed and ACL Anthology. In order to acquire multi-corpus data relevant to Named Entity Recognition (NER), we conducted searches using a set of carefully chosen keywords and query criteria.

Employing the selected keywords, we conducted searches across databases such as PubMed, yielding a substantial body of literature that spanned diverse aspects of the biomedical field. The databases and repositories retrieved encompassed BC4CHEMD [13], BC5CDR [14], BioNLP13, Ex-PTM, NCBI Disease [15], AnatEM, BC2GM, BioNLP11 [16], BioNLP09, CRAFT, JNLPBA, LINNAEUS, GENIA, ShARe/CLEFE, DDL, MedSTS, BIOSSES, ChemProt, i2b2-2010, Hoc, CoNLL-2003, SciERC, among others.

Data Selection Criteria. To ensure effective multi-corpus data transfer and enhance dataset quality, we prioritize entity consistency and consider similar entity types while balancing data quantity and quality.

Final Candidate Corpus. After executing the preceding procedures, we have curated a comprehensive and diverse repository of prospective datasets. This compilation comprises BC5CDR, BioNLP09, BioNLP11ID, BioNLP13CG, BioNLP13PC, NCBI-diseases, CRAFT, and BC4CHEMD, procured from PubMed and ACL Anthology.

3.3 Text Preprocessing

We use the BIO annotation format to label entities in the text. For example, for the entity "postural hypotension", its BIO annotation would be ["B-postural", "I-hypotension"]. In the text preprocessing phase, we convert the original text into the BIO annotation format, facilitating subsequent model training and evaluation.

3.4 Data Aggregation

Our transferring approach is based on a simple and practical method proposed by Johnson et al. [17]. It requires adding a single artificial token at the beginning of the input sentence to specify the desired target language, eliminating the need for complex private encoder-decoder structures.

Inspired by their work, we added two artificial tokens at the beginning and end of the input sentence to specify the desired target standard. For example, sentences from the candidate corpus are designed in (Fig. 2).

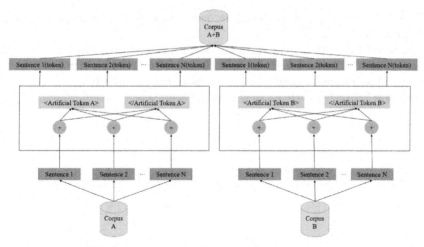

Fig. 2. Data processing for multi-corpus transferring.

These artificial tokens specify from which dataset a sentence originates. They are treated as regular symbols, or more specifically, as ordinary characters.

With their assistance, instances from different datasets can be seamlessly combined for joint training without additional effort. These two special markers are designed to carry standard-related information across long dependencies, influence the contextual representations of each character, and ultimately generate segment decisions that match the target standard. During testing, these markers are used to specify the desired segmentation standard. Similarly, they are not taken into account when computing performance scores.

3.5 Neural Network-Based Recognition Methods

BERT (Bidirectional Encoder Representations from Transformers) is a deep bidirectional pre-trained language model based on the Transformer architecture, introduced by Devlin et al. in 2018.

BiLSTM-CRF [18] is a promising deep learning-based methods in sequence labeling tasks, which have been proved achieving many SOTA results. Yuqi Si et al. integrate advanced neural network representation into clinical concept extraction and compare it to traditional word embedding. They tried several embedding methods on four concept extraction datasets. The results show that context embeddings pre-trained with large-scale clinical corpora achieve new best performance in all concept extraction tasks [19]. Namrata Nath et al. proposed a multi-label named entity recognition (NER) approach aimed at identifying entities and their attributes in clinical text. By introducing three architectures, BiLSTM n-CRF, BiLSTM-CRF-SMAX-TF, and BiLSTM nCRF-TF, the study was evaluated on the 2010 i2b2/VA and i2b2 2012 shared task datasets. The results showed that the different models achieved remarkable success in the NER task [20]. BiLSTM-CRF combines the advantages of Bidirectional Long Short-Term Memory (BiLSTM) and Conditional Random Field (CRF). It can effectively solve sequence labeling problems such as named entity recognition and part-of-speech tagging in the field of natural language processing.

The BERT-BiLSTM-CRF framework is adopted in this study, which combines the advantages of BERT as a feature extractor and BiLSTM-CRF as a sequence tagger to capture context information and label dependencies more accurately.

The BERT-BiLSTM-CRF model is shown in (Fig. 3).

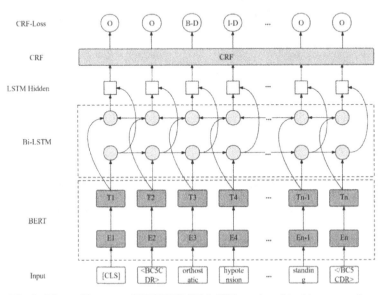

Fig. 3. The architecture of BERT-BiLSTM-CRF employed in this manuscript.

4   Evaluation

4.1   Datasets

In order to evaluate the method proposed in this paper, we conducted experiments with eight BioNER datasets, and detailed information about the datasets adapted in our evaluation are shown in Table 1.

We covert all datasets to BIO format, and since these datasets use various BioNER labels to annotate entities, we classify them into six classes: cells, chemicals, diseases, genes, proteins, and species. We standardized labels with the same meaning while retaining other labels.

Table 1. Biomedical NER datasets used in the experiments

Dataset	Size	Entity types & counts
BioNLP09	11356 sentences	Protein (14963)
BioNLP11ID	5178 sentences	Chemical (973), Protein (6551), Species (3471)
BioNLP13CG	6739 sentences	Chemical (2270), Disease (2582), Cell (3492), Species (1715), Gene (7908)
BioNLP13PC	5051 sentences	Cell (1013), Chemical (3989), Gene (10891)
NCBI-disease	7287 sentences	Disease (6881)
BC5CDR	13938 sentences	Chemical (15935), Disease (12852)
BC4CHEMD	107208 sentences	Chemical (84310)
CRAFT	21,000 sentences	Chemical (6053), Cell (5495), Species (6868), Gene (16064)

4.2 Evaluation Metrics

In the experimental design, we compared the performance difference between of multi-corpus transferring method and the single-corpus training method in NER tasks. Specifically, we used BERT-BiLSTM-CRF models as baseline models and compared them with the following methods:

Single-corpus training: training BERT-BiLSTM-CRF models using data from a single corpus.

Multi-corpus aggregation: training BERT-BiLSTM-CRF models after aggregating data from multi-corpus.

Multi-corpus transferring with artificial tokens: an aggregation method that puts artificial tokens before and after each sentence.

On the test set, we conducted comprehensive evaluations of all methods, focusing on precision, recall, and F1-score.

4.3 Parameter Setting

Our experimental parameters are shown in Table 2.

Table 2. Parameter setting in our experiment

Parameter Type	Parameter setting
Model	BioBERT-v1.1-pubmed
Train epoch	30
Maximum sentence length	128
Batch size	128
Eval step	100
Learn rate	3e−5
Hidden size	10

4.4 Result

In this section, we present and analyze the experimental results and compare our multi-corpus transferring method with aggregate methods.

Multi-corpus Transferring Experiment Result. We conducted a permutation and combinatorial data transferring study, which included different combinations of 8 major data sets. Specifically, we examined various combinations of BC5CDR and BioNLP09, BC5CDR and BioNLP11ID, BC5CDR and BioNLP13C, and so on. However, not all possible combinations have been exhaustively tested, and we have selected a few for our study. For example, we first test the combination effect of corpus without same entities. For example, there are 2 kind of entities, Chemical, Disease in BC5CDR while there are Protein in BioNLP09. No overlap between them. Then gradually increase the proportion of corpus with some same entities to explore the effect of corpus quantity on the results.

In this study, we first focus on the combination of corpus without same entities. We selected the BioNLP09 dataset and conducted transferring experiments with the BC5CDR, BioNLP13CG, BioNLP13PC, NCBI-disease and CRAFT dataset. The following Table 3 shows the transferring results of BioNLP09 with different data sets, both without and with artificial tokens.

The results show that for corpora that are no overlap entities, the method of directly aggregating without adding artificial tokens has a negative effect on all F1 scores. However, when we introduced artificial tokens, the multi-corpus transferring method improved the F1 score of the aggregated arrangement with the BioNLP09 corpus by about one percentage point without introducing negative effects. Compared with other methods, our multi-corpus transferring method achieves better results.

Table 3. Experimental results of multi-corpus transferring without same entities. Bold indicates better results than other methods. F1 (tokens) represents results with artificial tokens, F1 (No-tokens) represents results without artificial tokens. The abbreviations Bio09, Bio13CG, Bio13PC, BC5, and CR respectively stand for BioNLP09, BioNLP13CG, BioNLP13PC, BC5CDR, and CRAFT. Test data: BioNLP09.

Dataset	F1 (tokens)	F1 (No-tokens)
WordCharacterBERT [21]		0.8300
MO-MTM [22]		0.8476
MimicBERT [23]		0.8819
Ours		
Bio09		0.8819
Bio09 + BC5	**0.8847 (+0.0028)**	0.8237
Bio09 + CR	**0.8887 (+0.0028)**	0.8332
Bio09 + BC5 + Bio13CG	**0.8894 (+0.0075)**	0.7410
Bio09 + Bio13CG + Bio13PC	**0.8906 (+0.0087)**	0.7288
Bio09 + BC5 + Bio13CG + CR	**0.8943 (+0.0124)**	0.8411
Bio09 + BC5 + Bio13CG + Bio13PC	**0.8950 (+0.0131)**	0.8221
Bio09 + Bio13CG + Bio13PC + CR	**0.8952 (+0.0133)**	0.8209
Bio09 + Bio13CG + Bio13PC + CR + NC	**0.8925 (+0.0106)**	0.8189
Bio09 + BC5 + Bio13CG + Bio13PC + CR + NC	**0.8960 (+0.0141)**	0.8115

Next, we conducted the transferring experiment of corpus with some same entities, including six data sets BC4CHEMD, BC5CDR, BioNLP11ID, BioNLP13CG, BioNLP13PC and CRAFT. Various permutations of these datasets were aggregated and finally tested on four datasets: BC5CDR, BioNLP11ID, BioNLP13CG, and BioNLP13PC. Due to space limitations, only the results for BC5CDR and BioNLP11ID are presented here. Table 4 and Table 5 show the transferring test results for BC5CDR and BioNLP11ID respectively.

The results show that aggregation methods that do not use artificial tokens have a negative effect in most cases, resulting in a decrease in results. Using the multi-corpus transferring method, we find that the method is widely applicable to the result improvement of corpus with some same entities. In the summary results of the four data sets, by introducing artificial token methods, we achieved some level of performance improvement for most of the summary arrangements without introducing negative effects. In most aggregation arrangements, our approach is superior to other approaches.

Ablation Experiment. We performed ablation experiments on the BC5CDR, BioNLP09, BioNLP11ID, BioNLP13CG, BioNLP13PC, NCBI-disease, BC4CHEMD, and CRAFT data sets. First, we ran an experiment on each individual data set, comparing without and with artificial tokens, the results of which are shown in Table 6. In most datasets, the difference between the results with and without artificial tokens was not

Table 4. Experimental results of multi-corpus transferring with same entities. Bold indicates better results than other methods. F1 (tokens) represents results with artificial tokens, F1 (No-tokens) represents results without artificial tokens. The abbreviations Bio11ID, Bio13CG, Bio13PC, BC5, BC4, and CR respectively stand for BioNLP11ID, BioNLP13CG, BioNLP13PC, BC5CDR, BC4CHEMD and CRAFT. Test data: BC5CDR.

Dataset	F1 (tokens)	F1 (No-tokens)
AutoNER [24]		0.8000
BNPU [25]		0.5920
BERT-ES [26]		0.7370
Conf-NPU [27]		0.8010
SciBERT-Base Vocab [28]		0.8811
Ours		
BC5		0.8779
BC5 + Bio11ID	**0.8856 (+0.0045)**	0.8513
BC5 + CR	**0.8901 (+0.0090)**	0.8688
BC5 + Bio11ID + Bio13PC	**0.8863 (+0.0052)**	0.8712
BC5 + Bio11ID + CR	**0.8900 (+0.0089)**	0.8712
BC5 + Bio11ID + BC4	**0.8893 (+0.0082)**	0.8476
BC5 + Bio11ID + Bio13CG + CR	**0.8897 (+0.0086)**	0.8555
BC5 + Bio11ID + Bio13CG + Bio13PC + CR	**0.8885 (+0.0074)**	0.8510
BC4 + BC5 + Bio11ID + Bio13CG + CR	**0.8892 (+0.0081)**	0.8270
BC4 + BC5 + Bio11ID + Bio13CG + Bio13P + CR	**0.8908 (+0.0097)**	0.8276

Table 5. Experimental results of multi-corpus transferring with same entities. Bold indicates better results than other methods. F1 (tokens) represents results with artificial tokens, F1 (No-tokens) represents results without artificial tokens. The abbreviations Bio11ID, Bio13CG, Bio13PC, BC5, BC4, and CR respectively stand for BioNLP11ID, BioNLP13CG, BioNLP13PC, BC5CDR, BC4CHEMD and CRAFT. Test data: BioNLP11ID.

Dataset	F1 (Tokens)	F1 (No tokens)
D-MTM [22]		0.8173
MTM-CW [29]		0.8326
BioBERT [23]		0.8557
Ours		
Bio11ID		0.8481
Bio11ID + BC4	**0.8609 (+0.0052)**	0.7759
Bio11ID + CR	**0.8620 (+0.0063)**	0.8073
Bio11ID + BC5 + CR	**0.8610 (+0.0053)**	0.8192
Bio11ID + BC5 + Bio13CG + CR	**0.8699 (+0.0142)**	0.8127
Bio11ID + BC5 + Bio13PC + CR	0.8484	0.7999
Bio11ID + BC5 + Bio13CG + Bio13PC + CR	**0.8666 (+0.0109)**	0.7932

significant, suggesting that the inclusion of artificial tokens had no material effect on the results because we did not include these tokens in the score calculation. However, some datasets, such as BioNLP09, showed a slight performance improvement with the addition of artificial tokens, while BioNLP13PC showed a two percentage point performance decrease with the addition of artificial tokens.

These experimental results show that the effect of adding artificial tokens in ablation experiments on datasets varies from dataset to dataset. For most datasets, the introduction of artificial tokens did not seem to affect the results. However, in certain cases, such as BioNLP09 and BioNLP13PC, the inclusion of artificial tokens may have some impact on performance.

Table 6. Comparison of individual data sets with and without artificial tokens. F1 (tokens) represents results with artificial tokens, F1 (No-tokens) represents results without artificial tokens. Differ stands for difference between them.

Dataset	F1 (Tokens)	F1 (No tokens)	Differ
BCCDR	0.8821	0.8779	0.0042
BioNLP09	0.8830	0.8644	**0.0186**
BioNLP11ID	0.8488	0.8481	0.0007
BioNLP13CG	0.8679	0.8743	0.0064
BioNLP13PC	0.8797	0.9028	**0.0231**
NCBI-disease	0.8764	0.8833	0.0069
BC4CHEMD	0.9146	0.9133	0.0013
CRAFT	0.8575	0.8547	0.0028

In addition, we performed an ablation-comparison experiment that retained only the Chemical entity types in the BC5CDR, BioNLP11ID, BioNLP13CG, BioNLP13PC, BC4CHEMD, and CRAFT data sets, and excluded the others. Due to space limitations, only the results for BioNLP11ID and CRAFT are presented here. Table 7 and Table 8 in the following table represent the aggregation results of BioNLP11ID and CRAFT respectively.

The experimental results show that the performance of our method can be improved to some extent in most aggregate permutations of most datasets.

These experimental results underscore the universality of our approach, which can indeed play an important role in corpus transferring.

Table 7. Experimental results of multi-corpus transferring with only chemical entity. F1 (tokens) represents results with artificial tokens, F1 (No-tokens) represents results without artificial tokens. Bold indicates an increase or decrease of more than one percentage point compared to a single corpus. The abbreviations Bio11ID, Bio13CG, Bio13PC, BC5, and CR respectively stand for BioNLP11ID, BioNLP13CG, BioNLP13PC, BC5CDR, BC4CHEMD and CRAFT. Test data: BioNLP11ID.

Dataset (Only-Chemical)	F1 (Tokens)	F1 (No-tokens)
Bio11ID	–	0.6765
Bio11ID + BC5	0.7087 (**+0.0322**)	0.7103 (**+0.0338**)
Bio11ID + Bio13CG	0.7081 (**+0.0316**)	0.6917 (**+0.0152**)
Bio11ID + Bio13PC	0.6154 (**−0.0611**)	0.6861 (+0.0096)
Bio11ID + BC5 + CR	0.7031 (**+0.0266**)	0.6065 (**−0.0700**)
Bio11ID + Bio13CG + CR	0.6936 (**+0.0171**)	0.6200 (**−0.0565**)
Bio11ID + BC5 + Bio13CG + CR	0.7203 (**+0.0438**)	0.6316 (**−0.0449**)
Bio11ID + BC5 + Bio13PC + CR	0.7330 (**+0.0565**)	0.6367 (**−0.0398**)
Bio11ID + Bio13CG + Bio13PC + CR	0.7309 (**+0.0544**)	0.6070 (**−0.0695**)
Bio11ID + BC5 + Bio13CG + Bio13PC + CR	0.7220 (**+0.0455**)	0.6473 (**−0.0292**)

Table 8. Experimental results of multi-corpus transferring with only chemical entity. F1 (tokens) represents results with artificial tokens, F1 (No-tokens) represents results without artificial tokens. Bold indicates an increase or decrease of more than one percentage point compared to a single corpus. The abbreviations Bio11ID, Bio13CG, Bio13PC, BC5, and CR respectively stand for BioNLP11ID, BioNLP13CG, BioNLP13PC, BC5CDR, BC4CHEMD and CRAFT. Test data: CRAFT.

Dataset (Only-Chemical)	F1 (Tokens)	F1 (No-tokens)
CR		0.8020
CR + BC5	0.8268 (**+0.0248**)	0.8176 (**+0.0156**)
CR + Bio11ID	0.8333 (**+0.0313**)	0.8148 (**+0.0128**)
CR + Bio13CG	0.8383 (**+0.0363**)	0.7981 (−0.0039)
CR + BC5 + Bio13PC	0.8365 (**+0.0345**)	0.7723 (**−0.0297**)
CR + Bio11ID + Bio13PC	0.8224 (**+0.0204**)	0.7414 (**−0.0606**)
CR + Bio13CG + Bio13PC	0.8353 (**+0.0333**)	0.7675 (**−0.0345**)
CR + BC5 + Bio11ID + Bio13CG	0.8242 (**+0.0222**)	0.7371 (**−0.0649**)
CR + Bio11ID + Bio13CG + Bio13PC	0.8258 (**+0.0238**)	0.7288 (**−0.0732**)
CR + BC5 + Bio11ID + Bio13CG + Bio13PC	0.8444 (**+0.0424**)	0.7068 (**−0.0952**)

4.5 Discussion

In this paper, we present a simple but useful of multi-corpus transferring method for biomedical named entity recognition. It is focusing on the reusability of existing human annotated corpus. With the robust evaluation of our method, we find the following distinct features:

Artificial token, e.g., '<corpus> </corpus>', could benefit the corpus transferring comparing the direct combination of origin corpus. According to our ablation experiments, our multi-corpus transferring method showed significant improvements in the majority of combination results in two sets of experiments while direct transferring corpus for new entity recognition task resulted in an average decrease to the baseline in two sets of results.

No strict restriction for the corpus selection in our transferring. In real-world practice, it is very hard to find an exactly matching entities from external source and we could only identify a partial similar corpus in most cases. For example, in corpus BioNLP11ID and BC5CDR. Even in some corpus there is no absolute similar entities but the text with similar expressions would be also helpful for the performance enhancement. For instance. BioNLP09 and BC5CDR do not share similar entities, yet performing multi-corpus transferring on both of them still leads to performance improvement.

However, one drawback is in the case of low correlation between corpora, the multi-corpus transferring effect may not be obvious, and other strategies may need to be considered.

5 Conclusion

We conduct a study to solve the shortage of human annotated corpus in biomedical domain from data perspective. A practical method was proposed in this manuscript to reuse the existing public-available corpus to enhance the performance of biomedical named entity recognition. The evaluation results illustrate the multi-corpus transferring method presented in this paper would enhance the original BERT-BiLSTM-CRF method. The ablation results prove our method could outperform traditional data combination method.

Acknowledgements. This project was sponsored by Fundamental Research Funds for the Central Universities (B220201032, B220202076); and the Nanjing Science and Technology Innovation Project Selective Funding Program for Overseas Educated Scholars.

References

1. Frisoni, G., Moro, G., Carbonaro, A.: A survey on event extraction for natural language understanding: riding the biomedical literature wave. IEEE Access **9**, 160721–160757 (2021)
2. Spasic, I., Ananiadou, S., McNaught, J., Kumar, A.: Text mining and ontologies in biomedicine: making sense of raw text. Brief. Bioinform. **6**(3), 239–251 (2005)
3. Rodriguez-Esteban, R.: Biomedical text mining and its applications. PLoS Comput. Biol. **5**(12), e1000597 (2009)

4. Wang, Y., Yao, Q., Kwok, J.T., Ni, L.M.: Generalizing from a few examples: A survey on few-shot learning. ACM Comput. Surv. (CSUR) **53**(3), 1–34 (2020)
5. Devlin, J., Chang, M.-W., Lee, K., Toutanova, K.: BERT: pre-training of deep bidirectional transformers for language understanding. arXiv preprint arXiv:1810.04805 (2018)
6. Raffel, C., et al.: Exploring the limits of transfer learning with a unified text-to-text transformer. J. Mach. Learn. Res. **21**(1), 5485–5551 (2020)
7. Brown, T., et al.: Language models are few-shot learners. In: Advances in Neural Information Processing Systems, vol. 33, pp. 1877–1901 (2020)
8. OpenAI: GPT-4 technical report. arXiv e-prints arXiv:2303.08774 (2023)
9. Lee, J., et al.: BioBERT: a pre-trained biomedical language representation model for biomedical text mining. Bioinformatics **36**(4), 1234–1240 (2020)
10. Ganin, Y., et al.: Domain-adversarial training of neural networks. J. Mach. Learn. Res. **17**(1), 2096–2030 (2016)
11. Lee, J.Y., Dernoncourt, F., Szolovits, P.: Transfer learning for named-entity recognition with neural networks. arXiv preprint arXiv:1705.06273 (2017)
12. Giorgi, J.M., Bader, G.D.: Transfer learning for biomedical named entity recognition with neural networks. Bioinformatics **34**(23), 4087–4094 (2018)
13. Krallinger, M., Leitner, F., Rabal, O., Vazquez, M., Oyarzabal, J., Valencia, A.: CHEMDNER: The drugs and chemical names extraction challenge. J. Cheminformatics **7**(1), 1–11 (2015)
14. Li, J., et al.: BioCreative V CDR task corpus: a resource for chemical disease relation extraction. Database **2016** (2016)
15. Pyysalo, S., Ohta, T., Miwa, M., Tsujii, J.: Towards exhaustive protein modification event extraction. In: Proceedings of BioNLP 2011 Workshop, pp. 114–123 (2011)
16. Pyysalo, S., Ananiadou, S.: Anatomical entity mention recognition at literature scale. Bioinformatics **30**(6), 868–875 (2014)
17. Collier, N., Kim, J.-D.: Introduction to the bio-entity recognition task at JNLPBA. In: Proceedings of the International Joint Workshop on Natural Language Processing in Biomedicine and Its Applications (NLPBA/BioNLP), pp. 73–78 (2004)
18. Huang, Z., Xu, W., Yu, K.: Bidirectional LSTM-CRF models for sequence tagging. arXiv preprint arXiv:1508.01991 (2015)
19. Si, Y., Wang, J., Xu, H., Roberts, K.: Enhancing clinical concept extraction with contextual embeddings. J. Am. Med. Inform. Assoc. **26**(11), 1297–1304 (2019)
20. Nath, N., Lee, S.-H., Lee, I.: NEAR: named entity and attribute recognition of clinical concepts. J. Biomed. Inform. **130**, 104092 (2022)
21. Francis, S., Van Landeghem, J., Moens, M.-F.: Transfer learning for named entity recognition in financial and biomedical documents. Information **10**(8), 248 (2019)
22. Crichton, G., Pyysalo, S., Chiu, B., Korhonen, A.: A neural network multi-task learning approach to biomedical named entity recognition. BMC Bioinform. **18**(1), 1–14 (2017)
23. Banerjee, P., Pal, K.K., Devarakonda, M., Baral, C.: Knowledge guided named entity recognition for biomedical text. arXiv preprint arXiv:1911.03869 (2019)
24. Shang, J., Liu, L., Ren, X., Gu, X., Ren, T., Han, J.: Learning named entity tagger using domain-specific dictionary. arXiv preprint arXiv:1809.03599 (2018)
25. Peng, M., Xing, X., Zhang, Q., Fu, J., Huang, X.: Distantly supervised named entity recognition using positive-unlabeled learning. arXiv preprint arXiv:1906.01378 (2019)
26. Liang, C., et al.: BOND: BERT-assisted open-domain named entity recognition with distant supervision. In: Proceedings of the 26th ACM SIGKDD International Conference on Knowledge Discovery & Data Mining, pp. 1054–1064 (2020)
27. Zhou, K., Li, Y., Li, Q.: Distantly supervised named entity recognition via confidence-based multi-class positive and unlabeled learning. arXiv preprint arXiv:2204.09589 (2022)

28. Beltagy, I., Lo, K., Cohan, A.: SciBERT: a pretrained language model for scientific text. arXiv preprint arXiv:1903.10676 (2019)
29. Wang, X., et al.: Cross-type biomedical named entity recognition with deep multi-task learning. Bioinformatics **35**(10), 1745–1752 (2019)

A BART-Based Study
of Entity-Relationship Extraction
for Electronic Medical Records
of Cardiovascular Diseases

Yifan Guo[1], Hongying Zan[1(✉)], Hongyang Chang[2], Lijuan Zhou[1],
and Kunli Zhang[1]

[1] School of Computer and Artificial Intelligence, Zhengzhou University,
Zhengzhou, China
{iehyzan,ieljzhou,ieklzhang}@zzu.edu.cn
[2] The Chinese People's Liberation Army Unit 63893, Luoyang, China

Abstract. With the advancement of training techniques, models such as BERT and GPT have been pre-trained on massive unlabeled texts, enabling effective learning of semantic representations of sentences and incorporating a wealth of prior knowledge. Therefore, we utilized a pre-trained model based on BART, called Joint entity Relation Extraction with BART (JREwBART), for entity relation extraction in medical texts. Building upon the JREwBART model, we proposed the Pipeline entity Relation Extraction based on the BART and Biaffine Transformation (PRE-BARTaBT) model. We evaluated the performance of these two models on three Chinese medical datasets: SEMRC, CVDEMRC (Cardiovascular/Stroke Disease Electronic Medical Record entity and relation Corpus), and CMeIE. The experimental results demonstrate the effectiveness of both models. Compared to the state-of-the-art baseline model, Cas-CLN, JREwBART achieved an improvement of 0.71%, 1.64%, and 0.37% in terms of F1 score on the three datasets, respectively. PRE-BARTaBT showed F1 score improvements of 0.81%, 2%, and 0.26% on the same datasets, respectively.

Keywords: Entity relation extraction · Cardiovascular and stroke information extraction · Pre-trained models

1 Introduction

Entity-relationship extraction is one of the classic tasks in the direction of information extraction in Natural Language Processing (NLP), which refers to identifying and extracting entities and relationships between entities from semi-structured or unstructured text and presenting them in the form of structured triples. In Chinese medical entity-relationship extraction data, there are many problems of ternary entity overlapping and single corpus containing multiple ternary groups, which bring great challenges to Chinese medical information

H. Xu et al. (Eds.): CHIP 2023, CCIS 1993, pp. 82–97, 2024.
https://doi.org/10.1007/978-981-99-9864-7_6

extraction. Ternary entity overlap refers to the phenomenon of entity sharing between ternaries, which is divided into three types: non-overlapping type (Normal), single entity overlap (SEO) and entity pair overlap (EPO). The Normal type means that all the entities in the triples contained in the corpus participate in entity pair matching only once in this corpus, and the entity pairs in the triples have only one relationship in the whole corpus; the Single entity overlap type means that at least one entity participates in two or more entity pair matches in a corpus; and the Entity pair overlap type means that there are cases where a certain entity pair has more than one semantic relationship in a single corpus or multiple corpora.

To address the issue of entity overlap, we use the Joint Relation Extraction with BART-based Generation (JREwBART) model [3], which utilizes the BART model [11] for generating entity relations. It takes unstructured medical case text as the source input and constructs the target sequence using the indices of the triplet elements implied in the text. We fine-tune BART by incorporating strategies such as constrained decoding, encoding representation reuse, feature fusion, and beam search to enhance the performance of the model. The autoregressive decoding process that utilises the model's ability to generate the same character as many times as needed is used to solve the entity overlap problem and the multiple ternary problem described above. Although the JREwBART model significantly reduces the candidate words of the model classifier through constrained decoding, the randomly initialized weights responsible for relation classification in the classifier contribute to an average proportion of over 34% in the cardiovascular and cerebrovascular dataset used. These weight parameters are trained relatively independently and cannot effectively capture the information from the encoder-side input text through strategies such as encoding representation reuse and multi-layer encoding feature fusion. To address this issue, we propose the PRE-BARTaBT model, which optimizes and adjusts specific subtasks separately, following a pipeline approach. We utilize the JREwBART model as the framework for the entity recognition subtask, allowing the model to focus more on conveying the information required for entity recognition and reducing the impact of inconsistent task objectives on the model. By using the generated entity indices and entity type sequences, we extract the feature vectors of the entities from the encoded representation of the input sentence. These feature vectors are concatenated with the soft labels of the relations and then fed into a multi-head selection model and a biaffine transformation calculation to determine the relations between arbitrary entity pairs.

In order to effectively address the above issues, we have made the following contributions:

– For small-scale or datasets with a large number of relation types, we developed the PRE-BARTaBT model based on the JREwBART model. By utilizing a weight sharing strategy at the encoding layer, we enhanced the connection between the named entity and relationship classification subtasks, leading to further improvements in the model's performance.

– Experimental results demonstrate that our two models achieved excellent performance on three Chinese medical text datasets: SEMRC [8], CVDEMRC [5] and CMeIE [19,31]. In particular, the results on the CMeIE dataset indicate a significant improvement in our approach compared to other methods.

2 Related Work

In the field of entity-relationship extraction, [25,29] investigated the application of pre-trained models in the task of entity-relationship extraction and achieved promising results. [23] utilized the seq2seq model and achieved competitive or superior results compared to state-of-the-art methods on multiple named entity recognition datasets. The rapid development of the entity-relationship extraction task has also driven the research related to this task in the medical domain. The research on entity-relationship extraction in the medical domain has gone through a process similar to that of the research in the general domain, i.e., a gradual transition from machine learning-based approaches to deep neural network-based approaches, and approaches based on fine-tuning of pre-trained models.

2.1 Traditional Machine Learning Methods

Machine learning-based methods have demonstrated good performance in entity recognition, thus Savova et al. [17] proposed a knowledge extraction method for clinical texts by combining machine learning algorithms and rule-based methods in the form of pipeline [2,14,27,30] to extract information from clinical records and electronic medical records. Chang et al. [6] used a combination of rule-based and Maximum Entropy (ME) based methods to sort out the sequential relationships between events to assist doctors in clinical decision-making. Nikfarjam et al. [15] proposed a combination of machine learning and graph-based reasoning for different temporal relationships to assist doctors in clinical decision-making. Yang et al. [24] combined Conditional Random Field (CRF) and specific rules to extract relationships between events from the text of medical records. Seol et al. [18] combined CRF and Support Vector Machine (SVM) models to detect patient-related clinical events and their relationships, respectively.

2.2 Pre-trained Models Based Methods

With the development of pre-training technology, models represented by BERT [9], GPT [16], RoBERTa [13], etc. are pre-trained on super-large scale unlabelled text to learn the semantic representation of sentences, which contains a large amount of a priori knowledge; these pre-training models are stacked with the Transformer [20] model as a unit, and the model structure itself contains a multi-head self-attention mechanism, which can obtain the contextual representation information of the text and get rid of the dependence on manually constructed corpus features; in addition, the pre-training process is not specific to certain tasks, and only requires fine-tuning of the model in downstream tasks, thus it has strong generality in many NLP tasks. In view of the excellent performance of CasREL [22], TPLinker [21] and other models, some research works have introduced and improved them for the characteristics of more frequent overlapping of medical text entities and higher average number of ternary groups in a single sentence corpus, e.g., Chang et al. [4] have made the following improvements on the basis of CasREL: increase the number of candidate primary entities sampled, use the Conditional Layer Normalisation deep fusion of main entity feature information and sentence information and the use of encoder multilayer sentence feature representation weight fusion, etc., which improve the model's performance ability in Chinese medical text for the above two problems. The pre-trained models in the medical field include Bio-BERT [10], which is pre-trained on the text data of English papers in the medical field, Clinical-BERT [1], which extracts medical records from the MIMIC-III database to be the pre-training corpus for the model, BEHRT [12], which is embedded based on medical entities rather than words, and Chinese data based on Chinese medical Q&A, EHRs, and medical encyclopaedias. MC-BERT [28], which is trained by masking at the whole word and entity level, and so on.

3 PRE-BARTaBT Model Based on BART and Biaffine

There are a large number of single subject-to-multiple object cases in the text of electronic medical records of cardiovascular and cerebrovascular diseases, and the types of relationships between entities are more complex compared to the commonly used datasets in the general domain, resulting in problems such as a large number of triples in a single corpus and a more common overlap of entities in triples in the corpus.

We propose the PRE-BARTaBT model based on the JREwBART model, and its structure is illustrated in Fig. 1. Following a pipeline approach, the PRE-BARTaBT model decomposes the entity relation extraction task into two subtasks, namely entity recognition and relation classification. These subtasks are controlled by the entity recognition and relation classification modules, respectively.

3.1 Entity Recognition Module

Aiming at the characteristics of the electronic medical record data of cardiovascular and cerebrovascular diseases, such as the average number of ternary groups and the serious problem of entity overlapping of ternary groups, JREw-BART uses the seq2seq framework to complete the ternary group joint extraction through the generative method. Benefiting from the generative decoding method of BART, the model is able to decode a certain identical candidate word in the candidate word list multiple times, which makes the model unnecessary to design

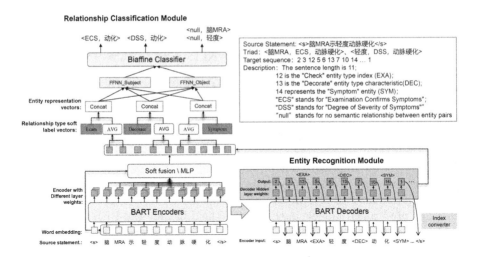

Fig. 1. PRE-BARTaBT model structure diagram.

complex sequence annotation strategies when dealing with the ternary entity overlapping problem.

The structure of the JREwBART model is shown in Fig. 2, the input sentence is fed into the encoder to get the sentence encoding information, and then soft fusion strategy is used to get the encoded representations of the sentence with different depths; a specific start token $<sos>$ is used as the input to the decoder, and then the decoder uses the encoded representation of the source statement and the embedded representation of the relation as the weights of entity and relation classifiers, respectively. The probability distribution of candidate words is obtained using the softmax function. The most probable candidate word "brain" is selected from them and added to the sequence headed by $<sos>$ as the input sequence of the decoder reasoning about the next word. This process is iterated until the decoder reasons out the end marker $<eos>$.

The overall logic of the model is to use the unstructured medical record text as the source input and the indexes of each element of the triad embedded in the text to form the target sequence, fine-tuning the BART while improving the model performance through strategies such as constrained decoding, coded representation reuse, feature fusion, and beam search. The problem of entity overlapping and multiple triples is addressed using an autoregressive decoding process in which the model is able to generate the same character as many times as needed.

In the PRE-BARTaBT model, the JREwBART model is employed for the entity recognition module. The model utilizes an encoder to obtain the feature vector H^E of the input sentence. The decoder takes $<sos>$ and H^E as inputs and performs inference until it generates the $<eos>$ marker. To adapt the model for entity recognition tasks, we replace the model's target sequence, which consists of elements of triples, with an indexed sequence formed by the entity and its relation type labels in the order of their occurrence in the encoder input text.

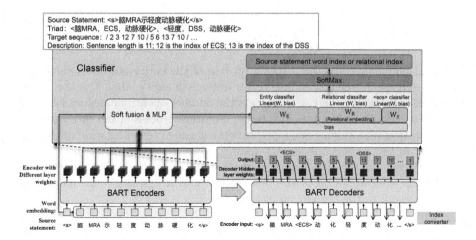

Fig. 2. JREwBART model structure diagram.

3.2 Relationship Classification Module

After obtaining the entities and entity types contained in the sentence through the generative model based on the pre-trained BART, we use the multiple head selection mechanism and biaffine attention to compute the semantic relationships that exist between the generated entities with each other. The feature coding layer of the relationship classification module is loaded with the model weights for entity recognition and then continues to be trained according to the task. Compared to re-training the BART coding layer, loading the trained model weights allows the model to make use of the entity information learnt in the entity recognition phase during the relationship classification computation and strengthens the connection between the two tasks.

Multi-head Selection Mechanism. The multi-head selection mechanism determines whether the "head" of each entity, referred to as the subject entity s_i, has a semantic relationship represented by relation r_j with the "head" of other entities, referred to as the object entity o_j. The results of this determination are recorded as (o_j, r_j). The multi-head selection mechanism is employed to address the issue of entity overlap.

Given an input sequence X, a set of relationships R, and a set of generated entity indices E, the model aims to identify the semantic relationship $r_{ij} \subseteq R$ between the entity feature vector $e_i, i \in \{0, 1, ..., n\}$ and the feature vector $e_j, j \in \{0, 1, ..., n\}$ of other entities under the condition that the i-th entity is recognized as the subject entity in the triple. The probability of the model discerning the semantic relationship r_{ij} between two entity feature vectors is calculated using the Eq. 1 to 5.

$$g_i = \frac{\sum softmax(t_i) \cdot T}{N} \qquad (1)$$

$$e_i = \left[\frac{h_0^{e_i} + h_{-1}^{e_i}}{2}; g_i\right], i \in \{0, 1..., n\} \tag{2}$$

Equation 1 represents the learning process of the entity label soft vector g_i, where t_i represents the embedding vector of the i-th entity label. T is the vector matrix of entity labels, and N represents the number of entity category labels in the dataset. Equation 2 represents the computation process of the entity feature representation vector, where h_i represents the encoded representation of the i-th character in the input sequence. $h_0^{e_i}$ and $h_{-1}^{e_i}$ respectively represent the encoded representations of the boundaries of the i-th entity in the input sequence. [;] denotes the concatenation of the two vectors, and n represents the number of entities present in the current input sentence.

$$s(e_j, e_i, r_{ij}) = V \cdot relu\left(U_{e_j} + W_{e_i} + b\right) \tag{3}$$

Equation 3 represents the calculation process of the relationship score, where U, V, and W represent the trainable parameter matrices, and b represents the bias of the linear function. The calculation of e_i follows Eq. 2.

$$p(head = e_j, label = r_{ij}|e_i) = \sigma(s(e_j, e_i, r_{ij})) \tag{4}$$

$$L_{rel} = \sum_{i=0}^{n}\sum_{j=0}^{m} -logP(head = e_j, label = r_{ij}|e_i) \tag{5}$$

Equation 4 represents the probability calculation process of the semantic relationship r_ij between the main entity e_i and other entities e_j, given a specific e_i. It utilizes the sigmoid function. In addition, we define the cross-entropy loss function of the relationship classification module under the multi-head selection mechanism as Eq. 5. Whereas n represents the number of entities generated by the entity recognition stage model, m denotes the number of triples where the entity feature vector e_i is considered as the subject entity.

Biaffine Attention. Dozat et al. [7] found that the Biaffine classifier can more accurately parse out the syntactic relationship between core and dependent words by using the Biaffine attention mechanism instead of the traditional MLP-based multilayer perceptual attention in the dependent syntactic analysis task; Yu et al. [26] introduced the Biaffine bisimulation attention mechanism into the named entity recognition task by using a Biaffine classifier instead of a bilinear classifier for the purpose of enhancing the interaction of the information between the entity's head and tail characters in the task of dealing with the named entity recognition.

In Eqs. 6 and 7, $FFNN\_subject(\cdot)$ and $FFNN\_object(\cdot)$ represent two separate feed-forward neural networks that operate on the main entity and the guest entity respectively. e_i and e_j are entity vector representations obtained through Eq. 2.

$$e_i' = FFNN\_subject(e_i) \tag{6}$$

$$e'_j = FFNN\_object\left(e_j\right) \tag{7}$$

$$s_{bia}\left(e'_i, e'_j\right) = e'_i U_{bia} e'_j + W_{bias}\left(e'_i \oplus e'_j\right) + b_{bia} \tag{8}$$

Equation 8 calculates the scores of the two entities on each semantic relationship, where $U_{bias} \in \mathbb{R}^{d \times |R| \times d}$ and $W_{bias} \in \mathbb{R}^{2d \times |R|}$, d represents the dimension of the feed-forward neural network layers and R represents the number of predefined relationships in the dataset. The softmax function is then applied to obtain the probability distribution of the two entities on the relation types. The cross-entropy loss function is used, as shown in Eq. 10, which is the same as Eq. 5.

$$P'\left(head = e_j | e_i\right) = softmax\left(s_{bia}\left(e'_i, e'_j\right)\right) \tag{9}$$

$$L'_{rel} = \sum_{i=0}^{n} \sum_{j=0}^{m} -log P'\left(head = e_j, label = r_{ij} | e_i\right) \tag{10}$$

4   Experiments

To validate the effectiveness of JREwBART and PRE-BARTaBT models, this paper conducts four sets of entity-relationship extraction experiments for cardiovascular and cerebrovascular diseases on two datasets, SEMRC and CVDEMRC; in order to validate the model's extraction performance on ternary groups, the experiments are completed and analysed in the complete dataset; in order to validate the model's performance against overlapping ternary groups of entities, and a single corpus containing multiple ternary groups, The dataset is cut accordingly and experiments and analyses are completed; in order to verify the model's generalisation ability in medical data, the publicly available multi-source medical text dataset CMeIE is selected for experiments and analyses.

4.1   Dataset

In this paper, the three datasets used were re-sized. The results of the dataset size statistics are shown in Table 1.

4.2   Baseline

For the experimental analysis of the proposed entity-relationship extraction model in the electronic medical record text of cardiovascular diseases, the following three models are selected as the control experimental group in this paper.

– An entity-relationship extraction model Lattice LSTM-Trans; using Lattice LSTM model as an encoder fusing state transfer networks.

Table 1. Database statistics.

Databases	Categories	Train set	Valid set	Test set
SEMRC	Corpus	7,304	913	917
	Triads	30,699	3,914	3,699
	Sub-relation	40	40	40
CVDEMRC	Corpus	4,856	614	607
	Triads	20,311	2,659	2,465
	Sub-relation	40	40	40
CMeIE	Corpus	17,924	4,482	5,602
	Triads	54,286	13,484	17,512
	Sub-relation	44	44	44

- CasREL [22] model based on pre-trained BERT model combined with stacked pointer network, converting multi-label classification task into binary classification task by stacking multi-layer pointer networks, and completing joint decoding of guest entities and relationships.
- A Cas-CLN [4] model based on a pre-trained RoBERTa [13] model combined with a cascaded pointer network and a conditional layer normalisation strategy, replacing BERT as an encoder to extract input text features using a RoBERTa model with stronger modelling capabilities and containing more prior knowledge, and using a conditional layer normalisation strategy to deeply fuse sentence feature representations and main entity feature vectors.

4.3   Pre-training Nodes

The pre-training models used in the controlled experimental group in this section are BERT and BART, and the pre-training nodes selected are BERT-base-Chinese, BERT-large-Chinese, BART-base-Chinese, and BART-large-Chinese. Because the accessible resources for pre-training the BERT model are relatively abundant, in order to verify the impact of different pre-training strategies on the cardiovascular entity relationship extraction task, pre-training nodes such as ERNIE, MC-BERT and RoBERTa were added to the experimental group of Cas-CLN models.

4.4   Main Results

The results of the JREwBART, PRE-BARTaBT and baseline models on the SEMRC and CVDEMRC datasets are shown in Table 2, where the results can be seen that the F1 values of the PRE-BARTaBT model on both datasets are somewhat improved compared to the other methods.

Analysis of the experimental results reveals that the results of the pre-trained model-based approach are significantly higher than those of the Lattice LSTM-Trans model on all datasets, which suggests that the a priori knowledge learnt

Table 2. Overall results of the model in the dataset.

Group	Configure	SEMRC			CVDEMRC		
		Pre (%)	Rec (%)	F1 (%)	Pre (%)	Rec (%)	F1 (%)
(a)	Lattice LSTM-Trans	60.25	23.37	33.68	61.37	24.16	34.67
(b)	CasREL$_{BERT-base}$	59.02	62.52	60.72	62.89	57.60	60.13
	CasREL$_{BERT-large}$	61.72	65.14	63.38	64.27	59.71	61.91
(c)	Cas-CLN$_{BERT-base}$	59.49	62.23	60.83	59.49	62.23	60.83
	Cas-CLN$_{ERNIE}$	58.75	63.34	60.96	63.40	59.88	61.59
	Cas-CLN$_{BERT-large}$	61.33	65.99	63.57	65.31	60.24	62.67
	Cas-CLN$_{RoBERTa}$	61.98	66.01	63.93	**66.09**	62.12	64.04
	Cas-CLN$_{MC-BERT}$	62.51	65.77	64.10	65.18	63.31	64.23
(d)	JREwBART$_{BART-base}$	61.92	65.80	63.80	65.13	62.01	63.53
	JREwBART$_{BART-large}$	62.33	66.37	64.28	66.01	62.69	64.31
(e)	PRE-BARTaBT$_{BART-base}$	58.78	**67.83**	62.98	60.08	**69.22**	64.33
	PRE-BARTaBT$_{BART-large}$	**62.78**	66.07	**64.38**	61.85	67.78	**64.67**

by pre-training from a large amount of unlabelled text enhances the model's semantic understanding of the input text when fine-tuned for the downstream task.

Compared to the Cas-CLN$_{BERT-large}$ model, JREwBART$_{BART-large}$ improves the results on the two datasets by 0.71% and 1.64%, respectively, potentially because the JREwBART uses autoregressive decoding to cope with the problem of ternary entity overlap without any restriction on the number of times, reducing the number of classifiers from the number of predefined relations to 1, and using the restricted decoding approach to significantly reduce the range of the classifiers' candidates to solve the problem of signal sparsity and at the same time improve the correctness of the model prediction. By comparing the improvement of the JREwBART$_{BART-large}$ model's results on the dataset with the size of the dataset (CVDEMRC dataset training corpus of 4,856 entries, with a 1.64% improvement in the results; SEMRC dataset training corpus of 7,304 entries, with a 0.71% improvement in the results), it can be seen that as the dataset size decreases, the more obvious the improvement is for the signal sparsity problem caused by cascading pointer annotation networks.

The PRE-BARTaBT$_{BART-large}$ model achieves improved F1 values compared to the JREwBART model on both datasets. It proves that PRE-BARTaBT's strategy of dividing the entity-relationship extraction task into two word tasks and by sharing the coding layer weights is effective. The reason for this improvement is that in the JREwBART model, although a constrained decoding strategy is used to reduce the candidate word range significantly, the indices corresponding to semantic relations still occupy over 34.35% of the probability distribution space of the candidate words. The weights of the classifier responsible for calculating the relation indices are learned through random initialization, which cannot capture the source sentence's feature representation learned by the encoder, resulting in a decrease in classifier performance. This negative impact affects the entire sequence generation process of the model. To mitigate the performance degradation caused by random initialization, the PRE-BARTaBT model divides the entity relation extraction task into two modules: named entity recognition and relation classification. During the constrained decoding process, only entity labels with fewer entities are generated, and the model strengthens the connection between the two subtasks by sharing the weights of the encoding layer. In this way, the model can focus more on the entity recognition task and utilize the shared encoding layer weights to enhance the performance of the relation classification task. Through this approach, the PRE-BARTaBT model effectively reduces the negative impact of random initialization on classifier performance and achieves overall improvement.

Table 3. Statistics of specific types and quantities of datasets.

Category	SEMRRC						CVDEMRC					
	Train set		Dev set		Test set		Train set		Dev set		Test set	
	Num	Pro	Num	Pro	Num	Pro	Num	Pro	Num	Pro	Num	Pro
1	2,681	36.71	344	37.68	343	37.40	1,687	34.74	221	35.99	213	35.09
2	1,288	17.63	173	18.95	174	18.97	862	17.75	110	17.92	106	17.46
3	752	10.30	81	8.87	76	8.29	487	10.03	60	9.77	69	11.37
4	647	8.86	82	8.98	81	8.83	506	10.42	61	9.93	65	10.71
≥ 5	1,936	26.51	233	25.52	243	26.50	1,314	27.06	162	26.38	154	25.37
NOR	2,788	38.17	392	42.94	385	41.98	1,754	36.12	279	45.44	272	44.81
SEO	4,000	54.76	499	54.65	496	54.09	2,665	54.88	326	53.09	327	53.87
EPO	2,205	30.19	101	11.06	101	11.01	1,747	35.98	58	9.45	56	9.23
Total	7,304	79.96	913	10.00	917	10.04	4,856	79.91	614	10.10	607	9.99
Triplet	30,699	80.13	3,914	10.22	3,699	9.66	20,311	79.85	2,659	10.45	2,465	9.69

4.5   Overlapping Triples of Different Types of Entities

The extraction results of the model for different types of entity overlap triples on the SEMRC dataset are shown in Fig. 3, where it can be seen that the extraction results of the Lattice LSTM-Trans model for the Non-Entity Overlap Type (Normal), Entity Pair Overlap (EPO), and Single-Entity Overlap Type (SEO) test corpora show a gradually decreasing trend, which indicates that the extraction difficulty of the model for these different types of overlapping triples are progressively more difficult to extract. As shown in Table 3, in the SEMRC dataset testing data, the proportion of Normal type triple corpus is 41.98%, the Entity Pair Overlap type (EPO) triple corpus is 11.01%, and the Single Entity Overlap type (SEO) triple corpus is 54.09%. Compared to the Cas-CLN model, the PRE-BARTaBT model only exhibits a decrease of 1.37% in extraction performance in Normal type triples, but demonstrates enhancements of 3.02% and 2.46% in SEO and EPO types, respectively. In comparison to the JREwBART model, although the PRE-BARTaBT model shows a downward trend of 4.92% in EPO type, the lower proportion of EPO type corpus and the increase of 4.37% and

2.49% in Normal type and SEO type respectively compensate for this. Thus, the overall performance of the PRE-BARTaBT model on the SEMRC dataset is superior to the other two models. The results show that the PRE-BARTaBT model can effectively alleviate the triple entity overlap problem in small-scale cardiovascular and cerebrovascular disease datasets, and can also obtain good results for non-entity overlap type triplets.

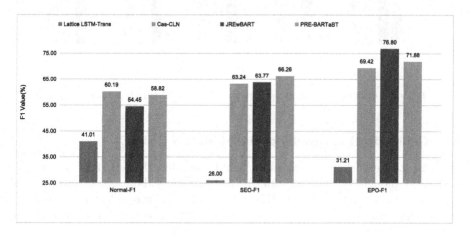

Fig. 3. Model Extraction Results for Different Entity Overlap Types on the SEMRC Dataset.

4.6   Different Number of Triads

In order to verify the extraction effect of the model on the corpus containing different numbers of triples, the corpus in the SEMRC dataset was divided into five subsets according to the number of triples contained, such as containing 1, 2, 3, 4 triples, and containing five or more triples. Figure 4 shows the model's extraction results on each subset. The PRE-BARTaBT model achieves the best results in all the corpus subsets except for the number of triples 4, especially when the number of triples is five or more, it still shows high extraction results. The proportion of the corpus with five or more ternary groups in the CVDEMRC and SEMRC constructed based on EHR data is more than 25%, which is the focus and difficulty in the research of CVD entity relationship extraction and it indicates the necessity of our work.

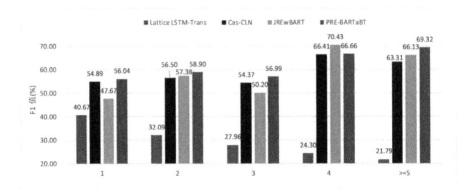

Fig. 4. Model extraction results for corpus containing different number of triples.

4.7   Generalization Results of the Model on CMeIE

In order to test the generalisation ability of the JREwBART and PRE-BARTaBT models for medical data, the Chinese medical dataset CMeIE, which was used for Task 2 of the CHIP-2020 evaluation, was selected for entity-relationship extraction experiments. The main results are shown in Table 4 below.

Table 4. Model results on the CMeIE dataset.

Data	Group	Models	Precision (%)	Recall (%)	F1 (%)
CMeIE	(a)	Lattice LSTM-Trans	**87.54**	15.86	26.86
	(b)	CasRELBERT-large	60.61	55.09	57.72
	(c)	Cas-CLNBERT-large	60.94	57.28	59.05
	(d)	JREwBARTBART-large	58.16	60.74	**59.42**
	(e)	PRE-BARTaBTBART-large	55.93	**63.12**	59.31

It can be seen from the experimental results that the JREwBART and PRE-BARTaBT models achieved a certain improvement in the results of extracting F1 values in the CMeIE dataset compared to the baseline Cas-CLN model, indicating that the two models have a certain degree of generalisation ability in medical data.

5   Conclusion

In this paper, we first propose applying JREwBART to the study of cardiovascular disease entity relationship extraction in electronic medical records (EMRs). Additionally, we introduce the PRE-BARTaBT model as an optimization of the JREwBART model. Extensive experiments are conducted to demonstrate the effectiveness of these models in addressing the issue of entity overlap. In JREw-BART, the model addresses the challenges of entity overlap and multiple triplets by utilizing the autoregressive decoding process, which allows for multiple generations of the same character. In PRE-BARTaBT, we employ JREwBART for entity recognition and enhance the extraction of semantic relations between two entities through the use of multi-head selection mechanisms and biaffine attention in the classification task. The pipeline approach has shown excellent performance in addressing overfitting issues in small-scale datasets. However, the independent nature of subtasks in the pipeline also introduces the problem of error propagation, which to some extent limits the extraction performance of the model. In future, we aim to design extraction algorithms that are more tailored to the data characteristics based on specific needs. Overall, our approach outperforms the baseline model CASCLN on the SEMRC, CVDEMRC, and CMeIE datasets. The results across different sentence types indicate that our model performs exceptionally well in complex and challenging scenarios.

Acknowledgements. This research was supported by the National Natural Science Foundation of China (Grant No. 62006211), the key research and development and promotion project of Henan Provincial Department of Science and Technology in 2023 (232102211041), Science and technology research project of Henan Provincial science and Technology Department in 2023 (232102211033) and Science and Technology Innovation 2030-"New Generation of Artificial Intelligence" Major Project under Grant No. 2021ZD0111000. We want to acknowledge the valuable data support provided by SEMRC, CVDEMRC, and CMeIE. We would like to thank the anonymous reviewers for their valuable comments and suggestions on the improvement of this paper.

References

1. Alsentzer, E., et al.: Publicly available clinical. In: Proceedings of the 2nd Clinical Natural Language Processing Workshop. Association for Computational Linguistics (2019)
2. Chan, Y.S., Roth, D.: Exploiting syntactico-semantic structures for relation extraction. In: Proceedings of the 49th Annual Meeting of the Association for Computational Linguistics: Human Language Technologies, pp. 551–560 (2011)
3. Chang, H., Xu, H., van Genabith, J., Xiong, D., Zan, H.: JoinER-BART: joint entity and relation extraction with constrained decoding, representation reuse and fusion. In: IEEE/ACM Transactions on Audio, Speech, and Language Processing (2023)
4. Chang, H., Zan, H., Guan, T., Zhang, K., Sui, Z.: Application of cascade binary pointer tagging in joint entity and relation extraction of Chinese medical text. Math. Biosci. Eng. **19**(10), 10656–10672 (2022)
5. Chang, H., Zan, H., Zhang, S., Zhao, B., Zhang, K.: Construction of cardiovascular information extraction corpus based on electronic medical records. Math. Biosci. Eng. **20**(7), 13379–13397 (2023)
6. Chang, Y.C., Dai, H.J., Wu, J.C.Y., Chen, J.M., Tsai, R.T.H., Hsu, W.L.: TEMPT-ING system: a hybrid method of rule and machine learning for temporal relation extraction in patient discharge summaries. J. Biomed. Inform. **46**, S54–S62 (2013)

7. Dozat, T., Manning, C.D.: Deep biaffine attention for neural dependency parsing. In: International Conference on Learning Representations (2016)

8. Hongyang, C., Hongying, Z., Yutuan, M., Kunli, Z.: Corpus construction for named-entity and entity relations for electronic medical records of stroke disease. J. Chin. Inf. Process. **36**(8), 37–45 (2022)

9. Devlin, J., Chang, M.W., Lee, K., Toutanova, K.: BERT: pre-training of deep bidirectional transformers for language understanding. In: Proceedings of NAACL-HLT, pp. 4171–4186 (2019)

10. Lee, J., et al.: BioBERT: a pre-trained biomedical language representation model for biomedical text mining. Bioinformatics **36**(4), 1234–1240 (2020)

11. Lewis, M., et al.: BART: denoising sequence-to-sequence pre-training for natural language generation, translation, and comprehension. In: Proceedings of the 58th Annual Meeting of the Association for Computational Linguistics, pp. 7871–7880. Association for Computational Linguistics (2020). https://doi.org/10.18653/v1/2020.acl-main.703. https://aclanthology.org/2020.acl-main.703

12. Li, Y., et al.: BEHRT: transformer for electronic health records. Sci. Rep. **10**(1), 7155 (2020)

13. Liu, Y., et al.: RoBERTa: a robustly optimized BERT pretraining approach. arXiv preprint arXiv:1907.11692 (2019)

14. Mintz, M., Bills, S., Snow, R., Jurafsky, D.: Distant supervision for relation extraction without labeled data. In: Proceedings of the Joint Conference of the 47th Annual Meeting of the ACL and the 4th International Joint Conference on Natural Language Processing of the AFNLP, pp. 1003–1011 (2009)

15. Nikfarjam, A., Emadzadeh, E., Gonzalez, G.: Towards generating a patient's timeline: extracting temporal relationships from clinical notes. J. Biomed. Inform. **46**, S40–S47 (2013)

16. Radford, A., Wu, J., Child, R., Luan, D., Amodei, D., Sutskever, I., et al.: Language models are unsupervised multitask learners. OpenAI Blog **1**(8), 9 (2019)

17. Savova, G.K., et al.: Mayo clinical Text Analysis and Knowledge Extraction System (cTAKES): architecture, component evaluation and applications. J. Am. Med. Inform. Assoc. **17**(5), 507–513 (2010)

18. Seol, J.W., Yi, W., Choi, J., Lee, K.S.: Causality patterns and machine learning for the extraction of problem-action relations in discharge summaries. Int. J. Med. Inform. **98**, 1–12 (2017)

19. Guan, T., Zan, H., Zhou, X., Xu, H., Zhang, K.: CMeIE: construction and evaluation of Chinese medical information extraction dataset. In: Zhu, X., Zhang, M., Hong, Yu., He, R. (eds.) NLPCC 2020. LNCS (LNAI), vol. 12430, pp. 270–282. Springer, Cham (2020). https://doi.org/10.1007/978-3-030-60450-9_22

20. Vaswani, A., et al.: Attention is all you need. In: Advances in Neural Information Processing Systems, vol. 30 (2017)

21. Wang, Y., Yu, B., Zhang, Y., Liu, T., Zhu, H., Sun, L.: TPLinker: single-stage joint extraction of entities and relations through token pair linking. In: Proceedings of the 28th International Conference on Computational Linguistics, pp. 1572–1582 (2020)

22. Wei, Z., Su, J., Wang, Y., Tian, Y., Chang, Y.: A novel cascade binary tagging framework for relational triple extraction. In: Proceedings of the 58th Annual Meeting of the Association for Computational Linguistics, pp. 1476–1488 (2020)

23. Xia, Y., Zhao, Y., Wu, W., Li, S.: Debiasing generative named entity recognition by calibrating sequence likelihood. In: Proceedings of the 61st Annual Meeting of

the Association for Computational Linguistics (Volume 2: Short Papers), pp. 1137–1148. Association for Computational Linguistics, Toronto (2023). https://doi.org/10.18653/v1/2023.acl-short.98. https://aclanthology.org/2023.acl-short.98

24. Yang, Y.L., Lai, P.T., Tsai, R.T.H.: A hybrid system for temporal relation extraction from discharge summaries. In: Cheng, S.M., Day, M.Y. (eds.) TAAI 2014. LNCS(LNAI), vol. 8916, pp. 379–386. Springer, Cham (2014). https://doi.org/10.1007/978-3-319-13987-6_35

25. Ye, D., Lin, Y., Li, P., Sun, M.: Packed levitated marker for entity and relation extraction. In: Proceedings of the 60th Annual Meeting of the Association for Computational Linguistics (Volume 1: Long Papers), pp. 4904–4917 (2022)

26. Yu, J., Bohnet, B., Poesio, M.: Named entity recognition as dependency parsing. arXiv preprint arXiv:2005.07150 (2020)

27. Zelenko, D., Aone, C., Richardella, A.: Kernel methods for relation extraction. J. Mach. Learn. Res. **3**, 1083–1106 (2003)

28. Zhang, N., Jia, Q., Yin, K., Dong, L., Gao, F., Hua, N.: Conceptualized representation learning for Chinese biomedical text mining. arXiv preprint arXiv:2008.10813 (2020)

29. Zhao, K., Xu, H., Cheng, Y., Li, X., Gao, K.: Representation iterative fusion based on heterogeneous graph neural network for joint entity and relation extraction. Knowl.-Based Syst. **219**, 106888 (2021)

30. Zhou, G., Su, J., Zhang, J., Zhang, M.: Exploring various knowledge in relation extraction. In: Proceedings of the 43rd Annual Meeting of the Association for Computational Linguistics (ACL 2005), pp. 427–434 (2005)

31. Zifa, G., et al.: Overview of chip 2020 shared task 2: entity and relation extraction in Chinese medical text. J. Chin. Inf. Process. **36**(6), 101–108 (2022)

Multi-head Attention and Graph Convolutional Networks with Regularized Dropout for Biomedical Relation Extraction

Mian Huang, Jian Wang$^{(\boxtimes)}$, Hongfei Lin, and Zhihao Yang

Dalian University of Technology, Dalian 116024, China
huangmian@mail.dlut.edu.cn, {wangjian,hflin,yangzh}@dlut.edu.cn

Abstract. Automatic extraction of biomedical relation from text becomes critical because manual relation extraction requires significant time and resources. The extracted medical relations can be used in clinical diagnosis, medical knowledge discovery, and so on. The benefits for pharmaceutical companies, health care providers, and public health are enormous. Previous studies have shown that both semantic information and dependent information in the corpus are helpful to relation extraction. In this paper, we propose a novel neural network, named RD-MAGCN, for biomedical relation extraction. We use Multi-head Attention model to extract semantic features, syntactic dependency tree, and Graph Convolution Network to extract structural features from the text, and finally R-Drop regularization method to enhance network performance. Extensive results on a medical corpus extracted from PubMed show that our model achieves better performance than existing methods.

Keywords: Regularized Dropout · Multi-head Attention · GCN · Biomedical Relation Extraction

1 Introduction

Biomedical relation extraction is an important natural language processing task, which aims to quickly and accurately detect the relations between multiple entities related to medicine from the mass medical information on the Internet, it plays an important role in clinical diagnosis [1], medical intelligence question and answer [2], and medical knowledge mapping [3]. This research can provide technical support for medical institutions and drug companies, and has great benefits for public health. At present, there are some knowledge bases of entities and relations, but more biomedical relations exist in cross-sentence documents, which brings challenges to the research of relation extraction.

With the rise of the neural network, the deep learning model has been widely used in medical relationship extraction tasks. The existing methods are mainly divided into two categories: semantic-based model and dependency-based model. Semantic-based models, such as Convolutional Neural Network (CNN), and Recurrent Neural Network (RNN), can obtain context information effectively by encoding text sequences. Ekbal

H. Xu et al. (Eds.): CHIP 2023, CCIS 1993, pp. 98–111, 2024.
https://doi.org/10.1007/978-981-99-9864-7_7

et al. [4] used the CNN model to classify relations by using the features extracted from the convolution kernel and max-pooling layer. As a feature extraction method, CNN has a good performance, but it is more suitable to capture local information features. To better capture long-distance information and reflect the importance of different information, the attention mechanism [5] attracts researchers' attention. Zhou et al. [6] proposed an attention-based Bi-directional Long Short-Term Memory (BI-LSTM) framework that automatically focuses on words that have a decisive effect on classification and captures important semantic information in sentences. At present, the attention-based Bi-LSTM model has become an important method for natural language processing tasks.

In order to fully mine the deep information in sentences, syntactic dependency structure is applied to the relation extraction task. Guo et al. [7] fused the attention mechanism based on the shortest dependency path with CNN and RNN to obtain keywords and sentence features; Zhang et al. [8] used Graph Convolutional Network to extract relations based on the Lowest Common Ancestor (LCA) rule of entities. Miwa and Bansal [9] encoded the Shortest Dependency Path (SDP) between two entities by using Tree LSTM. Peng et al. [10] divided the input graph into two directed acyclic graphs (Dags), and Song et al. [11] proposed the Graph Recurrent Network model (GRN) to obtain the semantic structure. In addition to using parsers to construct dependency graphs, researchers also begin to pay attention to and propose methods to construct dependency graphs automatically. Jin et al. [12] proposed a complete dependency forest model, to construct a weight map that adapts to terminal tasks, Guo et al. [13] proposed a "Soft pruning" strategy, the neural network of Attention-Guided graph is used to represent the graph better. Besides, Jin et al. [14] proposed a method to generate dependency forests consisting of the semantic-embedded 1-best dependency tree. Qian et al. [15] proposed an auto-learning convolution-based graph convolutional network to perform the convolution operation over dependency forests and Tang et al. [16] devised a cross-domain pruning method to equalize local and nonlocal syntactic interactions. In the general domain, Chen et al. [17] proposed to exploit the sequential form of POS tags and naturally fill the gap between the original sentence and imperfect parse tree. Zhang et al. [18] proposed a dual attention graph convolutional network with a parallel structure to establish bidirectional information flow.

Based on the above ideas, we propose a novel end-to-end model called Multi-head Attention and Graph Convolutional Networks with R-Drop (RD-MAGCN) for N-ary document-level relation extraction, which combines semantic information and syntactic dependency information. First, we interact the input representation and the relation representation with Multi-head Attention Layer to obtain the weighted context semantic representation of the text. To make full use of syntactic dependency information in cross-sentence extraction, we construct document-level syntactic dependency trees and encode them with GCN to solve the long-distance dependence problem. Then, Concatenate the two representations and feed them into the decoder. Finally, the network is enhanced by using the R-Drop mechanism and the biomedical relation is extracted.

The major contributions of this paper are summarized as follows.

- We propose a novel end-to-end model (RD-MAGCN) that effectively combines context semantic information and syntactic information.

- We introduce a regularization method for the randomness of dropout, which can enhance the performance of the network.
- We evaluate the performance of our model, the experimental results show that the performance of this model exceeds that of previous models.

2 Method

In this section, we introduce our proposed method. The input of our model is the long documents containing the relations between medical entities, and the output is a certain type of relation. There are four steps in our method: (1) preprocessing the corpus, including instance construction and other information extraction; (2) constructing document-level syntactic dependency tree; (3) building Attention and Graph convolution Networks for relation extraction; (4) utilizing R-Drop mechanism to enhance the network.

2.1 Data Preprocessing

For the texts in the corpus, we carry out a series of preprocessing processes. We first use the Stanford CoreNLP toolkit to parse each document in the corpus to obtain the syntactic parsing results and POS tags for each word. Then we construct instances for each pair of entities marked in the dataset, each instance contains the tokens of the text, the directed dependency edges of each word, the POS tags of each word, the absolute position of each entity, and the relation type used as the label.

POS tags and entity positions are used in the Input Representation Layer to enrich the text information, and the syntactic dependency information is used to build dependency trees and encodes them with GCN to capture long-range dependency information in the text.

2.2 Dependency Tree Construction

Syntactic analysis [19] is one of the important techniques in natural language processing, which is used to determine the dependencies between words in sentences. The dependency tree is a kind of syntactic analysis method, which mainly expresses the dependence relation between the words. In order to get the syntactic dependency feature of documents, we introduce a document-level dependency tree, in which the nodes represent words and the edges represent the intra-sentence and inter-sentence lexical dependency relations. As shown in Fig. 1, in this paper, we use the following three types of edges between nodes to construct the dependency trees:

1. Syntactic dependency edges: the results of parsing text by Stanford CoreNLP toolkit. They denote the dependencies between the words in a sentence.
2. Adjacent sentence edges: we connect the dependency roots of two adjacent sentences using the adjacent sentence edges. The dependency between two sentences is indicated by "next". By using adjacent sentence edges, the entire document can form a connected graph.
3. Self-node edges: each node in the dependency tree has a self-node edge, which allows the model to learn about the node itself during training.

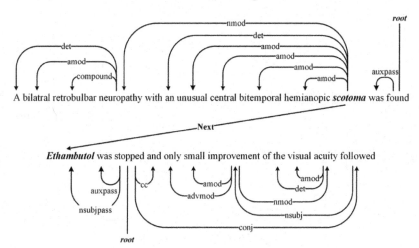

Fig. 1. An example of a constructed dependency tree consisting.

2.3 Model Structure

In this paper, we propose a novel model, Attention and Graph Convolutional Networks with R-Drop (RD-MAGCN), for N-ary document-level relation extraction. As shown in Fig. 2, the overall framework of our model consists of five parts: Input representation layer, Bi-LSTM layer, Multi-head Attention layer, GCN layer, and output layer. In addition, we utilize the R-Drop mechanism to enhance the networks and further improve the performance. The next few sections will describe the details of our model.

Input Representation Layer. For the specific domain of biomedical research, we introduce the Bio-BERT pre-trained language model [20] as the text representation encoder of Multi-head Attention Layer. However, since BERT and the improved pre-training models based on BERT use Word-Piece as the word segmentation method, and our dependency tree uses the entire words as nodes, we choose the ELMo pre-training model [21] to represent the input of GCN Layer. Furthermore, we enrich the representation of text with additional information, enabling the model to mine deeper semantics. POS tagging can strengthen the features of text, and position embedding can allow the model to locate the entities and better learn the information of the context near the entities. Therefore, our Input Representation Layer is divided into two parts, the embedding of Multi-head Attention layer is concatenated by Bio-BERT embedding, POS embedding, and position embedding:

$$w_1 = \left[w_{Bio-BERT}; w_{POS}; w_{position} \right] \tag{1}$$

The embedding of GCN Layer is concatenated by ELMo embedding, POS embedding, and position embedding:

$$w_2 = \left[w_{ELMO}; w_{POS}; w_{position} \right] \tag{2}$$

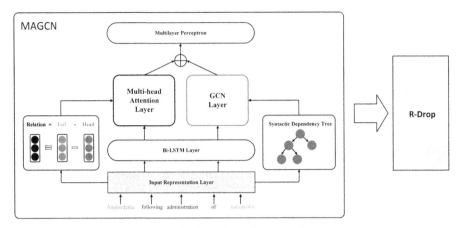

Fig. 2. Overview of our model.

Bi-LSTM Layer. RNN is very commonly used in NLP, it can capture the information of the previous text in the sentence, and LSTM utilizes the gating mechanism [22] to solve the problems of vanishing gradient, exploding gradient, and long-distance dependence that exist in RNN. Therefore, LSTM is suitable for handling document-level tasks. In this paper, we use two LSTMs, forward and backward, to encode two different input representations to obtain representations that contain both the preceding and the following information. We specify that the hidden state of the forward LSTM is h_t^f and the backward LSTM is h_t^b, the final hidden state is concatenated as:

$$h_t = \left[h_t^f ; h_t^b \right] \tag{3}$$

Multi-head Attention Layer. The attention mechanism has gradually become more and more important in NLP. The attention mechanism is the focus on the input weight distribution, which can enable the model to learn more valuable information and improve the performance of relation extraction. Following Li et al. [23], we build Multi-head Attention Layer that interacts with relation representations. Based on the idea of TransE [24], we regard relation representation as to the difference between entity representations:

$$w_{relation} = w_{tail} - w_{head} \tag{4}$$

When there are only two entities, the relation representation is denoted by the tail entity minus the head entity. When there are three entities such as drug, gene, and variety, we use the third entity representation (variety) minus the first entity representation (drug) as the relation representation.

We then use normalized Scaled Dot-Product Attention to compute a weighted score for the interaction of text with relation representations:

$$Attention(Q, K, V) = softmax\left(\frac{QK^T}{\sqrt{d}} \right) V \tag{5}$$

where Q indicates query, from the output of Bi-LSTM Layer, represented as sequences of text. K and V indicate key and value, from relation representation. d is the dimension of the vector and $\sqrt{d}$ is the scaling factor. The introduction of relation representation allows the model to give higher weight to text representations that are closer to the relation representation, which is helpful for relation extraction.

Eventually, concatenate the results of n heads:

$$h = [h_1; h_2; \ldots; h_n] \tag{6}$$

where n is set to 5 in our experiments. Multiple heads allow the model to learn relevant information from different representation subspaces. Finally, we perform max pooling to get the output h_{att} of Multi-head Attention Layer.

GCN Layer. GCN (Graph convolution Network) [25] is a natural extension of ConvNets on the graph structure, which can well extract the spatial structure features of images. The application of GCN to the syntactic dependency tree can extract the syntactic structure features of the text and solve the problem of long-distance separation of entities in document-level relation extraction.

In this paper, We convert the constructed document dependency tree into an adjacency matrix A, where $A_{i,j} = 1$ indicates that there is a dependency edge between word i and word j. Following Zhang et al. [8], we set the adjacency matrix as a symmetric matrix, i.e. $A_{i,j} = A_{j,i}$, and then we add self-node edges for each node, i.e. $A_{i,i} = 1$, for information about the node itself. Furthermore, we normalize the numerical values in the graph convolution to account for the large variation in node degrees in the dependency tree before adopting the activation function. At last, the graph convolution operation for node i at the l-th layer with the adjacency matrix of the dependency graph transformation can be defined as follows:

$$h_i^{(l)} = \rho\left(\frac{\sum_{j=1}^{n} A_{ij} W^{(l)} h_j^{(l-1)}}{d_i} + b^{(l)}\right) \tag{7}$$

where $h_i^{(l-1)}$ and $h_i^{(l)}$ denotes the input and the output of node i at the l-th layer. And the inputs of GCN Layer are the outputs of the Bi-LSTM Layer $h_1^{(0)}, \ldots, h_n^{(0)}$, then the outputs $h_1^{(L)}, \ldots, h_n^{(L)}$ are obtained through the graph convolution operation. W^l is the weight matrix, $b^{(l)}$ is the bias vector, $d_i = \sum_{j=1}^{n} A_{ij}$ is the degree of node i in the dependency tree for normalization, and ρ is the activation function.

Following Lee et al. [26], we also extract representations of entity nodes and concatenate them with representations of documents to highlight the role of entity nouns in the text structure and improve the performance of relation extraction. Similarly, we perform max pooling to get the output h_{GCN} of GCN Layer.

Output Layer. In this paper, our Output Layer is a two-layer perceptron. We concatenate the outputs of the two main modules to get h_{final} and then calculate as follow:

$$h_{final} = [h_{GCN}; h_{att}] \tag{8}$$

$$h_1 = ReLU\left(W_{h_1} h_{final} + b_{h_1}\right) \tag{9}$$

$$h_2 = ReLU\left(W_{h_2}h_1 + b_{h_2}\right) \tag{10}$$

In the end, we utilize the Softmax function to h_2 to determine the relation category:

$$o = Softmax(W_o h_2 + b_o) \tag{11}$$

2.4 R-Drop Mechanism

The dropout technique [27] accomplishes implicit ensemble by randomly hiding some neurons during neural network training. Liang et al. [28] introduce a simple regularization technique upon dropout, named as R-Drop. R-Drop works on the output of sub-models sampled by dropout. In each mini-batch training, each data sample undergoes two forward passes to obtain two sub-models. R-Drop forces two distributions of the same data samples outputted by two sub-models to be consistent with each other by minimizing the bidirectional Kullback-Leibler (KL) divergence between the two distributions. Finally, the two sub-models are used to jointly predict to achieve the effect of model enhancement. Results on multiple datasets show that R-Drop achieves good performance.

In this paper, we use the R-Drop mechanism to enhance our model. For the same batch of data, pass the model forward twice to get two distributions, denoted as $P_1(y_i|x_i)$ and $P_2(y_i|x_i)$. For each sub-model, we use cross-entropy as the loss function. Bidirectional KL divergence is then used to regularize the predictions of the two sub-models. Finally, the two are merged as the final loss function at the training steps:

$$L_{CE} = -logP_1(y_i|x_i) - logP_2(y_i|x_i) \tag{12}$$

$$L_{KL} = \frac{1}{2}(D_{KL}(P_1||P_2) + D_{KL}(P_2||P_1)) \tag{13}$$

$$L = L_{CE} + \alpha L_{KL} \tag{14}$$

where α is the weight coefficient, which we set to 0.5 in the experiments. In this way, R-Drop further regularizes the model space and improves the generalization ability of the model. This regularization method can be universally applied to different model structures, as long as there is randomness that can produce different outputs.

3 Experiments

3.1 Dataset

In this paper, we validate our method using the dataset introduced in Peng et al. [10], which contains 6987 drug-gene-mutation ternary relation instances and 6087 drug-mutation binary relation instances extracted from PubMed. The data we used were extracted by cross-sentence N-ary relation extraction, which extracts the triples in the biomedical literature. Table 1 shows the statistics of the data. Most instances are documents that contain multiple sentences. There are a total of 5 relation types for labels: "resistance or nonresponse", "sensitivity", "response", "resistance" and "None". Following Peng et al., we perform relation extraction for all instances according to binary classification and multi-classification, respectively, and obtain the results using a five-fold cross-validation method. In the case of binary classification, we classify all relation types as positive examples and "None" labels as negative examples.

Table 1. The statistics of the instances in the training set.

Data	Ternary	Binary
Single	2301	2728
Cross	4956	3359
Cross-percentage	70.1%	55.2%

3.2 Parameter Settings

This section describes the details of our model experiment setup. We tune the hyperparameters based on the results on the validation set, and the final hyperparameter settings are set as follows: the dimension of Bio-BERT pre-trained language model is 768, the dimension of ELMo pre-trained language model is 1024, the dimension of POS embedding obtained by StanfordNLP and position embedding are both 100. The dimension of the Bi-LSTM hidden layer and GCN layer are both 500, the number of heads of Multi-head Attention layer is 5, and the dimension is 1000. All dropouts in the model are set to 0.5. We train the model with a batch size of 16 and the Adam optimizer [29] with a learning rate: $lr = 1e - 4$.

We evaluate our method using the same evaluation metric as the previous research, that is the average accuracy of five cross-validations.

3.3 Baselines

In order to verify the effectiveness of the model in this paper, the model in this paper is compared with the following baseline models:

1. **Feature-Based** (Quirk and Poon, 2017) [3]: a model based on the shortest dependency path between all entity pairs;
2. **DAG LSTM** (Peng et al., 2017) [10]: contains linear chains and the graph structure of the Tree LSTM;
3. **GRN** (Song et al., 2018) [11]: a model for encoding graphs using Recurrent Neural Networks;
4. **GCN** (Zhang et al., 2018) [8]: a model for encoding pruned trees using Graph Convolutional Networks;

5. **AGGCN** (Guo et al., 2019) [13]: a model that uses an attention mechanism to build dependency forests and encodes it with GCN;
6. **LF-GCN** (Guo et al., 2020) [30]: a model for automatic induction of dependency structures using a variant of the matrix tree theorem;
7. **AC-GCN** (Qian et al., 2021) [15]: a model that learns weighted graphs using a 2D convolutional network;
8. **SE-GCN** (Tang et al., 2022) [16]: a model that uses a cross-domain pruning method to equalize local and nonlocal syntactic interactions;
9. **CP-GCN** (Jin et al., 2022) [14]: a model that uses dependency forests consisting of the semantic-embedded 1-best dependency tree and adopts task-specific causal explainer to prune the dependency forests;
10. **DAGCN** (Zhang et al., 2023) [18]: a model that uses a dual attention graph convolutional network with a parallel structure to establish bidirectional information flow.

3.4 Main Results

In the experiments, we count the test accuracies of ternary relation instances and binary relation instances in binary and multi-class, respectively. In the binary-class experiment, the intra-sentence and inter-sentence situations are counted separately. The results are shown in Table 2.

As can be seen from Table 2, the performance of neural network-based methods is significantly better than that of feature-based methods. Thanks to the powerful encoding ability of GCN for graphs, GCN-based methods generally outperform RNN-based methods. Except the ternary sentence-level in Binary-class, our model RD-MAGCN achieves state-of-the-art performance.

We first focus on the multi-class relation extraction task. On the ternary relation task, RD-MAGCN achieves an average accuracy of 90.2%, surpassing the previous state-of-the-art method CP-GCN by 5.3%. On the binary relation task, RD-MAGCN achieves an average accuracy of 90.3%, surpassing AC-GCN by 9.3%. This is a huge improvement, mainly due to the greater gain effect of the R-Drop mechanism on the model in multi-classification tasks.

For the binary-class relation extraction task, although our model RD-MAGCN does not have such a large increase as the multi-classification task, it almost still exceeds CP-GCN under different tasks. The above results show that our method of combining contextual semantic features and text structure features and enhancing the model with regularization methods is effective. Next, we will introduce the ablation study we have done for each module of the method.

Table 2. Compare with related work.

Model	Binary-class				Multi-class	
	Ternary		Binary		Ternary	Binary
	Intra	Inter	Intra	Inter	Inter	Inter
Feature-Based	74.7	77.7	73.9	75.2	–	–
DAG LSTM	77.9	80.7	74.3	76.5	–	–
GRN	80.3	83.2	83.5	83.6	71.7	71.7
GCN	85.8	85.8	83.8	83.7	78.1	73.6
AGGCN	87.1	87.0	85.2	85.6	79.7	77.4
LF-GCN	88.0	88.4	86.7	87.1	81.5	79.3
AC-GCN	88.8	88.8	86.8	86.5	84.6	81.0
SE-GCN	88.7	88.4	86.8	87.7	81.9	80.4
CP-GCN	**89.5**	89.1	87.3	86.5	84.9	80.1
DAGCN	88.4	88.4	85.9	86.2	84.3	78.3
RD-MAGCN	88.7	**89.5**	**87.8**	**88.6**	**90.2**	**90.3**

3.5 Ablation Study

In this section, we have proved the effectiveness of each module in our method. First, we investigate the role of the three main modules of R-Drop, Multi-head Attention Layer and GCN Layer. We define the following variants of RD-MAGCN:

w/o R-Drop: this variant denotes using the traditional single-model cross-entropy loss function instead of two sub-models ensembles at training steps.

w/o Attention: this variant denotes removing Multi-head Attention Layer and the corresponding inputs from the model.

w/o GCN: this variant denotes removing GCN Layer and the corresponding inputs from the model.

w/o $w_{relation}$: this variant denotes that Self-Attention is applied instead of introducing relation representation in Multi-head Attention Layer, that is, Q, K, and V all from text representation.

Table 3 shows the results of the comparison of RD-MAGCN with four variants.

It can be seen from Table 3: (1) The effect of the R-Drop regularization method to enhance the model is obvious, especially in the multi-class relation extraction task. Removing the R-Drop module has a performance loss of 4.9% and 6.5% in multi-class ternary and binary tasks, respectively. We speculate the reason is that in the binary classification task, due to its low difficulty, the constraint of KL divergence makes the distribution of the output of the two sub-models roughly the same, so the ensemble effect is not obvious. In multi-classification tasks, the ensemble effect will be better. (2) The performance of removing Multi-head Attention Layer model drops in each task, indicating the usefulness of interactive contextual semantic information. (3) The performance of removing GCN Layer model drops across tasks indicating the usefulness of syntactic structure information. Moreover, the performance of inter-sentence relation extraction drops more than that of intra-sentence relation extraction, indicating that GCN can capture long-distance structure features. (4) No introduction of relation representations in Multi-head Attention Layer degrades the results, indicating that the interaction of relation representations allows the model to pay more attention to the texts that are closer to the relation.

Table 3. The effect of the main modules of RD-MAGCN.

Model	Binary-class				Multi-class	
	Ternary		Binary		Ternary	Binary
	Intra	Inter	Intra	Inter	Inter	Inter
RD-MAGCN	**88.7**	**89.5**	**87.8**	**88.6**	**90.2**	**90.3**
w/o R-Drop	88.3	88.5	86.9	88.2	85.3	83.8
w/o Attention	86.3	86.2	84.7	84.6	86.9	86.0
w/o GCN	88.2	88.3	86.8	86.6	88.2	89.1
w/o $w_{relation}$	88.3	89.2	87.3	88.3	89.2	89.7

Next, we discuss the effects of the different input representations. We utilize the same model for the following types of inputs:

Table 4 shows the comparative performance of different input representations.

Original: The inputs to our proposed model. The input of Multi-head Attention module is the concatenation of Bio-BERT, POS and position embedding, and the input of the GCN module is the concatenation of ELMo, POS and position embedding.

Variant 1: The input of Multi-head Attention module is the concatenation of BERT, POS embedding, position embedding, and the input of the GCN module is the concatenation of ELMo, POS embedding, position embedding.

Variant 2: The input of Multi-head Attention module is the concatenation of Bio-BERT, POS embedding, and the input of the GCN module is the concatenation of ELMo, POS embedding.

Variant 3: The input of Multi-head Attention module is the concatenation of Bio-BERT, position embedding, and the input of the GCN module is the concatenation of ELMo, position embedding.

Variant 4: The input of Multi-head Attention module is Bio-BERT, and the input of the GCN module is ELMo.

From Table 4, we can see that: Bio-BERT, a domain-specific language representation model pre-trained on the large biomedical corpus, outperforms traditional BERT in the task of biomedical relation extraction. Bio-BERT enables a better understanding of complex biomedical literature. Besides, POS embedding and position embedding

Table 4. The effect of the input representation on performance.

Model	Binary-class				Multi-class	
	Ternary		Binary		Ternary	Binary
	Intra	Inter	Intra	Inter	Inter	Inter
RD-MAGCN	**88.7**	**89.5**	**87.8**	**88.6**	**90.2**	**90.3**
Variant 1	88.5	89.3	87.0	88.1	89.5	89.6
Variant 2	88.6	89.2	87.3	88.3	89.9	90.0
Variant 3	88.1	89.1	87.5	88.2	88.8	89.2
Variant 4	88.3	88.7	87.1	87.7	88.8	88.7

provide additional information for the model, which can help the model to better learn the semantics and structure of the text and locate the entities that appear in the text.

4 Conclusions

In this paper, we propose a novel end-to-end neural network named RD-MAGCN for N-ary document-level relation extraction. We extract weighted contextual features of the corpus via Multi-head Attention Layer that interacts with relation representations. We extract the syntactic structure features of the corpus through the syntactic dependency tree and GCN Layer. The combination of the two types of features can make the model more comprehensive. In addition, we ensemble the two trained sub-models through the R-Drop regularization method, and let the two sub-models jointly predict the relation type, which effectively enhances the performance of the model. Finally, we evaluate the model on multiple tasks of the medical dataset extracted from PubMed, where our RD-MAGCN achieves better results.

Our research improves the accuracy of biomedical relation extraction, which is helpful for other tasks in the medical field and the development of intelligent medicine. In future research, we will focus on applying more comprehensive techniques such as introducing medical knowledge graphs to study biomedical relation extraction more deeply.

References

1. Islamaj, R., Murray, C., Névéol, A.: Understanding PubMed user search behavior through log analysis. Database **6**(1), 1–18 (2009)
2. Yu, M., Yin, W., Hasan, S., Santos, C., Xiang, B., Zhou, B.: Improved neural relation detection for knowledge base question answering. In: Proceedings of the 55th Annual Meeting of the Association for Computational Linguistics, pp. 571–581 (2017)
3. Quirk, C., Poon, H.: Distant supervision for relation extraction beyond the sentence boundary. In: Proceedings of the European Chapter of the Association for Computational Linguistics, pp. 1171–1182 (2017)

4. Ekbal, A., Saha, S., Bhattacharyya, P.: A deep learning architecture for protein-protein inter-action article identification. In: Proceedings of the 23rd International Conference on Pattern Recognition (ICPR), pp. 3128–3133 (2016)

5. Vaswani, A., Shazeer, N., Parmar, N., et al.: Attention is all you need. In: Conference on Neural Information Processing Systems (NIPS), pp. 5998–6008 (2017)

6. Zhou, P., Shi, W., Tian, J., et al.: Attention-based bidirectional long short-term memory networks for relation classification. In: Proceedings of the 54th Annual Meeting of the Association for Computational Linguistics (Volume 2: Short Papers), pp. 207–212 (2016)

7. Guo, X., Zhang, H., Yang, H., et al.: A single attention-based combination of CNN and RNN for relation classification. IEEE Access 7(3), 12467–12475 (2019)

8. Zhang, Y., Qi, P., Manning, D.: Graph convolution over pruned dependency trees improves relation extraction. In: Conference on Empirical Methods in Natural Language Processing, pp. 2205–2215 (2018)

9. Miwa, M., Bansal, M.: End-to-end relation extraction using LSTMs on sequences and tree structures. In: Proceedings of the 54th Annual Meeting of the Association for Computational Linguistics (Volume 1: Long Papers), pp. 1105–1116 (2016)

10. Peng, N., Poon, H., Quirk, C., et al.: Cross-sentence N-ary relation extraction with graph LSTMs. Trans. Assoc. Comput. Linguist. 5(2), 101–115 (2017)

11. Song, L., Zhang, Y., Wang, Z., et al.: N-ary relation extraction using graph-state LSTM. In: Proceedings of the Conference on Empirical Methods in Natural Language Processing, pp. 2226–2235 (2018)

12. Jin, L., Song, L., Zhang, Y., et al.: Relation extraction exploiting full dependency forests. In: Proceedings of the Thirty-Fourth AAAI Conference on Artificial Intelligence (2020)

13. Guo, Z., Zhang, Y., Lu, W.: Attention guided graph convolutional networks for relation extraction. In: Proceedings of the 57th Annual Meeting of the Association for Computational Linguistics, pp. 241–251 (2019)

14. Jin, Y., Li, J., Lian, Z., et al.: Supporting medical relation extraction via causality-pruned semantic dependency forest. In: Proceedings of the COLING, pp. 2450–2460 (2022)

15. Qian, M., et al.: Auto-learning convolution-based graph convolutional network for medical relation extraction. In: Lin, H., Zhang, M., Pang, L. (eds.) CCIR 2021. LNCS, vol. 13026, pp. 195–207. Springer, Cham (2021). https://doi.org/10.1007/978-3-030-88189-4_15

16. Tang, W., Wang, J., Lin, H., et al.: A syntactic information-based classification model for medical literature: algorithm development and validation study. JMIR Med. Inform. 10(8), 378–387 (2022)

17. Chen, X., Zhang, M., Xiong, S., et al.: On the form of parsed sentences for relation extraction. Knowl.-Based Syst. 25(1), 109–184 (2022)

18. Zhang, D., Liu, Z., Jia, W., et al.: Dual attention graph convolutional network for relation extraction. IEEE Trans. Knowl. Data Eng. 10(11), 1–14 (2023)

19. Martin, J., Gompel, R.: Handbook of Psycholinguistics. 2nd edn. (2006)

20. Lee, J., Yoon, W., Kim, S., et al.: BioBERT: a pre-trained biomedical language representation model for biomedical text mining. Bioinformatics 36(4), 1234–1240 (2019)

21. Peters, M., Neumann, M., Iyyer, M., et al.: Deep contextualized word representations. In: Proceedings of the North American Chapter of the Association for Computational Linguistics, pp. 2227–2237 (2018)

22. Hochreiter, S., Schmidhuber, J.: Long short-term memory. Neural Comput. 9(8), 1735–1780 (1997)

23. Li, P., Mao, K., Yang, X., et al.: Improving relation extraction with knowledge-attention. In: Proceedings of the 2019 Conference on Empirical Methods in Natural Language Processing and the 9th International Joint Conference on Natural Language Processing (EMNLP-IJCNLP), pp. 229–239 (2019)

24. Bordes, A., Usunier, N., Weston, J., et al.: Translating embeddings for modeling multi-relational data. In: Proceedings of the International Conference on Neural Information Processing Systems, pp. 87–95 (2013)
25. Kipf, T., Welling, M.: Semi-supervised classification with graph convolutional networks. In: Proceedings of the International Conference on Learning Representations (2017)
26. Lee, K., He, L., Lewis, M., et al.: End-to-end neural coreference resolution. In: Proceedings of the Conference on Empirical Methods in Natural Language Processing (2017)
27. Hinton, G., Srivastava, N., Krizhevsky, A., et al.: Improving neural networks by preventing co-adaptation of feature detectors. Comput. Sci. $3(4)$, 212–223 (2012)
28. Liang, X., Wu, L., Li, J., et al.: R-Drop: regularized dropout for neural networks. In: Advances in Neural Information Processing Systems, vol. 34, no. 1, pp. 10890–10905 (2021)
29. Kingma, D., Ba, J.: Adam: a method for stochastic optimization. In: Proceedings of the 3rd International Conference for Learning Representations, San Diego (2015)
30. Guo, Z., Nan, G., Lu, W., et al.: Learning latent forests for medical relation extraction. In: Proceedings of the Twenty-Ninth International Joint Conference on Artificial Intelligence, pp. 3651–3675 (2020)

Biomedical Causal Relation Extraction Incorporated with External Knowledge

Dongmei Li[1] ⓘ, Dongling Li[1], Jinghang Gu[2], Longhua Qian[1(✉)], and Guodong Zhou[1]

[1] School of Computer Science and Technology, Soochow University, Suzhou 215006, Jiangsu, China
20224027005@stu.suda.edu.cn, {qianlonghua,gdzhou}@suda.edu.cn

[2] Department of Chinese and Bilingual Studies, The Hong Kong Polytechnic University, Hong Kong 999077, China

Abstract. Biomedical causal relation extraction is an important task. It aims to analyze biomedical texts and extract structured information such as named entities, semantic relations and function type. In recent years, some related works have largely improved the performance of biomedical causal relation extraction. However, they only focus on contextual information and ignore external knowledge. In view of this, we introduce entity information from external knowledge base as a prompt to enrich the input text, and propose a causal relation extraction framework JNT_KB incorporating entity information to support the underlying understanding for causal relation extraction. Experimental results show that JNT_KB consistently outperforms state-of-the-art extraction models, and the final extraction performance F1 score in Stage 2 is as high as 61.0%.

Keywords: Causal Relation Extraction · BEL Statement · Entity Information · External Knowledge

1 Introduction

In recent years, the biomedical text mining technology has made remarkable progress, especially in named entity recognition, relation extraction and event extraction [1–3]. Among them, causal relation extraction is one of the most complex tasks in biomedical text information mining [4]. It is critical to the analysis and understanding of complex biological phenomena in the biomedical field, which helps to reveal key information about biological processes, disease development, and drug action [5]. The task of biomedical causal relation extraction was proposed by BioCreative[1] community in 2015, aiming to extract causality statements from biomedical literature and generate corresponding Biological Expression Language (BEL) statements.

BEL [6] is a language that represents scientific discoveries in the field of biomedicine by capturing causal relationships between biomedical entities. Figure 1 illustrates the extraction of the BEL statements from biomedical texts and the simplified SBEL statements introduced in Sect. 3.2. BEL statements mainly includes three parts: BEL Term,

---

[1] https://biocreative.bioinformatics.udel.edu/.

© The Author(s), under exclusive license to Springer Nature Singapore Pte Ltd. 2024
H. Xu et al. (Eds.): CHIP 2023, CCIS 1993, pp. 112–128, 2024.
https://doi.org/10.1007/978-981-99-9864-7_8

Function type and Relation type [7]. We leave the three parts' details for BEL statement in the appendix.

However, in order to improve the expression efficiency in the biomedical literature, abbreviations or aliases are often used instead of complete full names [8], which increases the difficulty in understanding the meaning of entities. It is found that the function of entity is not only determined by context, but also closely related to the entity itself [9, 10].

Moreover, it is known that the integration of external knowledge in biomedical information extraction can make the encoder produce richer semantic representation in embedded space [11–13]. There are two main ways to integrate knowledge:

(1) Direct injection of external knowledge as word embedding. Li et al., 2020 [14] propose a BiLSTM network with the integration of KB information represented by the word embedding. Chen et al., 2018 [15] propose a approach for evaluating the semantic relations in word embeddings using external knowledge bases.
(2) Text concatenation of external knowledge. BioKGLM [16] propose to enrich a contextualized language model by integrating a large scale of biomedical knowledge graphs. Yuan et al., 2020 [17] propose a approach for knowledge graph construction based on unstructured biomedical domain-specific contexts.

Due to the absence of a large amount of entity information in experimental corpus, it is difficult to understand the function and meaning of entity [18, 19]. In this paper, we propose JNT_KB, which combines the original sentence and corresponding entity information in external biomedical knowledge base as the input of encoding model, and uses the joint model for causal relation extraction. The experimental results on BEL corpus show that JNT_KB effectively improves the overall performance of causal relation extraction.

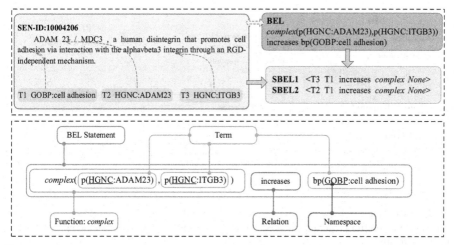

Fig. 1. A BEL statement example. The top part describes the process of converting a sentence into a BEL statement and SBEL statements with the corresponding subjects and object identified in the same color. The bottom part describes the components of the BEL statement.

2   Related Work

In this section, we reviews briefly related work to biomedical causal relation extraction, which can be broadly divided into two types: event-centric and entity-centric.

The event-centric approach aims to map events extracted from the biomedical literature onto entity functions and relations, which are then translated into BEL statements. Choi et al. [22] develop a system targeting generation of BEL statements by incorporating several text mining systems. However, the system is limited to identifying events involving specifically proteins and genes only. BELMiner [20] proposes a rule-based [21] causal relation extraction system to extract biological events and formalize them as BEL statements. But, the system suffers from rapid scaling of biomedical text. Lai et al., 2016 [23] use a SRL-based [24] approach to extract the events structure for BEL statements. But in the BioProp corpus [25], there are sentences without subject-verb-object structure, which decreases the performance of the approach.

The entity-centric approach directly extracts the entity functions and causality between entities, and then assembles them into BEL statements. Liu et al., 2019 [26] propose a deep learning-based approach to extract BEL statements with biomedical entities. But they do not tackle *complex* functions and nested relations. Following Liu et al., 2019 [26], Shao et al., 2021 [27] apply SBEL statements to enhances the expressivity of relations between entities, including the *complex* functions. In light of previous work, Li et al., 2023 [28] propose a joint learning model, which combines entity relation extraction and entity function detection to improve the performance of biomedical causal relation extraction. However, the recall rate of function detection subtask decreases significantly, due to the lack of entity information in the corpus.

Above all, they focus on text information between entities but ignore the semantic role of entity itself in biomedical causal relation extraction.

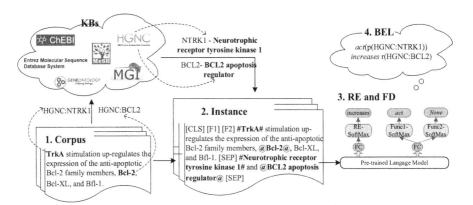

Fig. 2. An example for integration of external knowledge. We show the process of linking entity information from external knowledge bases, and use JNT_KB to obtain the predicted BEL statement finally.

3   Methodology

In this section, we introduce the details of JNT_KB. We first describe the system framework and the notations, including how to represent entities, relations and functions in BEL statements. Then we detail the two tasks: Relation Extraction (RE) task and Function Detection (FD) task, followed by the overall training objective. Last, we introduce the method for evaluating causal relation extraction tasks.

3.1   System Framework

As shown in Fig. 2, we construct the causal relation extraction framework with entity information, which consists of the following steps:

(1) Acquisition of external knowledge: Following Liu et al., 2019 [26] and Lai et al., 2019 [29], we identify entity mention from the sentence in the corpus and link it to entities in the namespace.
(2) Construction of instance: We get the full entity name from the external knowledge base (KBs) and concatenate it with the original sentence to construct a new input instance.
(3) Joint extraction of causality: Follwing JNT [28], we carry out RE and FD subtasks in the input instances based on BioBERT [5].
(4) BEL statement set: According to the relation type and function type, we assemble BEL statements predicted by JNT_KB.

3.2   Notations

JNT_KB is trained on a labeled BEL corpus leveraging the external knowledge base $\mathcal{K}$. Formally, let $\mathcal{S} = \{s_i\}_{i=1}^{|\mathcal{S}|}$ be a batch of sentences and $\mathcal{E}_i = \{e_{ij}\}_{j=1}^{|\mathcal{E}_i|}$ be all named entities in s_i, where e_{ij} is the j-th entity in s_i. For each sentence, we convert it to BEL statement, and then decompose to SBEL statement(s). We enumerate all quintuples (SBEL statements) $<e_{ij}, e_{ik}, r_{jk}^i, func_{ij}, func_{ik}>$ and link entity pairs (e_{ij}, e_{ik}) to their corresponding full name. Where e_{ij} and e_{ik} refer to entities corresponding to subject and object, and $func_{ij}$ and $func_{ik}$ represent the functions of the subject and object, and r_{jk}^i indicates the relation type between e_{ij} and e_{ik}. Then we obtain a tuple set $\mathcal{T}_i = \left\{ t_{jk}^i = (s_i, e_{ij}, e_{ik}, r_{jk}^i, func_{ij}, func_{ik}) | j \neq k \right\}$ for each sentence and the overall tuple set $\mathcal{T} = \mathcal{T}_1 \cup \mathcal{T}_2 \cdots \cup \mathcal{T}_{|\mathcal{S}|}$ for this batch.

3.3   RE and FD Task

RE task aims at finding a single interaction or regulatory relation between two or multiple biomedical entities. FD task aims at expressing the status information of the entitys in BEL statements. Figure 3 describes an example of RE and FD task, and gives the process of biomedical causal relation extraction. We input the instance to BERT's word segmentation tool [30] to generate the input sequence represented by word segmentation. We use BioBERT to encode each sentence s_i and obtain a hidden states sequence $H = \{c, f1, f2, h_1, h_2, \cdots, h_N\}$, where N denotes the number of tokens in the sentence [25].

The goal of RE and FD tasks are equivalent to maximizing the output $y = softmax(f(\cdot))$, where $f(\cdot)$ indicates a classifier [31, 32].

As shown in Fig. 3, in practice, three *softmax* classifiers are used to classify relation type, subject function type and object function type respectively, in respect to relation label set $L_r = \{l_1, l_2, \cdots, l_{m_r}\}$ and function label set $L_f = \{l_1, l_2, \cdots, l_{m_f}\}$. . The classifiers' outputs $[y_r, y_{f1}, y_{f2}]$ can be formulated as:

$$y_r = softmax(W_r c + b_r)$$
$$y_{f1} = softmax(W_f f1 + b_f)$$
$$y_{f2} = softmax(W_f f2 + b_f) \tag{1}$$

where $W_r \in \mathbb{R}^{d_z \times m_r}$, $W_f \in \mathbb{R}^{d_z \times m_f}$, d_z is the dimension of the BioBERT embeddings, $m_r = 3$ (relation types: increases, decreases, no_relation), $m_f = 7$ (function types: *complex, pmod, deg, tloc, sec, act, None*), b_r, b_f are the bias. The gold label corresponding to the predicted output $[y_r, y_{f1}, y_{f2}]$ is $[\hat{y}_r, \hat{y}_{f1}, \hat{y}_{f2}]$.

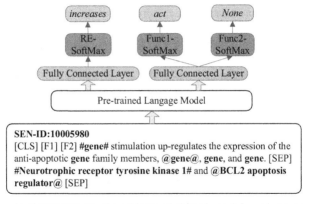

Fig. 3. An example of JNT_KB. For the subject and object in each input instance, we add special symbols "#" and "@" at the beginning and end of the entities, and the full name of the corresponding entity is also identified with the same special symbol.

Overall Training Objective. We train the relation and function representations of the entity pairs based on entity information.

In practice, we use the cross-entropy loss [5, 33] of RE and FD tasks as follows:

$$\mathcal{L} = -\sum_{i=1}^{|S|}\sum_{n=1}^{N}(\sum_{m=1}^{m_r}\hat{y}_{m,r}\log y_{m,r} + \sum_{m=1}^{m_f}w_m\hat{y}_{m,f1}\log y_{m,f1} + \sum_{m=1}^{m_f}w_m\hat{y}_{m,f2}\log y_{m,f2}) \tag{2}$$

where N is the length of the input token sequence, $w_m \in \mathbb{R}^{m_f}$ is the weight of the m-th function type. Empirically, we assign different weights to different function types in the loss of entity functions [7, 26]. The overall training objective of JNT_KB adopts the Adam algorithm [31] to optimize the loss and the loss function is used to update model parameters.

4 Experiment

In this section, experimental corpus, hyperparameter setting and experimental results will be introduced.

4.1 Experimental Corpus

Databases such as NCBI[2], PubMed, and UMLS provide researchers with rich and reliable biomedical resources, and API interfaces make these resources easier for developers to use and integrate into their own applications.

BEL corpus is labeled with four entity types: GENE, DISEASE, CHEMICAL and BPRO, and obtains biomedical entity nicknames from some external knowledge base. In order to disambiguate biomedical entities, six namespaces are defined in the BEL corpus, corresponding to six different external knowledge bases, including HGNC[3], MGI[4], EGID[5], GOBP[6], ChEBI[7] and MeSH[8]. We leave the details of external knowledge bases in the appendix.

By linking the namespace to the external knowledge base, we obtain entity information more efficiently and accurately, and reduce the possibility of introducing error information. Moreover, we leave the BEL corpus statistics in the appendix.

4.2 Experimental Setting

Our Method. We take the JNT model proposed by Li et al., 2023 [28] as the benchmark model, which has achieved good performance in BEL extraction task.

We term a variant of JNT_KB in order to explore whether entity names in the external knowledge base contain richer information than entity mentions in the corpus:

(1) JNT_KB using the joint model with the entity full name.
(2) JNT_ENT using the joint model with the entity mention in the original sentence.

Model Hyperparameter Settings. In practice, our model is consistent with the JNT model when setting the super parameters. It can highlight the impact of entity information on the model and is used to ensure the fairness of comparison.

Specifically, the maximum sequence length does not exceed 128 for the model containing 107M parameters, and we set the batch size to 16. For the BEL corpus, we train JNT_KB for 3 epochs with a linear warmup and linear decay learning rate schedule and a peak learning rate of $1e-5$. And the development set ratio is 0.1. Empirically, we set the class weight of function type to $[1, 3]$[9].

---

[2] https://www.ncbi.nlm.nih.gov/.
[3] https://www.genenames.org/.
[4] https://www.informatics.jax.org/.
[5] https://www.ncbi.nlm.nih.gov/Web/Search/entrezfs.html.
[6] http://geneontology.org/.
[7] https://www.ebi.ac.uk/chebi/init.do.
[8] https://www.nlm.nih.gov/mesh/meshhome.html.
[9] The weight is a hyper-parameter manually tuned on the development set.

Evaluation Levels and Stage. The official evaluation defines six evaluation levels: Term, Function, Relation, BEL, Function Secondary and Relation Secondary level for BEL statements. We show the details of the BEL evaluation levels in the appendix. The performance is measured in terms of standard P/R/F1 [26].

We evaluate the BEL statement extraction task on the test set in two stages [28]: Stage 1 and Stage 2, as shown in Table 1. Neither entity type nor entity position is provided in Stage 1, only entity type but no entity position is provided in Stage 2.

Table 1. The evaluation stage.

Evaluation stage	Entity type	Entity position	Operation
Stage1	×	×	We construct entity recognition and alignment as, i.e. Gnormplus [34], tmChem [35] and Dnorm [36]
Stage2	√	×	We find the unaligned entities through dictionary search [37]

4.3 Experimental Result

Stage 2 Performance Comparison. Stage 2 performance comparison aims to demonstrate that integrating entity full name into the model can indeed improve the extraction performance.

We compare the performance among JNT_KB, JNT_ENT and JNT in Stage 2 predicted on the test set. Table 2 lists the performance comparison under the seven evaluation levels.

According to Table 2, we can know that:

(1) In the FD subtasks, according to FS and Func evaluation level, the JNT_KB model improves its performance significantly. Although the precision is reduced, the final harmonic average F1 score is still better than the other two models. It indicates that integrating entity information can effectively improve the recall rate of FD subtasks, and entity information in external knowledge base contain more information affecting FD subtasks than entity mentions.

(2) In relation to RE subtasks, according to RS, Rel and BEL(Rel) evaluation level, the performance improvement of JNT_KB model is smaller than that of FD subtask, but it also improves the recall rate of relation extraction tasks.

(3) JNT_KB model has better performance than the other two models on BEL evaluation level. By analyzing the increase of F1 score from BEL(Rel) to BEL of the three models respectively, JNT increases by 3.6%, JNT_ENT increases by 4.4% and JNT_KB increases by 6.4%. It shows that the integration of entity information can significantly improve the performance of FD subtasks, thus improving the overall performance of BEL statement extraction.

Stage 1 Performance Comparison. Stage 1 performance comparison aims to explore the effect of noisy data on the model without gold entities.

As shown in Table 3, we compare the performance difference between the JNT_KB and JNT models in Stage 1.

Table 2. Performance comparison among JNT, JNT_ENT and JNT_KB in Stage 2, and the standard deviation of F1 score of the five training sessions is shown in parentheses.

Evaluation level	JNT			JNT_ENT			JNT_KB		
	P	R	F1	P	R	F1	P	R	F1
Term	**98.5**	85.7	91.7(±1.03)	98.4	86.2	91.9(±1.97)	**98.5**	**87.0**	**92.4**(±1.34)
FS	**96.2**	27.7	42.9(±3.72)	85.5	45.8	59.5(±5.02)	76.5	**57.3**	**65.4**(±3.09)
Func	**84.2**	29.2	43.2(±5.60)	72.6	47.2	**57.1**(±4.19)	65.1	**50.5**	56.9(±3.12)
RS	**100.0**	89.1	94.2(±0.72)	99.8	**89.6**	**94.4**(±1.30)	**100.0**	89.5	**94.4**(±1.15)
Rel	82.5	66.9	73.8(±1.01)	**84.0**	68.3	75.3(±1.87)	83.2	**71.9**	**77.1**(±1.96)
BEL(Rel)	59.1	47.9	52.9(±0.95)	**60.7**	49.0	54.2(±0.98)	59.1	**50.8**	**54.6**(±1.53)
BEL	62.9	51.3	56.5(±1.09)	65.4	53.1	58.6(±1.93)	**65.7**	**57.0**	**61.0**(±1.53)

Table 3. Performance comparison between JNT and JNT_KB in Stage 1.

Evaluation level	JNT			JNT_KB		
	P	R	F1	P	R	F1
Func	**66.1**	18.4	28.7(±1.8)	49.6	**42.3**	**45.6**(±3.8)
Rel	**50.9**	44.9	**47.6**(±1.2)	43.4	**49.6**	46.3(±0.2)
BEL(Rel)	**34.8**	30.7	**32.6**(±1.4)	29.9	**34.2**	31.8(±0.6)
BEL	**39.6**	35.2	**37.2**(±1.2)	34.4	**39.5**	36.8(±1.0)

(1) At the Func evaluation level, the recall rate of JNT_KB model is significantly higher than that of JNT model, reaching 42.3%, while the precision is low. However, the F1 score of JNT_KB model is 16.9% points higher than that of JNT model. This indicates that the JNT_KB model has certain advantages in the FD subtask.
(2) At the Rel and BEL(Rel) evaluation level, the recall rate performance of JNT_KB model is higher than that of JNT model. However, due to the low precision of JNT_KB model, the final F1 score is 1.3% points lower than JNT model in Rel evaluation level.
(3) In terms of BEL evaluation level, the F1 score of JNT_KB model is 0.4% points lower than that of JNT model. This indicates that the JNT_KB model is more dependent on the entity recognition results and more sensitive to the generated noise, which to some extent affects its performance on the BEL evaluation standard.

Performance Comparison with Other Systems. We compare the performance of the system proposed in this paper with that of other systems.

In order to ensure the consistency of standards, only six official evaluation levels at the BEL level are compared. We compare F1 scores of each evaluation level in Stage 1 and Stage 2 respectively.

From the results shown in Table 4:

(1) In Stage 1, the performance of JNT_KB was slightly lower than that of JNT model. The F1 scores of the two evaluation levels (FS and Func) of JNT_KB at the function level are the highest, and the F1 scores of the two evaluation level (RS and Rel) at the relation level are second or third only to the optimal performance. This indicates that the integration of entity information can still improve the performance of FD in Stage 1, but the final BEL statement extraction performance is slightly lower than that of JNT because it has little impact on relation extraction.

(2) In Stage 2, JNT_KB achieves the current optimal performance at the BEL evaluation level. Although the performance in Term and RS evaluation levels is slightly lower than the current optimal performance, the performance in FS, Func and Rel evaluation levels is far higher than the second-best system performance.

(3) Based on the performance differences between the two subtasks, it is found that JNT_KB system can significantly improve the performance of FD subtask stably, and has relatively little impact on the performance of RE subtask. It shows that more information related to entity function is implied in the external knowledge introduced.

4.4 Discussion and Analysis

In this section, we first conduct studies to explore how entity information in external knowledge base contribute to the performance of FD subtasks. Then we give a analysis on how entity information impact the performance with some examples.

The performance evaluation results of various function types of JNT and JNT_KB in Stage 2 are listed in Table 5.

As shown in Table 5:

(1) The recall rates of all function types in JNT_KB are significantly improved, especially the recall rate of *act* and *complex* types, which account for a large number, far exceeds JNT.

(2) In terms of precision, the precision scores of *act*, *sec* and *tloc* in JNT_KB are lower than JNT, but not to a low value. In addition, the improvement effect of recall rate is obvious, and the overall performance of the final function detection is better than JNT.

An Example Shows Why Recall Rates in FD Subtasks Increase. Take the sentence (SEN-ID: 10005980) "TrkA stimulation up-regulates the expression of the anti-apoptotic Bcl-2 family members, Bcl-2, Bcl-XL, and Bfl-1." for example. In JNT_KB model, we link the entity "TrkA" to the external knowledge base and obtain its full name "neurotrophic receptor tyrosine kinase 1". Almost all kinases in BEL corpus have *act* function, so that JNT_KB can correctly identify the function of the entity.

Table 4. Performance comparison with other systems.

System	Term	FS	Func	RS	Rel	BEL
(a)Stage 1						
BELMiner [20]	62.9	55.4	42.6	73.3	**49.2**	**39.2**
Event-based [22]	34.0	10.0	8.6	41.4	25.1	20.2
BelSmile [23]	45.5	–	13.3	–	28.7	27.8
Att-BiLSTM [26]	58.6	34.3	17.7	62.3	31.6	21.3
SBEL-BERT [27]	59.8	59.6	28.5	72.2	40.4	30.1
JNT [28]	68.4	41.5	28.7	**82.6**	47.6	37.2
JNT_KB	**70.3**	**64.1**	**45.6**	82.4	46.3	36.8
(b)Stage 2						
BELMiner [20]	82.4	56.5	30.0	82.4	65.1	25.6
Event-based [22]	54.3	26.1	20.8	61.5	43.7	35.2
BelSmile [23]	52.7	–	23.7	–	38.6	37.6
Att-BiLSTM [26]	**97.2**	34.8	26.6	**96.5**	65.8	46.9
SBEL-BERT [27]	94.2	63.2	47.9	95.8	74.3	54.8
JNT [28]	91.7	42.9	43.2	94.2	73.8	56.6
JNT_KB	92.4	**65.4**	**56.9**	94.4	**77.1**	**61.0**

Table 5. We compare the performance of the Func evaluation level of JNT and JNT_KB in Stage 2.

Evaluation level	Percentage	JNT			JNT_KB		
		P	R	F1	P	R	F1
act	36.8	**73.5**	21.5	33.2	51.9	**55.6**	53.6
complex	41.4	80.0	6.2	11.4	**100.0**	33.8	50.5
deg	6.9	**100.0**	60.0	75.0	**100.0**	76.0	86.1
pmod	5.7	69.3	33.3	45.0	**88.4**	66.7	75.9
sec	4.6	**100.0**	80.0	88.9	82.4	80.0	81.0
tloc	4.6	**98.2**	40.0	**56.8**	73.1	40.0	51.6
Func	100.0	**84.2**	29.2	43.2	65.1	**50.5**	**56.9**

The Introduction of Entity Information from External Knowledge Base Reduces the Precision of FD Subtasks. Take this sentence (SEN-ID: 10004324) "CTLA4-Ig fusion protein effectively blocked allergen-induced production of IL-5 and IL-13 in bronchial explants from atopic asthmatics." for example. IL5 and IL13 have no function in this sentence. But in the JNT_KB model, they are recognized as having *sec* function.

In BEL corpus, most interleukins have *sec* function, so the full names of IL5 and IL13 in this sentence will mislead JNT_KB.

According to the analysis, adding the external knowledge information provides JNT_KB with rich knowledge information, but it also brings noise to FD subtasks. The experimental results show that JNT_KB benefits more from external knowledge information, thus cancelling out some noise interference.

5   Conclusion

In this paper, we present JNT_KB, a framework for causal relation extraction task to improve the performance of BEL statement extraction via using entity information from external knowledge base. We demonstrate the effectiveness of our method on BEL corpus, including RE and FD subtasks. The experiment results show that JNT_KB outperforms all baselines at the BEL evaluation level in Stage 2, especially in FD subtasks, which means that JNT_KB better expresses the status information of entitys in BEL statements. But, we still discuss here the limitations of the proposed JNT_KB:

Firstly, we don't consider the self-relations in the causal relation extraction, but there is a special relationship between an entity and itself, i.e. 'p(HGNC:CTNNB1, *pmod*(P, S, 37)) increases *deg*(p(HGNC:CTNNB1))'.

Secondly, we need to consider FD subtasks in the few-shot setting, including *deg*, *pmod*, *sec* and *tloc* function types.

Findly, although JNT_KB performs well on the BEL corpus, for the massive biomedical literature, we need more knowledge information to enhance the BEL corpus.

Funding. This research is supported by the National Natural Science Foundation of China [61976147; 2017YFB1002101] and the research grant of The Hong Kong Polytechnic University Projects [#1-W182].

Appendix

A Description for BEL Statement
According to the components of BEL statement, which mainly includes three parts: BEL Term, Function type and Relation type. Next, the three parts are described in detail.

Term. Biomedical entities in BEL statements are represented by BEL terms, which mainly includes two categories. a() represents enrichment degree of proteins, and p() represents cell cycle or disease process.

Function. Table 6 describes the BEL function types involved in this paper.

The *complex* function type may modify one or more BEL terms, where the order of BEL terms does not affect the expression of function information. The *act* function type integrates *cat*, *kin*, *act* and *tscript* to express the functions of entity catalysis and activation.

Table 6. BEL function types

Function type	Abbreviation	Definition	Function example
complexAbundance	*complex*	Represents the enrichment degree of molecular complex of entities or molecular complex of multiple entities mixed	*complex*(p(MGI:Itga8),p(MGI:Itgb1))
proteinModification	*pmod*	Represents covalent modification of a protein	p(MGI:Cav1,*pmod*(P))
degradation	*deg*	Represents the frequency or enrichment of physical degradation	*deg*(a(CHEBI: 'hyaluronic acid'))
translocation	*tloc*	Represents a change of position for an entity	*tloc*(p(MGI:Stk16))
cellSecretion	*sec*	The specific direction of entity position movement is from intracellular to extracellular, i.e. the secretion process	*sec*(p(MGI:Il6))
molecularActivity	*act*	Represents the frequency of events caused by the activity of the protein	*act*(p(MGI:Prkd1))

Relation. The relationship in the BEL statement represents the causal relationship that exists between the subject and the object. We use two causal relationship types: increases and decreases.

"A *increases* B" indicates that an increase in A will cause an increase in B, or a decrease in A will cause a decrease in B. "A *decreases* B" indicates that an increase in A causes a decrease in B, or a decrease in A causes an increase in B.

B BEL Corpus. As shown in Table 7, there are fewer relation types *decreases* than *increases*. It also shows that *act* function type occupies the largest proportion in BEL, far more than *complex* function type which occupies the second place.

C External Knowledge Base. As shown in Table 8, different namespaces correspond to different biomedical knowledge bases.

(1) The HGNC (HUGO Gene Nomenclature Committee) database, which is a basic and authoritative database, provides official and authoritative naming of human genes, so that the physical information is reliable and standard.
(2) MGI (MGI Mouse Genome Informatics) integrates almost all the mouse gene information and provides a relatively perfect description to each gene. For example, the full name of the entity MGI: Hras in the laboratory mouse gene database is "Harvey rat sarcoma virus oncogene," which stands for Harvey rat sarcoma virus oncogene.
(3) EntrezGene IDs is a search engine used by NCBI to syndicate searches of numerous biomedical databases. NCBI numbers different genes, Rnas, and proteins with unique numbers that are EntrezGene numbers.
(4) Gene Ontology Resource is the largest source of gene function information in the world. It is stored in human-readable and machine-readable forms and records the detailed information of each entity, such as entity name, definition, association, etc.
(5) ChEBI collects a large number of chemical entities related to biomedicine, recording in detail the basic information of each chemical entity and the specific chemical structure formula and other rich data.
(6) The MeSH database not only contains the introduction of disease type entities, but also constructs the entity tree structure of the system according to the relevant subject terms.

Table 7. Corpus statistics

Statistics	BEL	
	Training Set	Test Set
Sentence	6353	105
BEL statement	11,066	202
SBEL statement	10,097	223
Relation Type	10,097	203

(*continued*)

Table 7. (*continued*)

Statistics	BEL	
	Training Set	Test Set
increases	7,382	150
decreases	2,715	53
Function Type	7,759	87
act	5,497	32
complex	971	36
tloc	71	4
pmod	832	5
deg	137	6
sec	251	4

Table 8. The correspondence between the external knowledge base and the namespaces, and the number of entities covered in the training set and test set of the BEL corpus.

Knowledge Base	Entity Type	Name-space	Training Set	Test Set
HUGO Gene Nomenclature Committee	GENE	HGNC	12,594	161
MGI Mouse Genome Informatics	GENE	MGI	5,704	146
Entrez Gene IDs	GENE	EGID	139	0
Gene Ontology resource	BPRO	GOBP	1,578	23
Chemicals of Biological Interest	CHEMICAL	CHEBI	779	27
Medical Subject Heading	DISEASE	MESHD	242	11
Total			21,036	368

D Evaluation Levels

The BEL evaluation level is the most important because it is designed to evaluate the performance of complete BEL statement extraction. Table 9 introduces different evaluation levels of BEL statement.

Table 9. BEL statement evaluation levels

Evaluation Levels	Abbreviation	Description
Term	–	Evaluate whether entity names, types, and namespaces are correct in terms of predictions
Function	Func	Evaluate the type of functionality and the correct terminology for it
Function-Secondary	FS	Evaluate whether the type of functionality predicted is correct, regardless of terminology
Relation	Rel	Evaluate whether the master and guest entities in the relation triplet and the relationship type are correct, regardless of the corresponding entity function
Relation-Secondary	RS	Evaluate whether any two elements of the relation triplet are correctly predicted, again regardless of the entity function
BEL Statement	BEL	Evaluate whether the full BEL statement of the prediction is correct
BEL Statement w/o function	BEL(Rel)	Evaluates the correctness of BEL statements generated only from the predicted relation triples (regardless of the function type of the entity)

References

1. Cho, M., Ha, J., Park, C., Park, S.: Combinatorial feature embedding based on CNN and LSTM for biomedical named entity recognition. J. Biomed. Inform. **103**, 103381 (2020). https://doi.org/10.1016/j.jbi.2020.103381
2. Hong, L., Lin, J., Li, S., et al.: A novel machine learning framework for automated biomedical relation extraction from large-scale literature repositories. Nat. Mach. Intell. **2**(6), 347–355 (2020). https://doi.org/10.1038/s42256-020-0189-y
3. Zhao, W., Zhang, J., Yang, J., He, T., Ma, H., Li, Z.: A novel joint biomedical event extraction framework via two-level modeling of documents. Inf. Sci. **550**, 27–40 (2021). https://doi.org/10.1016/j.ins.2020.10.047
4. Akkasi, A., Moens, M.F.: Causal relationship extraction from biomedical text using deep neural models: a comprehensive survey. J. Biomed. Inform. **119**, 103820 (2021). https://doi.org/10.1016/j.jbi.2021.103820
5. Lee, J., et al.: BioBERT: a pre-trained biomedical language representation model for biomedical text mining. Bioinformatics **36**(4), 1234–1240 (2020). https://doi.org/10.1093/bioinformatics/btz682
6. Slater, T., Song, D.: Saved by the bel: ringing in a common language for the life sciences. Drug Discov. World Fall **2012**, 75–80 (2012)
7. Liu, S., Shao, Y., Qian, L., Zhou, G.: Hierarchical sequence labeling for extracting bel statements from biomedical literature. BMC Med. Inform. Decis. Mak. **19**(2), 55–65 (2019). https://doi.org/10.1186/s12911-019-0758-3

8. Perera, N., Dehmer, M., Emmert-Streib, F.: Named entity recognition and relation detection for biomedical information extraction. Front. Cell Dev. Biol. 673 (2020). https://doi.org/10.3389/fcell.2020.00673
9. Li, Q., Li, S., Zhang, X., Xu, W., Han, X.: Programmed magnetic manipulation of vesicles into spatially coded prototissue architectures arrays. Nat. Commun. 11(1), 232 (2020). https://doi.org/10.1038/s41467-019-14141-x
10. Liu, F., Vulić, I., Korhonen, A., Collier, N.: Learning domain-specialised representations for cross-lingual biomedical entity linking. In: Annual Meeting of the Association for Computational Linguistics, pp. 565–574 (2021). abs/2105.14398
11. Sun, C., et al.: Chemical–protein interaction extraction via gaussian probability distribution and external biomedical knowledge. Bioinformatics 36(15), 4323–4330 (2020)
12. Zhao, W., Zhao, Y., Jiang, X., He, T., Liu, F., Li, N.: A novel method for multiple biomedical events extraction with reinforcement learning and knowledge bases. In: 2020 IEEE International Conference on Bioinformatics and Biomedicine (BIBM), IEEE Contribution, pp. 402–407 (2020). https://doi.org/10.1109/bibm49941.2020.9313214
13. Zhao, W., Zhao, Y., Jiang, X., He, T., Liu, F., Li, N.: Efficient multiple biomedical events extraction via reinforcement learning. Bioinformatics 37(13), 1891–1899 (2021). https://doi.org/10.1093/bioinformatics/btab024
14. Li, Z., Lian, Y., Ma, X., Zhang, X., Li, C.: Bio-semantic relation extraction with attention-based external knowledge reinforcement. BMC Bioinform. 21, 1–18 (2020)
15. Chen, Z., He, Z., Liu, X., Bian, J.: Evaluating semantic relations in neural word embeddings with biomedical and general domain knowledge bases. BMC Med. Inform. Decis. Mak. 18, 53–68 (2018). https://doi.org/10.1186/s12911-018-0630-x
16. Fei, H., Ren, Y., Zhang, Y., Ji, D., Liang, X.: Enriching contextualized language model from knowledge graph for biomedical information extraction. Brief. Bioinform. 22(3), bbaa110 (2021)
17. Yuan, J., et al.: Constructing biomedical domain-specific knowledge graph with minimum supervision. Knowl. Inf. Syst. 62, 317–336 (2020). https://doi.org/10.1007/s10115-019-01351-4
18. Zhang, Z., Han, X., Liu, Z., Jiang, X., Sun, M., Liu, Q.: ERNIE: enhanced language representation with informative entities. In: Proceedings of the 57th Annual Meeting of the Association for Computational Linguistics, pp. 1441–1451 (2019)
19. Lai, T., Ji, H., Zhai, C., Tran, Q.H.: Joint biomedical entity and relation extraction with knowledge-enhanced collective inference. In: Joint Conference of the 59th Annual Meeting of the Association for Computational Linguistics and the 11th International Joint Conference on Natural Language Processing, ACL-IJCNLP 2021, pp. 6248–6260. Association for Computational Linguistics (ACL) (2021)
20. Ravikumar, K., Rastegar-Mojarad, M., Liu, H.: BELMiner: adapting a rule-based relation extraction system to extract biological expression language statements from bio-medical literature evidence sentences. Database 2017, baw156 (2017)
21. Ravikumar, K., Wagholikar, K.B., Liu, H.: Towards pathway curation through literature mining–a case study using PharmGKB. In: Biocomputing 2014, pp. 352–363. World Scientific (2014)
22. Choi, M., Liu, H., Baumgartner, W., Zobel, J., Verspoor, K.: Coreference resolution improves extraction of biological expression language statements from texts. Database 2016, baw076 (2016). https://doi.org/10.1093/database/baw076
23. Lai, P.T., Lo, Y.Y., Huang, M.S., Hsiao, Y.C., Tsai, R.T.H.: BelSmile: a biomedical semantic role labeling approach for extracting biological expression language from text. Database 2016, baw064 (2016). https://doi.org/10.1093/database/baw064
24. Tsai, R.T.H., Lai, P.T.: A resource-saving collective approach to biomedical semantic role labeling. BMC Bioinform. 15(1), 1–12 (2014). https://doi.org/10.1186/1471-2105-15-160

25. Chou, W.C., Tsai, R.T.H., Su, Y.S., Ku, W., Sung, T.Y., Hsu, W.L.: A semi-automatic method for annotating a biomedical proposition bank. In: Proceedings of the Workshop on Frontiers in Linguistically Annotated Corpora 2006, pp. 5–12 (2006)
26. Liu, S., Cheng, W., Qian, L., Zhou, G.: Combining relation extraction with function detection for bel statement extraction. Database **2019**, bay133 (2019)
27. Shao, Y., Li, H., Gu, J., Qian, L., Zhou, G.: Extraction of causal relations based on SBEL and BERT model. Database **2021**, baab005 (2021)
28. Li, D., Wu, P., Dong, Y., et al.: Joint learning-based causal relation extraction from biomedical literature. J. Biomed. Inform. **139**, 104318 (2023)
29. Wang, X., Zhang, Y., Ren, X., et al.: Cross-type biomedical named entity recognition with deep multi-task learning. Bioinformatics **35**(10), 1745–1752 (2019). https://doi.org/10.1093/bioinformatics/bty869
30. Geng, Z., Yan, H., Qiu, X., Huang, X.: fastHan: a BERT-based multi-task toolkit for Chinese NLP. In: Annual Meeting of the Association for Computational Linguistics, pp. 99–106 (2021)
31. Kingma, D.P., Ba, J.: Adam: a method for stochastic optimization. In: 3th Inter-national Conference on Learning Representations, ICLR 2021 (2021)
32. Mower, J., Cohen, T., Subramanian, D.: Complementing observational signals with literature-derived distributed representations for post-marketing drug surveillance. Drug Saf. **43**, 67–77 (2020). https://doi.org/10.1007/s40264-019-00872-9
33. Ye, W., Li, B., Xie, R., Sheng, Z., Chen, L., Zhang, S.: Exploiting entity bio tag embeddings and multi-task learning for relation extraction with imbalanced data. Drug Saf. **43**(1), 67–77 (2020)
34. Wei, C.H., Kao, H.Y., Lu, Z., et al.: GNormPlus: an integrative approach for tagging genes, gene families, and protein domains. BioMed Res. Int. **2015** (2015)
35. Leaman, R., Wei, C.H., Lu, Z.: TmChem: a high performance approach for chemical named entity recognition and normalization. J. Cheminform. **7**(1), 1–10 (2015). https://doi.org/10.1186/1758-2946-7-s1-s3
36. Leaman, R., Islamaj Doğan, R., Lu, Z.: Dnorm: disease name normalization with pairwise learning to rank. Bioinformatics **29**(22), 2909–2917 (2013). https://doi.org/10.1093/bioinformatics/btt474
37. Altaweel, M.: The market for heritage: evidence from ebay using natural language processing. Soc. Sci. Comput. Rev. **39**(3), 391–415 (2021). https://doi.org/10.1177/0894439319871015

Biomedical Relation Extraction via Syntax-Enhanced Contrastive Networks

Wei Du[1], Jianyuan Yuan[1], Xiaoxia Liu[2], Hongfei Lin[3], and Yijia Zhang[1(✉)]

[1] School of Information Science and Technology, Dalian Maritime University,
Dalian 116026, Liaoning, China
{duwei,jianyuany,zhangyijia}@dlmu.edu.cn

[2] Department of Neurology and Neurological Sciences, Stanford University,
Stanford, CA 94305, USA
xxliu@stanford.edu

[3] School of Computer Science and Technology, Dalian University of Technology,
Dalian 116024, Liaoning, China
hflin@dlut.edu.cn

Abstract. Extracting biomedical relations from biomedical literature automatically is essential for discovering new biomedical knowledge. However, in the biomedical domain, some texts with different types have semantic similarities, which makes the differences between these types not obvious. Furthermore, lengthy and complex sentences in biomedical literature can impact the model's ability to comprehend the long-range grammatical structure of the text. We propose a contrastive network for extracting biomedical relations that are syntax-enhanced. The model successfully highlights the distinctions between types that are semantically similar by drawing point clusters of the same kind together in the embedding space and pushing clusters of different types farther apart. Meanwhile, this model can enhance the correlation between biomedical entities while increasing the number of positive pairs and making the classification effect between different types more obvious through syntactic enhancement. Compared with other methods, the experimental findings obtained on two publicly accessible biomedical datasets demonstrate that the approach we proposed performs the state-of-the-art.

Keywords: Biomedical Relation Extraction · Contrastive Learning · Biomedical Literature

1 Introduction

With the quick increase of biomedical literature, it has become the main carrier for biomedical relation extraction research. Although there is a lot of biomedical relation in a large number of scientific literature, manual extraction has become a very time-consuming and labor-intensive work. How to automatically, swiftly, and reliably gather and extract relation facts from biological documents is thus a fundamental challenge for researchers in this discipline.

H. Xu et al. (Eds.): CHIP 2023, CCIS 1993, pp. 129–144, 2024.
https://doi.org/10.1007/978-981-99-9864-7_9

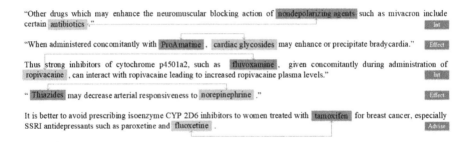

Fig. 1. There are five instances of sentences with labels for the biomedical entities and keywords.

The task of extracting relations in the biomedical domain draws on the advancements made in a range of research fields, including bioinformatics and natural language processing. Understanding the relation between entities in biomedical texts and identifying them is the primary objective of the task. This includes analyzing various types of interactions, such as drug-drug interactions and chemical-protein interactions [24]. In order to build a biochemical knowledge base and uncover novel biomedical information, it is imperative to quickly and effectively extract these interactions.

In biomedical datasets, there exist semantic commonalities among categories. Specifically, in biomedical datasets, the types are different, but the semantics of the text is similar. Meanwhile, the number of labeled instances of some types with semantic similarity is very limited, which leads to a lack of sufficient data for model training. The first two example statements between two biomedical entities have an "enhanced" relation, shown in Fig. 1. This will affect the performance of the model in these two classes. Meanwhile, many biomedical texts are characterized by lengthy and complex sentences that can pose a challenge for models to capture all of the relevant information they contain. For example, the fifth example sentence in Fig. 1 is a long and difficult sentence. The biomedical entities are distributed in two different clauses. This leads to insufficient relevance between the two biomedical entities.

We propose a biomedical relation extraction model based on a syntax-enhanced contrastive network(SECN). The model pulls the point clusters of the same types together in the embedding space. In addition, make the clusters of different types farther away. This makes the similarity between the same types and the difference between different types more obvious.

The positive sample during the training period consists of the original sample and the expanded sample after syntactic enhancement. The model should then be trained to differentiate between both positive and negative specimens. To use label information effectively, we employ comprehensive oversight.

The main contribution of the paper is as outlined below:

– We propose a syntax-enhanced contrastive network for biomedical relation extraction, which effectively narrows the distance between similar relation types and expands the distance between dissimilar types in the embedding space. By enhancing the capacity of the model to discriminate between different types, the proposed approach effectively alleviates the influence of text with similar semantics on the model's predictions.

- The model incorporates deep syntactic dependency information to enhance the relevance between biomedical entities, and further improve the model's ability to comprehend the long-range grammatical structure of the text. Meanwhile, this model can increase the positive logarithm, making the classification effect between different types more obvious.

- We performed experiments on two widely used biomedical datasets. Experimental findings show that when compared to other suggested methods, our method can produce outcomes that are state-of-the-art.

2   Related Work

2.1   Biomedical Relation Extraction

Recent developments in relation extraction tasks have shown promising results from various neural network-based approaches, which are now widely used in biomedical research.

For the purpose of extracting biomedical relations, Liu et al. [12] utilized a convolutional neural network (CNN) model, showcasing its efficiency in delivering excellent performance. In this model, the words in the sentences of the biomedical dataset serve as inputs to the CNN, which can effectively capture local features. Liu et al. [11] introduced a model for biomedical relation extraction tasks, which is the dependency convolutional neural network (DCNN) model. By utilizing the dependency parse tree, the DCNN model can effectively capture the interdependency between words. Masaki et al. [1] applied an attention-based CNN model to biomedical relation extraction tasks. Each word in a biomedical sentence has a varying impact on the final classification outcome in relation extraction.

Recurrent neural networks (RNNs) are used at the word and character levels in the approach put forth by Kavuluru et al. [6] to extract drug interactions. Lim et al. [10] proposed a method using recurrent neural networks to automatically extract drug interactions in the literature. This method decomposes the text into a syntax tree and uses RNN to recursively process the tree structure to extract biomedical interaction relations.

Wang et al. [20] used dependency parsing to model the relation between drugs in text and used the LSTM network to capture contextual information in text sequences. Zhang et al. [25] utilized the shortest dependency path to determine the grammatical relations within a sentence, and extracted keywords located between two entities.

Sun et al. [16] improved biomedical relation extraction by integrating attention and ELMo representations with bidirectional LSTM networks. Zhang et al. [23] proposed a model for extracting CPI that utilized depth context representation and a multi-head attention mechanism.

BERT (Bidirectional Encoder Representation of Transformer) is a pre-training language model. The BERT model was utilized by Peng et al. [15] to study biomedical relation extraction. The development of information extraction research in this area was greatly aided by this paradigm, which made it possible to extract entities and relationships from huge quantities of biological texts. Lee et al. [9] extracted biomedical relations using the BioBERT model. A BERT Att classifier model to extract CPI was suggested by Sun et al. [18]. This approach employs attention mechanisms to direct the extraction of interactions and capsule networks to record the semantic characteristics of those interactions. A classic keyword-based strategy and a grammar-enhanced model were both identified by Liu et al. [13]. The model uses graph-based grammar to build a syntactic tree and type keywords to guide the model to extract specific types of relations.

2.2 Contrastive Learning

An increased emphasis has been placed on the research aspect of natural language processing over the years due to contrastive learning. Chen et al. [2] proposed a method named SIMCLR that incorporates data augmentation techniques to improve contrastive learning. The Momentum Contrast (MoCo) was proposed by He et al. [4]. To improve image representations, Chen et al. [3] used self-supervised contrastive learning. Trinh et al. [19] proposed the Selfie model, which fills in missing parts of masked images using contrast predictive encoding loss by leveraging the masked language model.

The learning process can be enhanced by supervised contrastive learning, which uses the labeled data's existing knowledge and information. Khosla et al. [7] proposed the SupCon method, which extends batch self-supervised contrastive learning to supervised tasks.

3   Methods

3.1   Model Framework

The SECN architecture is depicted in Fig. 2. Three components make up the model: the BioBERT representations module, syntax enhancement module, and contrastive learning module. The sentences in the biomedical dataset are input into the model. We first utilize BioBERT to produce superior context representations for these sequences. Then syntactic dependency graphs and graph convolution neural networks are introduced to enhance the association between biomedical entities. Finally, the expanded representation of the syntactic dependency graph is compared with the original representation to obtain the contrastive loss.

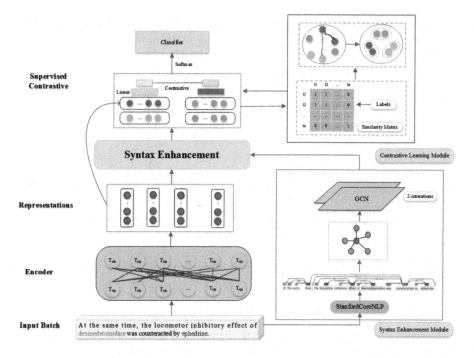

Fig. 2. The architecture of SECN.

3.2   BioBERT Representations Module

Pre-trained models have demonstrated their effectiveness in various NLP tasks, leading to their widespread use in the field. BioBERT has shown excellent performance in biomedical relation extraction compared with BERT model. Therefore, we utilize BioBERT to obtain the distribution of the input data.

We represent the text in the biomedical dataset as $S = \{s_1, s_2, e_1, ..., e_2, s_n\}$. n represents the length of the sequence. e_1 and e_2 are the two entities.

To represent a sentence in the biomedical corpus, the sentence is first tokenized into individual words. An embedding, indicated by the token "[CLS]", is included at the start of a sentence in the biomedical corpus to capture the general significance of the phrase. To signify the presence of entities within a sentence, the paper introduces specific tokens, namely "$" and "#", which are inserted on either side of each entity.

In the context of the biomedical corpus, a sentence S containing two entities e_1 and e_2 can be processed using the BioBERT model. The sentence's output vector representation is denoted as H_c. The entity is represented as a final vector H_c' by an activation function (AF) and a fully connected (FC) layer.

$$H_c' = W_0 \left(\tan h \left(H_c \right) \right) + b_0 \tag{1}$$

where w_0 denotes weight matrices. b_0 denotes bias vectors.

To generate the vector representations of e_1 and e_2, we calculate the averages from H_u to H_v and from H_y to H_z, respectively. The final entity vector representations, denoted as H_{e1} and H_{e2}, are obtained by further processing the averaged vectors through an AF and an FC layer. The mathematical expressions for the computation of the H_{e1} and H_{e2} are as follows:

$$H_{e1} = W_1 \left[\tan h \left(\frac{1}{v - u + 1} \sum_{t=u}^{v} H_t \right) \right] + b_1 \qquad (2)$$

$$H_{e2} = W_2 \left[\tan h \left(\frac{1}{z - y + 1} \sum_{t=y}^{z} H_t \right) \right] + b_2 \qquad (3)$$

where W_1 and W_2 denote weight matrices. b_1 and b_2 denote bias vectors.

The final output of the sentence is represented as:

$$f^s = W_3 \left[\text{concat} \left(H_c^{'}, H_{e1}, H_{e2} \right) \right] + b_3 \qquad (4)$$

3.3   Syntax Enhancement Module

In the model, we introduce a syntactic dependency graph and graph convolution neural network. The utilization of a syntactic dependency graph enables the effective acquisition of syntactic information present within a sentence, and further improves the model's ability to comprehend the long-range grammatical structure of the text.

Graph convolution neural networks can effectively extract topological information from the syntactic dependency graphs and use it to enhance the relevance between the entities. To acquire the syntax dependence metadata of the biomedical text, we first parse the text in the dataset using the StanfordCoreNLP syntax parser. This is followed by a two-dimensional matrix representation of the syntax dependency graph. The horizontal and vertical coordinates correspond to each label in the sentence, and the position corresponding to the two labels with dependent paths is set to the number 1. This means that the two words in the sentence are directly interdependent. Finally, the syntax dependency graph is input into the GCN to obtain the topology information of the syntax dependency graph.

Learn more in-depth topology information through GCN to enhance the relevance between biomedical entities. Meanwhile, the sentence representation after the introduction of the syntactic dependency graph is compared with its semantic representation. After all data augmentation is performed, we obtain 2N samples.

To obtain the adjacency matrix A for a given sentence in a biomedical dataset, we first convert each node dependency A_i of the dependency tree to a numerical index. In addition, we add self-connections to the adjacency matrix by setting $A_{i,i} = 1$ for all nodes i. The adjacency matrix A can be used to capture the structural information of the dependency tree. Analyzing Sentence Structure and

Extracting Useful Information from Biomedical Datasets via graph convolutional network model. After constructing the adjacency matrix, we feed it along with the sentence feature representation into the GCN. The GCN model can learn important features and relations between dependent nodes. The completed result of the final hidden layer is calculated using the following formula:

$$H^{l+1} = \sigma \left(\tilde{D}^{-\frac{1}{2}} \tilde{A} \tilde{D}^{-\frac{1}{2}} H^l W^l \right) \tag{5}$$

where the degree matrix $\tilde{D}$ is present. σ is an activation function.

To extract the syntactic characteristics f^g of a given sentence S from a biomedical dataset, this model employs a double-layer GCN. Its calculation algorithms are as follows:

$$\hat{A} = \tilde{D}^{-\frac{1}{2}} \tilde{A} \tilde{D}^{-\frac{1}{2}} \tag{6}$$

$$f^g = \hat{A} \sigma \left(\hat{A} H_0 W_4 \right) W_5 \tag{7}$$

where W_4 and W_5 denote weight matrices.

3.4 Contrastive Learning Module

The discipline of natural language processing has recently begun to pay increasing attention to contrastive learning. This approach has shown outstanding performance in training deep neural network models without the need for human-labeled data. Contrastive learning methods have emerged as a popular approach for learning effective representations by comparing different samples. The goal is to identify the similarities and differences between similar inputs and dissimilar inputs, which are referred to as positive and negative pairs, respectively.

In this study, we use supervised contrastive learning, which is able to exploit labeled information to obtain more positive examples. By incorporating labeled information, our proposed supervised contrastive learning approach can learn better representations for downstream tasks in natural language processing. We adopt a contrastive loss to optimize the similarity between representations of examples that belong to the same classes while minimizing the similarity between representations of examples from distinct categories. In the embedding space, clusters from different samples are separated by supervised contrastive learning, while samples from the same type are closer together. This makes the similarity between the same types stronger, and the difference between different types is more obvious.

In addition to the input data, supervised contrastive learning also takes into account the class labels associated with the data. This enables the model to learn representations that better capture the similarities and differences between inputs. The contrastive loss function seeks to learn representations of dissimilar samples that are far from each other and those of comparable samples that are close to each other. The following are the calculating formulas:

$$L^{sup} = \sum_{i=1}^{2N} L_i^{sup} \tag{8}$$

$$L_i^{sup} = \frac{-1}{2N_{y_i} - 1} \sum_{j=1}^{2N} l_{i \neq j} l_{y_i = y_j} Log_{i,j}^{sup} \tag{9}$$

$$Log_{i,j}^{sup} = log \frac{\exp\left(\frac{s_{i,j}}{\tau}\right)}{\exp\left(\frac{s_{i,j}}{\tau}\right) + \sum_{k=1}^{2N} l_{i \neq k} \exp\left(\frac{s_{i,k}}{\tau}\right)} \tag{10}$$

where N represents the batch size of the training examples. Between the characteristic representation of the i-th example and the j-th example, $s_{i,j}$ stands for cosine similarity.

In multi-label n-classification tasks, the cross-entropy loss function is calculated for a batch of data by adding the logarithmic loss over all the labels and samples in the batch. The method of calculation is as follows:

$$L_C = \frac{1}{N} \sum_{j=1}^{N} \sum_{c=1}^{n} -y_{j,c} \log \hat{y}_{j,c} \tag{11}$$

where $\hat{y}_{j,c}$ stands for the model's predictions for the class c possibility.

We suggest a combined loss function that encompasses both cross-entropy and contrastive loss to integrate these two loss functions. While maintaining the effectiveness of the cross-entropy loss, the joint loss function's mission is to increase the discriminative capacity of learned representations.

$$L_{CL} = \lambda L_C + (1 - \lambda) L_i^{sup} \tag{12}$$

where λ denotes the trainable parameter.

4   Experiments

4.1   Datasets

For the purpose of assessing the suggested model, our team utilized the DDI extraction 2013 dataset [5] and ChemProt dataset [8]. These datasets are open-source datasets, which are more authoritative and representative.

DDI Extraction 2013 Dataset. Sentences from the biomedical databases MedLine(ML) and DrugBank(DB) are part of the collection known as the DDI corpus. It contains summaries from the MedLine dataset and manually curated text from the DrugBank dataset, providing a wide variety of biomedical text styles for analysis. Information on the quantity of annotated sentences and drug-drug interactions is provided by the corpus statistics, which are displayed in Table 1. The high-quality annotations in this corpus make it a valuable resource for training and evaluating models for DDI extraction.

ChemProt Dataset. The task of CPI extraction involves identifying whether a sentence or document contains a chemical-protein pairing that specifies a CPR (chemical-protein relation) type, and if so, categorizing it into one of six different interaction types. The abstracts of scientific papers often describe interactions between chemical and protein pairings, and correctly identifying these interactions can be critical for drug discovery and development. Table 2 shows the relation types and numbers in the CPI dataset.

4.2   Parameter Settings

The model in this study is implemented using the PyTorch development framework, and the code is implemented using the Python development language. Table 3 shows the specific hyper-parameter settings.

To evaluate the effectiveness of the model we have developed, examine the precision, recall, and micro-F1 results. By combining the contributions from all classes, micro-averaged metrics can be utilized to determine the average metric. When working with datasets that are unbalanced and have a wide range of sample sizes between classes, this method is advantageous.

Table 1. Statistics for the DDI dataset.

Relation	Training set		Test set	
	DB	ML	DB	ML
Advice	818	8	214	7
Mechanism	1257	62	278	24
Effect	1535	152	298	62
Int	178	10	94	2
Negative	22217	1555	4381	401
Total	26005	1787	5265	496

4.3   Experimental Results

DDI2013 and ChemProt test sets were used to assess SECN's performance.

Table 4 displays the comparison outcomes between the suggested model and various baseline methods in the DDI dataset. The comparative findings clearly

Table 2. Statistics for the CPI dataset.

Relation	Training set	Development set	Test set
CPR:3	768	550	665
CPR:4	2251	1094	1661
CPR:5	173	116	195
CPR:6	235	199	293
CPR:9	727	457	644
False	15306	9404	13485
Total	19460	11820	16943

Table 3. The setting of hyperparameters.

Parameter Name	Value
Sentence feature dimension	768
Max sentence length	512
Number of hidden layers of BioBERT	12
Batch size	8
Dropout rate	0.1
Epoch	10
Learning rate	2e−5
Number of hidden layers of GCN	16
Weight decay	5e−4

indicate that our model outperforms each of the competing models. The values of the three evaluation indicators of the proposed model are 83.4%, 81.7%, and 82.5%, respectively. Compared to other models, the performance of the proposed model in Int type and Effect type suggests that our approach effectively alleviates the issue of semantic similarity in DDI texts.

Table 5 shows that the performance on the CPI dataset, and the values of the three evaluation indicators of the proposed model are 78.0%, 79.1%, and 78.6%, respectively, demonstrating that our model performs more effectively compared to the baseline methods. Meanwhile, it is evident that our model significantly improves the classification accuracy of various CPI relation extraction missions.

4.4   Ablation Study

On biomedical datasets, we performed ablation experiments. Table 6 presents the findings from these trials, which sought to ascertain the effect of eliminating each module on model performance.

SECN w/o SE: The model's F1-score decreased by 0.7% and 0.6% in the DDI dataset and CPI dataset, respectively, after the syntactic augmentation had been

Table 4. Performance comparison on the DDI dataset.

Model	F1-score on each type				P	R	F1
	Advice	Mechanism	Effect	Int			
CNN	77.7	70.2	69.3	46.4	75.7	64.7	69.8
DCNN	78.2	70.6	69.9	46.4	77.2	64.4	70.2
ACNN	–	–	–	–	76.3	63.3	69.1
RNN	–	–	–	–	78.6	63.8	72.1
ASDP-LSTM	80.3	74.0	71.8	54.3	74.1	71.8	72.9
ATT-BLSTM	85.1	77.5	76.6	57.7	78.4	76.2	77.3
AGCN	86.2	78.7	74.2	52.6	78.2	75.6	76.9
BERT	–	–	–	–	–	–	78.8
BioBERT	–	–	–	–	79.9	78.1	79.0
Yang et al. [22]	–	–	–	–	78.5	79.7	79.2
R-BioBERT [21]	88.2	84.1	80.9	53.2	81.8	80.7	81.3
EMSI-BERT	86.8	86.6	80.7	56.0	–	–	82.0
Liu et al. [13]	–	–	–	–	83.0	81.1	82.0
Our model	88.7	85.6	81.2	59.4	83.4	81.7	82.5

Table 5. Performance comparison on the CPI dataset.

Model	F1-score on each type					P	R	F1
	CPR:3	CPR:4	CPR:5	CPR:6	CPR:9			
LSTM	–	–	–	–	–	59.1	67.8	63.1
Lu et al. [14]	–	–	–	–	–	65.4	64.8	65.1
Zhang et al. [23]	59.4	71.8	65.7	72.5	50.1	70.6	61.8	65.9
Bi-LSTM	64.7	75.3	68.1	79.3	55.7	67.0	72.0	69.4
Yang et al. [22]	–	–	–	–	–	69.7	69.8	69.7
BERT	–	–	–	–	–	74.5	70.6	72.5
BioBERT	–	–	–	–	–	77.0	75.9	76.5
R-BioBERT	72.5	82.2	78.2	82.3	66.8	77.9	76.9	77.4
Sun et al. [17]	71.5	81.3	70.9	79.9	69.9	77.1	76.1	76.6
BERT-Att-Capsule	72.9	78.6	72.7	77.9	64.4	77.8	71.7	74.7
Our model	72.5	83.2	78.8	86.2	69.3	78.0	79.1	78.6

removed. These results indicate that syntactic enhancement is effective for the performance of SECN.

SECN w/o CL: When we remove supervised contrastive learning from SECN, the F1-score on the DDI dataset and CPI dataset decreases by 0.9% and 0.7%, respectively. These results indicate the crucial role of supervised contrastive learning in enhancing the performance of biomedical relation extraction.

SECN w/o SE w/o CL: When we remove both the syntactic dependency graph and supervised contrastive learning from our model, the F1-score in DDI dataset and CPI dataset drops to 81.3% and 77.4%, respectively.

According to the experimental findings, the syntactic dependency graph and supervised contrastive learning are essential modules of our suggested approach and have a large impact on how effectively biomedical relation extraction performs.

Table 6. Ablation study of the model.

Model	DDI 2013			ChemProt		
	P	R	F1	P	R	F1
Our Model(SECN)	83.4	81.7	82.5	78.0	79.1	78.6
SECN w/o SE	83.3	80.5	81.8	78.9	77.1	78.0
SECN w/o CL	82.9	80.3	81.6	78.3	77.6	77.9
SECN w/o SE w/o CL	81.8	80.7	81.3	77.9	76.9	77.4
BioBERT	79.9	78.1	79.0	77.0	75.9	76.5

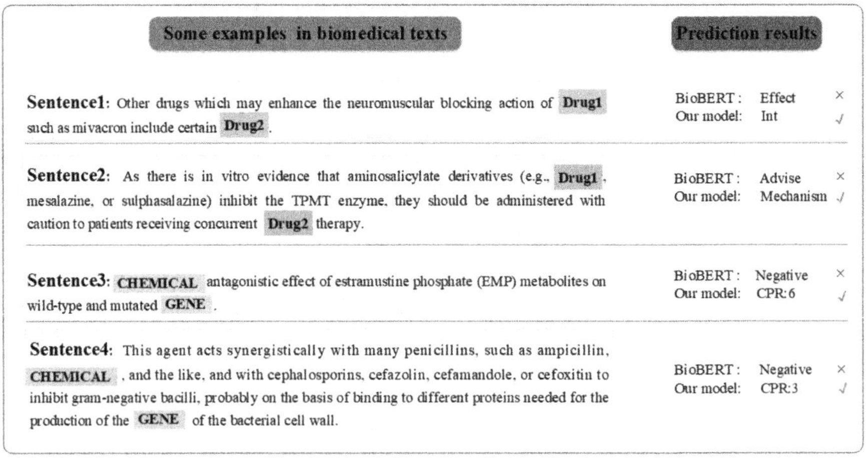

Fig. 3. Four cases predicted by BioBERT and our model.

4.5   Case Study

Comparison research is performed between the prediction outcomes produced by the model we designed and the widely used BioBERT model in order to assess the effectiveness of our approach. We selected four examples, as shown in Fig. 3.

For sentence 1, the BioBERT model made an incorrect prediction because the effect and Int types are semantically similar. In contrast, the distance between instances of the identical category within the embedding space is shortened by the contrastive learning module in our model, while the distance between examples of different categories is increased. Our model makes correct predictions because it can enhance the similarity between classes and the difference between classes.

Sentence 2 is a difficult sample in the DDI dataset. The long text leads to insufficient context connection and relevance between entities. The BioBERT model made the wrong prediction. The model proposed by us can effectively enhance the relevance between entities by adding a syntactic dependency graph and graph neural network, thereby our model makes correct predictions.

For sentence 3, contrastive learning can effectively enhance the difference between the class with few samples and other classes in the embedding space. Our model makes correct predictions.

Sentence 4 is a long and difficult sentence in the CPI dataset. Our model can effectively enhance the correlation between context and entities so it makes correct predictions.

4.6   Visualization

To provide a more intricate analysis of our proposed model, we have generated visualizations of the classification results. These visualizations depict the distribution of different classes and the distances between them.

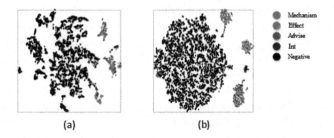

(a)   (b)

Fig. 4. Visualization of labels of DDI dataset. (a) is the classification visualization of the BioBERT model, and (b) is the classification visualization after adding supervised contrastive learning.

As shown in Fig. 4, in the DDI label classification, we observed that the distance between each type is significantly large, indicating that our model is

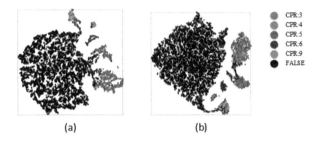

CPR:3
CPR:4
CPR:5
CPR:6
CPR:9
FALSE

(a)   (b)

Fig. 5. Visualization of labels of CPI dataset. (a) is the classification visualization of the BioBERT model, and (b) is the classification visualization after adding supervised contrastive learning.

able to effectively differentiate between different types. Additionally, we noticed that the distance between the same types is relatively small, indicating that our model can accurately cluster similar instances together. Meanwhile, the model can effectively distinguish between Effect type and Int type, indicating that the model in this study can effectively alleviate the problems caused by semantic similarity.

As shown in Fig. 5, in CPI label classification, our model alleviates the situation in which the same type is far away. The aforementioned improvement has a favorable effect on the model's ultimate classification performance. The classification outcomes show that SECN effectively shortens the gap between examples of the precise same type while lengthening it between instances of distinct kinds inside the embedding space.

5   Conclusion

In this study, we introduce a syntax-enhanced contrastive network for the extraction of biomedical interactions. The model we proposed increase the distance between instances of various types and concurrently decrease the distance between instances of identical types by contrastive learning. This approach effectively enhances the discriminative capability of the model. Meanwhile, our model employs syntactic dependencies to enhance the relevance between biomedical entities and improve their precision in the prediction of long and complex biomedical texts. Experiments are conducted on a biomedical dataset, and the results demonstrate that the incorporation of contrastive learning and syntactic information enhancement significantly enhances the performance of the model.

We intend to the continue investigating contrastive learning's potential and experimenting with different data augmentation methods in our subsequent research.

Acknowledgment. This work is supported by grant from the Natural Science Foundation of China (No. 62106034).

References

1. Asada, M., Miwa, M., Sasaki, Y.: Extracting drug-drug interactions with attention CNNs. In: BioNLP 2017, pp. 9–18 (2017)
2. Chen, T., Kornblith, S., Norouzi, M., Hinton, G.: A simple framework for contrastive learning of visual representations. In: International Conference on Machine Learning, pp. 1597–1607. PMLR (2020)
3. Chen, X., He, K.: Exploring simple Siamese representation learning. In: Proceedings of the IEEE/CVF Conference on Computer Vision and Pattern Recognition, pp. 15750–15758 (2021)
4. He, K., Fan, H., Wu, Y., Xie, S., Girshick, R.: Momentum contrast for unsupervised visual representation learning. In: Proceedings of the IEEE/CVF Conference on Computer Vision and Pattern Recognition, pp. 9729–9738 (2020)
5. Herrero-Zazo, M., Segura-Bedmar, I., Martínez, P., Declerck, T.: The DDI corpus: an annotated corpus with pharmacological substances and drug-drug interactions. J. Biomed. Inform. **46**(5), 914–920 (2013)
6. Kavuluru, R., Rios, A., Tran, T.: Extracting drug-drug interactions with word and character-level recurrent neural networks. In: 2017 IEEE International Conference on Healthcare Informatics (ICHI), pp. 5–12. IEEE (2017)
7. Khosla, P., et al.: Supervised contrastive learning. In: Advances in Neural Information Processing Systems, vol. 33, pp. 18661–18673 (2020)
8. Kringelum, J., Kjaerulff, S.K., Brunak, S., Lund, O., Oprea, T.I., Taboureau, O.: ChemProt-3.0: a global chemical biology diseases mapping. Database **2016** (2016)
9. Lee, J., Yoon, W., Kim, S., Kim, D., Kim, S., So, C.H., Kang, J.: BioBERT: a pre-trained biomedical language representation model for biomedical text mining. Bioinformatics **36**(4), 1234–1240 (2020)
10. Lim, S., Lee, K., Kang, J.: Drug drug interaction extraction from the literature using a recursive neural network. PLoS ONE **13**(1), e0190926 (2018)
11. Liu, S., Chen, K., Chen, Q., Tang, B.: Dependency-based convolutional neural network for drug-drug interaction extraction. In: 2016 IEEE International Conference on Bioinformatics and Biomedicine (BIBM), pp. 1074–1080. IEEE (2016)
12. Liu, S., Tang, B., Chen, Q., Wang, X.: Drug-drug interaction extraction via convolutional neural networks. Comput. Math. Methods Med. **2016** (2016)
13. Liu, X., Tan, J., Fan, J., Tan, K., Hu, J., Dong, S.: A syntax-enhanced model based on category keywords for biomedical relation extraction. J. Biomed. Inform. **132**, 104135 (2022)
14. Lu, H., Li, L., He, X., Liu, Y., Zhou, A.: Extracting chemical-protein interactions from biomedical literature via granular attention based recurrent neural networks. Comput. Methods Programs Biomed. **176**, 61–68 (2019)
15. Peng, Y., Yan, S., Lu, Z.: Transfer learning in biomedical natural language processing: an evaluation of BERT and ELMo on ten benchmarking datasets. arXiv preprint arXiv:1906.05474 (2019)
16. Sun, C., et al.: A deep learning approach with deep contextualized word representations for chemical-protein interaction extraction from biomedical literature. IEEE Access **7**, 151034–151046 (2019)
17. Sun, C., et al.: Chemical-protein interaction extraction via Gaussian probability distribution and external biomedical knowledge. Bioinformatics **36**(15), 4323–4330 (2020)
18. Sun, C., Yang, Z., Wang, L., Zhang, Y., Lin, H., Wang, J.: Attention guided capsule networks for chemical-protein interaction extraction. J. Biomed. Inform. **103**, 103392 (2020)

19. Trinh, T.H., Luong, M.T., Le, Q.V.: Selfie: self-supervised pretraining for image embedding. arXiv preprint arXiv:1906.02940 (2019)
20. Wang, W., Yang, X., Yang, C., Guo, X., Zhang, X., Wu, C.: Dependency-based long short term memory network for drug-drug interaction extraction. BMC Bioinform. **18**(16), 99–109 (2017)
21. Wu, S., He, Y.: Enriching pre-trained language model with entity information for relation classification. In: Proceedings of the 28th ACM International Conference on Information and Knowledge Management, pp. 2361–2364 (2019)
22. Yang, C., Deng, J., Chen, X., An, Y.: SPBERE: boosting span-based pipeline biomedical entity and relation extraction via entity information. J. Biomed. Inform. **145**, 104456 (2023)
23. Zhang, Y., Lin, H., Yang, Z., Wang, J., Sun, Y.: Chemical-protein interaction extraction via contextualized word representations and multihead attention. Database **2019** (2019)
24. Zhang, Y., et al.: Neural network-based approaches for biomedical relation classification: a review. J. Biomed. Inform. **99**, 103294 (2019)
25. Zhang, Y., Zheng, W., Lin, H., Wang, J., Yang, Z., Dumontier, M.: Drug-drug interaction extraction via hierarchical RNNs on sequence and shortest dependency paths. Bioinformatics **34**(5), 828–835 (2018)

Entity Fusion Contrastive Inference Network for Biomedical Document Relation Extraction

Huixian Cai[1], Jianyuan Yuan[1], Guoming Sang[1], Zhi Liu[1], Hongfei Lin[2],
and Yijia Zhang[1(✉)]

[1] School of Information Science and Technology, Dalian Maritime University, Dalian 116026,
Liaoning, China
{caihuixian,jianyuany,sangguoming,lzdlmu,zhangyijia}@dlmu.edu.cn
[2] School of Computer Science and Technology, Dalian University of Technology,
Dalian 116024, Liaoning, China
hflin@dlut.edu.cn

Abstract. In recent years, the field of biomedical information has experienced remarkable growth. Consequently, the extraction of semantic relationships between biological entities from unstructured biomedical documents has gained increasing significance. Recent research has often employed sequential or graph models to predict relationships among biological entities in scientific articles. However, these models may not fully harness contextual information, resulting in the absence of entity reference details that can influence relationship judgments. In this paper, we introduce the **EFCI** model: Entity Fusion Contrastive Inference Network. Comprising an Entity Information Exchange Fusion module and a Contrast Enhanced Inference module. This model facilitates the interaction of essential information from the contextual context of both the head and tail entities through the information exchange fusion module. It consolidates this information into a feature matrix and subsequently employs the contrast enhancement inference module to capture implicit dependency relationships between entity pairs. This expansion extends the coverage of relational triples compared to prior studies. Additionally, the model enhances its inference capabilities and effectively addresses the issue of imbalanced label distribution in biomedical literature. Our comprehensive experiments demonstrate significant performance improvements of our model compared to the baseline model, showcasing its competitive advantage across two biomedical datasets: BIORED and CDR.

Keywords: Biomedical literature · Document level relationship extraction · Information exchange fusion · Contrast Enhanced Inference

1 Introduction

The relationships between biomedical entities hold significant importance in advancing the field of biomedical science. In recent years, the maturation of artificial intelligence technology has spurred an increasing number of scholars to concentrate on extracting these relationships. While earlier research primarily centered on extracting entity relationships from individual sentences, the exponential growth of biomedical literature has

H. Xu et al. (Eds.): CHIP 2023, CCIS 1993, pp. 145–163, 2024.
https://doi.org/10.1007/978-981-99-9864-7_10

given rise to a multitude of relationships spanning across multiple sentences. Simple sentence-level relation extraction is no longer adequate to meet the evolving research requirements. Consequently, several studies have broadened their scope to the document level. This approach allows for the extraction of highly valuable biomedical information that can better serve the research community within the biomedical field.

In contrast to sentence-level relationship extraction, extracting biomedical entity relationships at the document level presents several significant challenges. Firstly, entities are distributed extensively throughout the document, spanning various positions. This necessitates capturing complex interactions between entities and the document that extend across sentences. Furthermore, the same entity may appear multiple times within the document in varying contexts, demanding the need for contextual referencing. Lastly, the dataset may display an extremely unbalanced distribution of positive and negative cases. The direct utilization of long-tail data for training may lead to overfitting of head data and underfitting of tail categories.

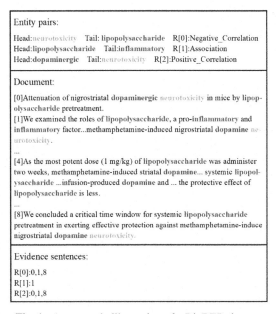

Fig. 1. An example illustration of a BioRED dataset.

In a document, an entity may have multiple references, and the head entity in one entity pair may be the tail entity in another entity, resulting in a relatively large span that poses significant challenges to relation extraction. As exemplified by the mention of "Dopaminergic" in Fig. 1, context references are essential to identify entity relationships. The head entity "Dopaminergic" has several references in the article, and the expressions are not identical, such as "dopamine" across different sentences. They all refer to the same chemical entity Number D004298, which has a positive correlation with the tail entity "Neurotoxicity" (Disease or Phenotypic Feature) as inferred from the context. However, previous studies have not focused on the differential weighting of reference pairs in the target entity pairs, which can lead to different relationships being extracted depending on the importance of reference pairs.

Document-level relationship extraction in the biomedical field remains a formidable challenge, particularly in terms of efficiently acquiring context representation for references to diverse entity pairs while keeping computational costs in check. Given the abundance of specialized terminology within a biomedical article, accurately discerning relationships among these entities demands substantial computational resources, resulting in heightened time complexity. Furthermore, the precise identification and prioritization of relevant contexts for specific entity pairs within an article present a unique challenge compared to sentence-level extraction. The sheer volume of entity pairs for classification, coupled with the intricacies of their associated relation types, compounds the complexity of the task. Existing document-level extraction methods within the biomedical domain often fall short in fully harnessing both local and global information to bolster connections between entities and facilitate the extraction of relationships among biological entities.

To alleviate the existing bottleneck in document-level relationship extraction, we present the EFCI model as a solution. Our approach involves several key components. Firstly, the Entity Information Exchange module is employed to gather essential information from both entity heads and tails. It facilitates comprehensive interactions and generates context representations. Subsequently, the Entity Information Fusion module assigns specific weights to each mentioned entity pair, consolidating the resulting reference pairs into a feature matrix. Thirdly, the feature matrix is fed into our Inference module, which enhances the model's capacity to uncover potential dependencies between entities. This extension goes beyond the existing relational triples, effectively capturing dependencies between entity mentions. Nevertheless, one of the root causes of the long-tail problem lies in the underutilization of label correlations. To address the issue of label imbalance in biomedical documents, we introduce a combination of Focus Loss and Cross-Entropy Loss within our contrastive learning framework. The Focus Loss adapts the weights of various sample categories, thereby enhancing the model's recognition ability for minority categories. Concurrently, the Cross-Entropy Loss aggregates positive examples within the batch, while negative examples extend beyond the batch. This encourages negative examples to make a more significant contribution to the overall loss across the entire training dataset, thereby promoting the learning of long-tail labels.

In this paper, we introduce the EFCI model aimed at bolstering contextual reference information and addressing the issue of missing critical information. To enhance the model's reasoning capabilities, the principal contributions of this paper can be succinctly summarized as follows:

- We propose the Entity Information Exchange Fusion module to obtain the reference representation of the head and tail entities in the document, effectively obtain the reference representation of the context and generate the feature matrix, thus enhancing interpretability.
- We employ the Contrast Enhanced Inference module to efficiently capture the dependency between entity pairs, enhance the relational inference ability, and cover more

relational triples. At the same time, comparative learning is introduced to solve the problem of label imbalance in biomedical data sets.

- Our model outperforms current state-of-the-art relational extraction methods on two open source biological datasets.

2 Related Work

The task of relation extraction (RE) can be divided into sentence-level and document-level based on the granularity. Early approaches of RE focused on single sentences and only attempted to extract entity relationships within each sentence, mainly by identifying relationships between entities through interaction in the input sequence (Zeng et al., 2014; Wang et al., 2016; Ji et al., 2017; Zhang et al., 2017; Guo et al., 2020). Experimental results have shown that this method can effectively address the task of sentence-level RE. However, in real-world scenarios, many relational facts are contained in entity pairs across different sentences in the document, and there are often complex relationships among multiple entities. Wu et al. (2022) introduced contrastive learning into sentence perception in open-domain paragraph retrieval to address the problem of contrastive conflicts.

2.1 Document-Level Relation Extraction (DLRE)

In recent years, research in relation extraction has been extended to the document level. There are two types of models currently being used to address this issue: graph-based and sequence-based models. Graph neural networks are more effective in establishing relationships between entities for document-level relational reasoning compared to traditional CNN and RNN models. The construction of a graph is a key component of these models, and the graph can be categorized into a heterogeneous or homogeneous graph based on whether the types of edges in the graph need to be distinguished. To better capture the characteristics in documents, scholars such as Quirk and Poon (2017) have constructed document-level graphs by using entities as nodes and dependencies as edges. EoG (2019) established various types of edges between different types of nodes to determine the amount of information flowing into the nodes, better fitting the heterogeneous interaction relationship between documents.

Building upon this, Nan et al. (2020) proposed the Latent Structure Refinement (LSR) model, which improves upon the use of hard rules to encode connections between nodes. Instead, LSR automatically learns knowledge through the hidden state of neighboring nodes and captures more non-neighbor information through fully connected states. In January 2021, Tang et al. proposed the Multi-Granularity Heterogeneous Graph (MHG) model to capture complex interactions between entities and enhance the reasoning power of the model. The MHG model defines four node types (mention, entity, sentence, and document) with different granularity and eight types of edges based on heuristic rules. R-GCN with a gating mechanism is used to propagate relational information and reason on the graph, and entity awareness attention is introduced to further aggregate inference information in supporting sentences.

Additionally, building upon the sequence model, Shaw, Uszkoreit, and Vaswani et al. (2018) added an attention bias check at the relative position in the input token.

Wang et al. (2019) adjusted the relative position around the entity, and Xu et al. (2021) further incorporated the dependence relationship between entity pairs in the self-attention mechanism to better guide the model in extracting relevant text. Recognizing the internal semantic dependencies and the complex logical structures of documents, Yang et al. (2021) proposed a document-level entity relation extraction model BSRU-ATTCapsNet, which combines a bidirectional simple recurrent network and capsule network to achieve better results.

The bidirectional simple recurrent network can fuse representations of the relationships between multiple sentences, model the shortest dependent path, assign different weights to relationship features learned from each path through attention mechanisms, optimize the entity relationship representation of the complex logical structure within the document, and improve parallelization efficiency. The capsule network, on the other hand, optimizes learning of entity relationships in terms of spatial and directional relationship representations.

2.2 Contrastive Learning

Although contrastive learning has been widely used in computer vision, its application in biomedical natural language processing, particularly in relation extraction tasks, poses challenges in designing an efficient data augmentation method to construct positive examples. In 2021, Su et al. proposed using contrastive learning as a pre-training step, leveraging linguistic knowledge in selecting text data and an external knowledge base to construct large-scale data for facilitating contrastive learning. To address contrastive conflicts in sentence perception for open-domain paragraph retrieval, Wu et al. (2022) introduced contrastive learning. Similarly, Li et al. (2022) applied unsupervised contrastive learning to phrase representation and topic mining and improved phrase representation on topics by selecting negative samples from cluster-assisted contrast learning, reducing noise in the process.

For the multi-label problem, Zhou et al. (2020) proposed the adaptive threshold loss, which replaces the global threshold with a learnable threshold class. The threshold classes are learned through the adaptive threshold loss, which is a rank-based loss that pushes the logical value of a positive class above the threshold and pushes the logical graph of a negative class below the threshold during model training. This technique eliminates the need for threshold adjustment and also allows the threshold to be adjusted for different entity pairs. By learning adaptive thresholds that depend on entity pairs, the decision errors caused by using global thresholds can be reduced.

Based on ATL (Adaptive Threshold Loss), Tan et al. (2022) proposed the adaptive focus loss (AFL) as an enhancement for long-tail classes. AFL consists of two parts: the positive loss and the negative loss. Unlike the original ATL, where all positive logic is sorted with the SoftMax function, AFL aims to focus more on low-confidence classes, which allows for better optimization of long-tail categories.

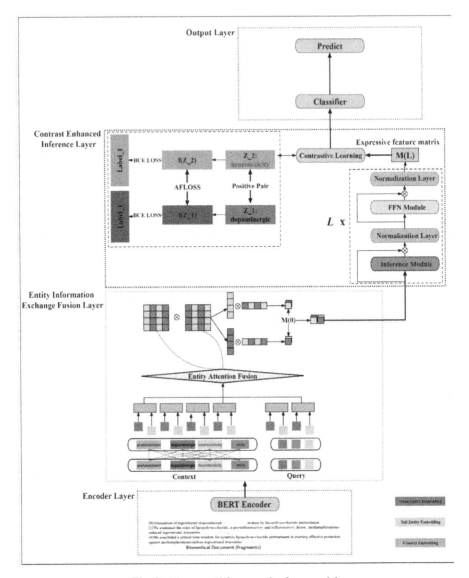

Fig. 2. The overall framework of our model.

3 Methodology

In this section, we will introduce the task definition for document-level relationship extraction in the biomedical field. We will introduce our model from the following four aspects: Encoder Layer; Entity Information Exchange Fusion Layer; Contrast Enhanced Inference Layer; Output Layer. In Fig. 2 a presentation of our model overview is provided.

3.1 Problem Formulation

In this section, we will introduce the relevant formulas of document-level relationship extraction in the biomedical field. Give a document D that contains a set of entities $\{e_i\}_{i=1}^n$, the task aims to extract the relation between entity pairs (e_h, e_t). Where the e_h, e_t is to represent subject and object. An entity may appear multiple times in a document, so there may be multiple pairs of mentions for each entity pair $\{m_j^i\}_{j=1}^{N_{e_i}}$. If there is a relationship between entity pairs (e_h, e_t), it is represented by a reference pair between them.

3.2 Model Architecture

Encoder Layer

For a given document D of length l, we have $D = [x_t]_{t=1}^l$, where x_t is the word at location t. Continuing our previous work on classifying relationships, we use special tags * to mark the mentioned start and end positions. Then the contextual embedding of the document is obtained through the pre-trained language model (PrLM):

$$H = PrLM\left([x_1, ..., x_l]\right) = [h_1, ..., h_l] \tag{1}$$

where $H \in R^{l \times d}$ and d is the hidden dimension of the PrLM.

Entity Information Exchange Fusion Layer

To obtain the reference representation of the context, we use the Entity Information Exchange module to select header and tail mention in the encoder. The reference pairs are then weighted by an integration, which demonstrates that the reference between different pairs of entities has varying effects on them. Both participants are implemented by a single-layer Bert encoder.

Attention Module

According to previous studies (Xu et al.), context information is critical for relational classification tasks, we refer to the context pool method proposed by Zhou et al. (2021) For each mention pairs, we first aggregate the attention output for its mentions by mean pooling:

$$A_h = \sum_{j=1}^{N_{e_i}} (a_{m_h}) \tag{2}$$

where $a_{m_h} \in R^{H \times L}$ is the self-attention weight at the position of mention m_h, H is the number of attention heads, and L is the document length.

Then the context query can be calculated as:

$$Q^{(h,t)} = \sum_{i=1}^{H} (A_h^i \cdot A_t^i) \tag{3}$$

$$C^{(h,t)} = H^T q^{(h,t)} \tag{4}$$

$$G_h = tanh(W_s h_{e_h} + W_c c^{(h,t)}) \tag{5}$$

where $A_h^i \in \mathbf{R}^{H \times L}$ is the aggregated attention output for head entity h, likewise for t. $Q^{(h,t)} \in \mathbf{R}^L$ is the mean-pooled attention weight for entity pair (e_h, e_t) and $\mathbf{H} \in \mathbf{R}^{l \times d}$ is the contextual embedding of the whole document. Then the context vector $C^{(h,t)} \in \mathbf{R}^d$ is fused with the entity representations. And where $G_h \in \mathbf{R}^d$ is the context-enhanced representation of head entity h for entity pair (e_h, e_t). We obtain the object representation G_t in the same manner.

Entity Information Exchange Module
According to the work of Zhou et al. (2021), we use grouped bilinear functions for feature fusion. The mention embedding G_s will be split into k equal-sized groups, such like $G_h = \left[G_h^1, G_h^2, G_h^3, ...G_h^k \right]$, we get the following formula:

$$G_t = \left[G_t^1, G_t^2, G_t^3, ...G_t^k \right] \tag{6}$$

$G_h = \left[G_h^1, G_h^2, G_h^3, ...G_h^k \right]$ is referred to as the representation of the selected header, where $|k|$ is the number of the head entity's mentions. By analogy G_t is the reference representation of the selected tail entity.

Inspired by the attention flow layer of BIDAF model, we use bidirectional attention to model the interaction between query and context, and introduce a mutual attender to obtain the context representation of header and tail references respectively:

$$Head = MultiHeadAttentionLayer[G_h, G_t, G_t] \tag{7}$$

$$Tail = MultiHeadAttentionLayer[G_t, G_h, G_h] \tag{8}$$

The interaction instrument makes the head and tail references sufficiently mutually attentive to produce contextual representations. In fact, the head or tail references are selected from the same distribution, and the head entity in a pair of entities may be the tail entity of another entity, so the above two multi-headed concerns are actually the same, so we use a shared multi-headed concern layer to implement this part. In addition, this setup introduces fewer parameters and thus reduces computational costs.

Entity Information Fusion Module
The merge instrument plays a crucial role in weighing the representations of mention pairs and fusing them together. Specifically, we first construct representations of reference pairs using the representations of the head and tail mentions, along with other relevant features. Let h = Head denote the i-th mention of the head entity; In the same way, t = Tail denote the j-th mention of the tail entity. We define the formula of mention pairs (e_h, e_t) to the representation as:

$$P_{ij} = \left[G_h^k; G_t^k; G_h^k * G_t^k; d_{ij} \right] \tag{9}$$

where $*$ denotes the element-wise multiplication, d_{ij} stands for relative distance embedding referring to pairs. To obtain the relative distance embedding, we first calculate the relative distance between references, and then divide the distance into the interval {1, 2,...} where each interval is assigned a trainable embedding. Overlap feature($h_i * h_j$) and relative distance (d_{ij})

Let $p = (p_{11}, p_{12}, ...)$ be the representation of mentioned pairs. We use merge instrument when referring to representations of pairs:

$$P = MultiHeadAttentionLayer(P, P, P) \tag{10}$$

By utilizing the Merge instrument, each reference pair is assigned a weight based on the self-attention of all reference pairs. This process enables us to identify and highlight the references with the highest weight distribution, allowing for more interpretable predicted results.

Contrast Enhanced Inference Layer

Enhanced Inference

We concatenate the representation of entity pairs into an eigenvector $M^{(0)}$, $M^{(0)} = [P_{h,t}]_{N*N}$ where each row $M_{h,*}^{(0)}$ represents a head entity e_h and each column $M_{*,t}^{(0)}$ represents a tail entity e_t.

Our inference module explores implicit relationships between entities by learning more expressive entity pair representations. The inference module consists of L inference layers and classifiers, each of which contains four components: an inference multi-head self-attention module, an FFN module and two normalizing sublayers. The Inference polycephalic self-attention module is a variant of the traditional polycephalic self-attention module, which is equipped with four attention heads that model each of the four common reasoning patterns and can cover more relational triples. Since all inferential head self-attention modules are calculated in the same way, let's take the first entity pair as an example:

$$F_i^{(l,1)} = W_d\left[M_{h,i}^{(l)}; M_{i,t}^{(l)}\right] + b_d, i = 1, 2, \ldots, N \tag{11}$$

where W_d and b_d are the training parameters, [;] Represents the join operation, and then we get the output matrix $M_{h,t}^{(l,1)}$ for the first entity pair (e_h, e_t):

$$M_{h,t}^{(l,1)} = Attention(Q, K, V), where\ Q = M_{h,t}^{(l)}, K = V = \left[M_{h,t}^{(l)}; F_1^{(l,1)}; \ldots; F_N^{(l,1)}\right] \tag{12}$$

It should be noted that the upper corner of $M_{h,t}^{(l,1)}$ and $F_i^{(l,1)}$ represents the index value of the inference layer, and the lower corner represents the entity index. We then add all the outputs of the bull self-attention module to get the output of the bull self-attention module:

$$\widetilde{M}_{h,t}^{(l)} = LN(M^{(l)} + W_O[M_{h,t}^{(l,1)}; \ldots; M_{h,t}^{(l,4)}] + b_O) \tag{13}$$

where W_O and b_O are model parameters, $LN(\cdot)$ are layer normalized functions.

Finally, the output of the inference layer $l + 1$ is calculated:

$$M^{(l+1)} = LN(\widetilde{M}^{(l)} + FNN\left(\left(\widetilde{M}^{(l)}\right)\right), where\ \widetilde{M}^{(l)} = [\widetilde{M}^{(l)}]_{N*N} \tag{14}$$

After repeating the above process for L times, we can get a more expressive eigenmatrix $M^{(L)}$.

Contrastive Predicting Output Layer
Given that each target entity pair may have multiple mention pairs in a document, we apply a classification scheme based on multiple instances learning to aggregate the predictions of all target mention pairs. To do so, we utilize a multilayer perceptron (MLP) to project the reference pair representation onto the fraction of each relation. Finally, we employ the *LogSumExp* function to consolidate the relational scores from the corresponding mention pairs:

$$m\left(head_i, tail_j\right) = W_f^{(2)} ReLU\left(W_f^{(1)} M_{h,t}^{(l)}\right) + b \tag{15}$$

We use contrastive learning to address the issue of label distribution imbalance. Firstly, our loss consists of two parts, the first part is for positive classes, and the second part is for negative classes. During the training process, the label space is divided into two subsets: the positive class subset P_T and the negative class subset N_T. The positive class subset P_T contains the relations that exist in the entity pair (e^{head}, e^{tail}), and if there is no relation between (e^{head}, e^{tail}), P_T is empty ($P_T=\oslash$). On the other hand, the negative class subset NT contains the relation classes that do not belong to the positive classes, $N_T = R\backslash P_T$. Moreover, we incorporate cross-entropy loss for each positive class, which is computed as follows:

$$P(r_i|e^{head}, e^{tail}) = \frac{exp(l_{r_i}^{(head,tail)}) + exp(g(head, tail))}{exp(l_{r_i}^{(head,tail)}) + exp(l_{TH}^{(head,tail)}) + exp(g(head, tail)} \tag{16}$$

$$P\left(r_{TH}|e^{head}, e^{tail}\right) = \frac{exp(l_{r_{TH}}^{(head,tail)})}{\sum_{r_j \in N_T \cup \{TH\}} exp(l_{r_j}^{(head,tail)})} \tag{17}$$

where the logit of r_i is ranked with the logit of threshold class TH individually.

$$scores\left(e^{head}, e^{tail}\right) = \sum(1 - P(r_i))^{\gamma} log(P(r_i)) log \sum_{1 \leq i,j \leq k} exp\left(g\left(head_i, tail_j\right)\right)$$
$$+ log(P(r_{TH})) \tag{18}$$

4   Experiment

4.1   Datasets

We conducted an evaluation of our model using document-level relational extraction datasets for two benchmark biomedical domains. Additional details can be found in Table 1.

- **BioRED:** (Luo et al. 2022) In a set of 600 PubMed abstracts, the authors pioneered a biomedical Relationship Extraction dataset (BioRED) that includes six conceptual types: genes; Chemical; Disease; A variant; Species; CellLine. It covers eight document-level relationship pairs that are often discussed in the research. Furthermore, each relationship is categorized based on whether it describes new discoveries or previously established background knowledge, which allows automated algorithms to differentiate between novel and existing information. Notably, our work represents the first application of this dataset to the task of document and relationship extraction in the biomedical domain since its publication.

Table 1. The details of the datasets.

Datasets		Docs	Relations	entities	mentions	Relations'	sentences
BIORED	Train	400	9	3.8	304	10.8	11.9
	Dev	100					
	Test	100					
CDR	Train	500	2	7.6	–	11.9	9.7
	Dev	500					
	Test	500					

- **CDR**: (Li et al. 2016) Is a human-annotated chemical disease relationship extraction dataset in the biomedical field. Consists of 1500 PubMed abstracts and divides it into three equally sized collections for training, development, and testing. The task of this dataset is to predict the binary interaction between Chemicals and the concept of Diseases.

4.2   Data Pre-processing

We implemented our model with the PyTorch version of the Huggingface Transformers (Wolf et al., 2019). In the experiment on BIORED and CDR, we use the SciBERT (Beltagy, Lo, and Cohan 2019) model as the document encoder. AdamW (Loshchilov and HutTer, 2019) as an optimizer. Our model was trained on an NVIDIA 3080 GPU with 16 GB of memory. Following the ATLOP model work, we use F1 measures as evaluation metrics for the document-level relation extraction performance. For BIORED and CDR datasets, the training takes 15.4 min and 17.2 min respectively. Table 2 lists some basic hyperparameters.

Table 2. Hyperparameters Setting.

Pretraining model/Dataset	SciBERT/BIORED	SciBERT/CDR
Hyperparameters	Value	Value
Batch Size	4	4
Learning Rate	2e-5	2e−5
Epoch	40	40
Seed	66	66
Document Encoder	BERT	BERT
Max_grad_norm	1.0	1.0
Num_class	9	2

4.3 Main Results

The Results of BIORED Dataset

Table 3 details the main results of the comprehensive experiment of the EFCI model on the BIORED dataset, which was first used in the experiment.

Both the LSR model and the GAIN model are graphical structures based on structural reasoning. The LSR model enhances relational reasoning between sentences by automatically inducing latent document level diagrams; The GAIN model aggregates potential references to the same entity by capturing complex interactions between different references. However, considering only the two-hop relationship, it should be easier to reason, but the experimental results show that the role of the reasoning module is not obvious.

Table 3. The main results in BIORED dataset.

Dataset	BIORED		
Method	P	R	F1
EncAttAgg (Jiang et al., 2020)	70.3	69.4	68.8
LSR (Nan et al., 2020)	–	–	66.3
GAIN (Zeng et al., 2020)	–	–	70.2
SSAN (Xu et al., 2021)	–	–	69.6
ATLOP (Zhou et al., 2020)	71.7	72.3	71.8
DHGCN (Sun et al., 2022)	–	–	77.1
DGI (Wang et al., 2023)	–	–	76.9
Ours	**77.5**	**75.8**	**78.2**

Sequential models such as ATLOP and SSAN encode more global dependency information, especially location-related information, into the model. However, such approaches ignore the complex interactions between different references. Potential references of the same entity contain many entities information, which has important implications for our relational extraction task.

Our model solves these problems well, and the experimental results are better than other methods. Our model is 5.6 above the F1 score of the best baseline (ATLOP) in the BIORED dataset. And the accuracy rate and recall rate are significantly improved. Since we are placing greater emphasis on improving the recall rate of smaller categories, it is possible that the algorithm may become overly focused on predicting those categories, which could result in sacrificing the predictive performance of larger categories, thereby affecting the overall recall rate. Consequently, the improvement in the recall rate may not be substantial.

The results of CDR Dataset
Table 4 details the main results of the integrated experiments of the EFCI model and other models on the CDR dataset, which is superior to other models in previous work.

Our model achieved an F1 score 4.2 points higher than the baseline model (ATLOP) also outperformed other representative models by a significant margin. It's evident that, in comparison to the sequential model, the graph model exhibits improved utilization of context information in biomedical documents. However, it falls short in capturing the intricate relationships between contexts. Our model, on the other hand, places a strong emphasis on interactions between references, enabling more effective learning of CID relationship extraction.

Table 4. The main results in CDR dataset.

Dataset	CDR		
Method	P	R	F1
EncAttAgg (Jiang et al., 2020)	59.9	70.9	64.9
GCNN (Sahu et al., 2019)	52.8	66.0	58.6
EoG (Christopoulou et al., 2019)	62.1	65.2	63.6
SSAN (Xu et al., 2021)	–	–	65.8
MGSN (Liu et al., 2021)	69.0	66.7	67.8
GLRE (Wang et al., 2020)	65.1	72.2	68.5
ATLOP (Zhou et al., 2020)	–	–	69.4
HANN (Zhao et al., 2022)	68.0	69.5	68.8
DHGCN(Sun et al., 2022)	–	–	73.1
SAIS(Xiao et al., 2022)	–	–	74.5
DGI(Wang et al., 2023)	–	–	72.9
REGREx (Dao et al., 2023)	68.8	65.2	66.8
RDDCP(Dong et al., 2023)	–	–	71.6
Ours	**72.8**	**72.5**	**73.7**

4.4 Ablation Study

In this section, to further analyze the EFCI model, we also conducted ablation studies in the datasets BIORED and CDR to illustrate the effectiveness of different modules and mechanisms in EFCI. We show the results of the ablation study in Table 5. First, we explore the impact of the Entity Information Exchange Fusion module on the EFCI model, when this module was removed from the EFCI model, F1 scores dropped by 2.5.

Then Subsequently, we systematically dissected the various components within the Entity Information Exchange Fusion module, meticulously evaluating their impact on the experiment. As we proceeded, we assessed the influence of the Entity Information Exchange module by removing it from the model, resulting in a discernible decrease of 1.7 in the F1 score. Following this, we eliminated the Entity Information Fusion module, leading to a reduction of 1.1 in the F1 score. Further exploration saw the removal of the Contrast Enhanced Inference module, resulting in a substantial drop of 2.1 in the F1 score. Lastly, the removal of the Contrastive Learning module led to a reduction of 0.9 in the F1 score.

Table 5. Ablation Study of the EFCI model in BIORED dataset.

Model	F1
Full Model	78.2
o-Entity Information Exchange Fusion module	75.7
o-Entity Information Exchange	76.5
o-Entity Information Fusion	77.1
o-Contrast Enhanced Inference module	76.1
o-Enhanced Inference	76.4
o-Contrastive learning(AFLoss+BCELoss)	77.3

Nevertheless, during our investigation into the impact of the Enhanced Inference on the model, we observed a noteworthy decline in the model's relationship extraction capability, specifically by 1.8, upon the removal of the module. Interestingly, our inference module exhibits a remarkable proficiency in identifying implicit relationships. However, its performance may not be as strikingly apparent due to the inherent clarity of relationships within the medical dataset. It is conceivable that the module would yield even more impressive results when applied to more versatile, general-purpose datasets.

As we systematically removed specific components from the model, we observed varying degrees of decline in F1 scores. The comprehensive data from our ablation experiments on the CDR dataset are meticulously presented in Table 6. Notably, we discern that the Entity Information Exchange Fusion module's impact surpasses that of the Contrast Enhanced Inference module. This observation may be attributed to the relatively straightforward relationships within the CDR dataset. Our reasoning model encounters challenges in deducing the underlying relationships, thus resulting in less substantial gains. In essence, these experiments underscore the robustness of our model,

Table 6. Ablation Study of the EFCI model in CDR dataset.

Model	F1
Full Model	73.7
-Entity Information Exchange Fusion module	70.9
-Entity Information Exchange	72.1
-Entity Information Fusion	71.4
-Contrast Enhanced Inference module	72.8
-Enhanced Inference	73.0
-Contrastive learning(AFLoss + BCELoss)	72.4

revealing that it excels particularly when dealing with complex semantic relationships. This further solidifies its position as a formidable contender in the realm of extracting biomedical entity relationships.

4.5 Case Study

As shown in the Fig. 3, we select an article from the BIORED dataset for case analysis, there are eight entities (including three categories) distributed in different sentences in the article. Therefore, the task requires the machine to read the entire document to infer the relationship.

Document:
[0]Attenuation of methamphetamine-induced nigrostriatal dopaminergic neurotoxicity in mice by lipopolysaccharide pretreatment.
[1]Immunological activation has been proposed to play a role in methamphetamine-induced dopaminergic terminal damage.
[2]In this study, we examined the roles of lipopolysaccharide, a pro-inflammatory and inflammatory factor, treatment in modulating the methamphetamine-induced nigrostriatal dopamine neurotoxicity.
[3]Lipopolysaccharide pretreatment did not affect the basal body temperature or methamphetamine-elicited hyperthermia three days later.
[4]Such systemic lipopolysaccharide treatment mitigated methamphetamine-induced striatal dopamine and 3,4-dihydroxyphenylacetic acid depletions in a dose-dependent manner.
[5] As the most potent dose (1 mg/kg) of lipopolysaccharide was administered two weeks, one day before or after the methamphetamine dosing regimen, methamphetamine-induced striatal dopamine and 3,4-dihydroxyphenylacetic acid depletions remained unaltered.
[6]Moreover, systemic lipopolysaccharide pretreatment (1 mg/kg) attenuated local methamphetamine infusion-produced dopamine and 3,4-dihydroxyphenylacetic acid depletions in the striatum, indicating that the protective effect of lipopolysaccharide is less likely due to interrupted peripheral distribution or metabolism of methamphetamine.
[7]We concluded a critical time window for systemic lipopolysaccharide pretreatment in exerting effective protection against methamphetamine-induced nigrostriatal dopamine neurotoxicity.

Entity:
A dopaminergic / dopamine(ChemicalEntity)
B inflammatory(DiseaseOrPhenotypicFeature)
C neurotoxicity(DiseaseOrPhenotypicFeature)
D 3,4-dihydroxyphenylacetic acid(ChemicalEntity)
E methamphetamine (ChemicalEntity)
F mice(OrganismTaxon)
G dopaminergic terminal damage(DiseaseOrPhenotypicFeature)
H lipopolysaccharide(ChemicalEntity)

Relation labels:
R0 <lipopolysaccharide,inflammatory> **Association**
R1 <lipopolysaccharide,neurotoxicity> **Negative_Correlation**
R2 <lipopolysaccharide,3,4-dihydroxyphenylacetic acid> **Association**
R3 <lipopolysaccharide,dopaminergic> **Association**
R4 <lipopolysaccharide,methamphetamine> **Negative_Correlation**

Fig. 3. Case study on BIORED test set.

To judge the relationship between entities, it is necessary to combine the context and mention relevant information to enhance the entities. "*dopaminergic*" is a chemical entity, "*dopamine*" is its reference, and "*dopaminergic terminal damage*" is a characteristic of the disease. The baseline model did not correctly predict the relationship between entity "*lipopolysaccharide*" and "*dopaminergic*", misjudged the relationship between "*lipopolysaccharide*" and "*dopaminergic terminal damage*", in fact, there is no relationship. However, our model successfully predicted that the relationship between them is "Association". Mention is extremely important for predicting significant relationships. It can be seen that our model better combines the context, fuses the head and tail entity information at the same time, and correctly assigns high weights to reference pairs.

We conducted a visual analysis of both the baseline model ATLOP and our proposed model to assess the relationship between entity pairs based on attention weights. As shown in the Fig. 4, the attention weight of our model to methamphetamine, 3,4-dihydroxyphenylacetic acid, inflammatory et al. is significantly higher than that of the baseline model. In addition, for the prediction of the relationship between A and B, our model does not assign too much weight, while the baseline model assigns a high weight, believing that this entity pair is strongly correlated, which is different from the real result. This further illustrates the accuracy of our model.

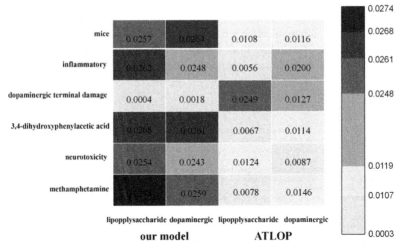

Fig. 4. Compare our model to the baseline model for visual analysis.

5   Conclusion and Future Work

In this research, we introduce a document-level relationship extraction method tailored for biomedical applications. Our approach centers around the development of the EFCI model, which serves to amplify contextual information between entity mentions. The core components of our method involve the utilization of the Entity Information Exchange Fusion module. This module facilitates comprehensive information exchange between the contextual head and tail entities and reference pairs. Subsequently, the fusion module amalgamates this information and refines it to extract the pertinent reference pairs, ultimately constructing the feature matrix. This feature matrix is then channeled into the inference layer, where we employ multi-head attention to unearth latent relationships among biological entities. Finally, we employ contrastive learning to address label imbalance concerns, thereby enhancing the model's performance in long-tail classification. This approach not only bolsters the model's inference capabilities but also enhances its interpretability.

There remains ample room for improvement in our future work. We can extend the application of this method to more specialized and expansive datasets to validate its effectiveness conclusively. Moreover, we must confront the challenge of striking the right balance between recall and precision when handling long-tailed labels. Lastly, we can explore the incorporation of multi-hop reasoning to augment contextual semantic information, which will be the primary focus of our forthcoming research endeavors.

Acknowledgment. This work is supported by grant from the Natural Science Foundation of China (No. 62072070).

References

Zeng, D., Liu, K., Lai, S., Zhou, G., Zhao, J.: Relation classification via convolutional deep neural network. In: Proceedings of COLING 2014, the 25th International Conference on Computational Linguistics: Technical Papers, pp. 2335–2344 (2014)

Wang, L., Cao, Z., de Melo, G., Liu, Z.: Relation classification via multi-level attention CNNs. In: Proceedings of the 54th Annual Meeting of the Association for Computational Linguistics (Volume 1: Long Papers), pp. 1298–1307 (2016)

Ji, Y., Tan, C., Martschat, S., Choi, Y., Smith, N.A. Dynamic entity representations in neural language models. In: Proceedings of the 2017 Conference on Empirical Methods in Natural Language Processing, 1830–1839. Association for Computational Linguistics, Copenhagen (2017). https://doi.org/10.18653/v1/D17-1195, https://www.aclweb.org/anthology/D17-1195

Zhang, Y., Zhong, V., Chen, D., Angeli, D., Manning, C.D.: Position-aware attention and supervised data improve slot filling. In: Proceedings of the 2017 Conference on Empirical Methods in Natural Language Processing, pp. 35–45 (2017)

Guo, Z., Nan, G., Lu, W., Cohen, S.B.: Learning latent forests for medical relation extraction. In: Proceedings of IJCAI (2020)

Quirk, C., Poon, H.: Distant supervision for relation extraction beyond the sentence boundary. In: Proceedings of the 15th Conference of the European Chapter of the Association for Computational Linguistics: Volume 1, Long Papers, pp. 1171–1182 (2017)

Nan, G., Guo, Z., Sekulic, I., Lu, W.: Reasoning with latent structure refinement for document-level relation extraction. In: Proceedings of the 58th Annual Meeting of the Association for Computational Linguistics, pp. 1546–1557 (2020)

Shaw, P., Uszkoreit, J., Vaswani, A.: Self-attention with relative position representations. In: Proceedings of the 2018 Conference of the North American Chapter of the Association for Computational Linguistics: Human Language Technologies, Volume 2 (Short Papers), pp. 464–468. Association for Computational Linguistics, New Orleans (2018). https://doi.org/10.18653/v1/N18-2074, https://www.aclweb.org/anthology/N18-2074

Wang, H., et al.: Extracting multiple-relations in one-pass with pre-trained transformers. In: Proceedings of the 57th Annual Meeting of the Association for Computational Linguistics, pp. 1371–1377. Association for Computational Linguistics, Florence (2019b). https://doi.org/10.18653/v1/P19-1132, https://www.aclweb.org/anthology/P19-1132

Xu, B., Wang, Q., Lyu, Y., Zhu, Y., Mao, Z.: Entity structure within and throughout: modeling mention dependencies for document-level relation extraction. In: Thirty-Fifth AAAI Conference on Artificial Intelligence, AAAI 2021, Thirty-Third Conference on Innovative Applications of Artificial Intelligence, IAAI 2021, The Eleventh Symposium on Educational Advances in Artificial Intelligence, EAAI 2021, Virtual Event, 2–9 February 2021, pp. 14149–14157. AAAI Press (2021a)

Zhou, W., Huang, K., Ma, T., Huang, J.: Document-level relation extraction with adaptive thresholding and localized context pooling. In: Proceedings of AAAI (2021)

Luo, L., Lai, P.-T., Wei, C.-H., Arighi, C.N., Lu, Z.: BioRED: a rich biomedical relation extraction dataset. Brief. Bioinform. (2022). https://doi.org/10.1093/bib/bbac282

Li, J., et al.: BioCreative V CDR task corpus: A resource for chemical disease relation extraction. Database **2016**, baw068 (2016)

Wolf, T., et al.: Hugging face's transformers: state-of-the-art natural language processing. ArXiv arXiv-1910 (2016)

Beltagy, I., Lo, K., Cohan, A.: SciBERT: a pre-trained language model for scientific text. In: EMNLP-IJCNLP (2019)

Loshchilov, I., Hutter, F.: Decoupled weight decay regularization. In: ICLR (2019)

Jiang, P., Mao, X.L., Bian, B., Huang, H.: Improving document-level relation extraction via contextualizing mention representations and weighting mention pairs. In: 2020 IEEE International Conference on Knowledge Graph (ICKG), pp. 305–312. IEEE (2020)

Zeng, S., Xu, R., Chang, B., Li, L.: Double graph based reasoning for document-level relation extraction. In: Proceedings of the 2020 Conference on Empirical Methods in Natural Language Processing, EMNLP, pp.1630–1640 (2020)

Gu, J., Sun, F., Qian, L., Zhou, G.: Chemical-induced disease relation extraction via convolutional neural network. Database **2017**, bax024 (2017)

Nguyen, D.Q., Verspoor, K.: Convolutional neural networks for chemical-disease relation extraction are improved with character-based word embeddings. In: Proceedings of the BioNLP 2018 Workshop, pp. 129–136 (2018)

Verga, P., Strubell, E., McCallum, A.: Simultaneously self-attending to all mentions for full-abstract biological relation extraction. In: Proceedings of the 2018 Conference of the North American Chapter of the Association for Computational Linguistics: Human Language Technologies, Volume 1 (Long Papers), pp. 872–884 (2018)

Sahu, S.K., Christopoulou, F., Miwa, M., Ananiadou, S.: Inter-sentence relation extraction with document-level graph convolutional neural network. In: Proceedings of the 57th Annual Meeting of the Association for Computational Linguistics, pp. 4309–4316 (2019)

Liu, X., Tan, K., Dong, S.: Multi-granularity sequential neural network for document-level biomedical relation extraction. Inf. Process. Manage. (2021). https://doi.org/10.1016/j.ipm.2021.102718

Tan, Q., He, R., Bing, L., Ng, H.T.: Document-level relation extraction with adaptive focal loss and knowledge distillation. In: ACL (Findings) 2022, pp. 1672–1681 (2022). https://doi.org/10.18653/v1/2022.findings-acl.132, https://aclanthology.org/2022.findings-acl.132

Improving BERT Model Using Contrastive Learning for Biomedical Relation Extraction. https://aclanthology.org/2021.bionlp-1.1

Sentence-aware Contrastive Learning for Open-Domain Passage Retrieval. https://aclanthology.org/2022.acl-long.76

UCTopic: Unsupervised Contrastive Learning for Phrase Representations and Topic Mining. https://aclanthology.org/2022.acl-long.426

Sun, Q., et al.: Dual-channel and hierarchical graph convolutional networks for document-level relation extraction. Expert Syst. Appl. **205**, 117678 (2022). https://doi.org/10.1016/j.eswa. 2022.117678. ISSN 0957-4174

Xiao, Y., Zhang, Z., Mao, Y., Yang, C., Han, J.: SAIS: supervising and augmenting intermediate steps for document-level relation extraction. In: Proceedings of the 2022 Conference of the North American Chapter of the Association for Computational Linguistics: Human Language Technologies, pp. 2395–2409. Association for Computational Linguistics, Seattle (2022)

Wang, H., Qin, K., Duan, G., Luo, G.: Denoising graph inference network for document-level relation extraction. Big Data Min. Anal. **6**(2), 248–262 (2023). https://doi.org/10.26599/BDMA. 2022.9020051

Pham Thi, Q.T., Dao, Q.H., Nguyen, A.D., et al.: Document-level chemical-induced disease semantic relation extraction using bidirectional long short-term memory on dependency graph. Int. J. Comput. Intell. Syst. **16**, 131 (2023). https://doi.org/10.1007/s44196-023-00305-7

Dong, Y., Xu, X.: Relational distance and document-level contrastive pre-training based relation extraction model. Pattern Recognit. Lett. **167**, 132–140 (2023). https://doi.org/10.1016/j.pat rec.2023.02.012. ISSN 0167-8655

Zhao, W., Zhang, J., Yang, J., Jiang, X., He, T.: Document-level chemical-induced disease relation extraction via hierarchical representation learning. IEEE/ACM Trans. Comput. Biol. Bioinf. **19**(5), 2782–2793 (2022). https://doi.org/10.1109/TCBB.2021.3086090

Chapter-Level Stepwise Temporal Relation Extraction Based on Event Information for Chinese Clinical Medical Texts

Wenjun Xiang(ID), Zhichang Zhang(✉)(ID), Ziqin Zhang(ID), and Deyue Yin(ID)

College of Computer Science and Engineering, Northwest Normal University,
Lanzhou, China
zzc@nwnu.edu.cn

Abstract. Temporal relation extraction of medical events for Chinese clinical medical texts is an important natural language processing task, which is the basis of many intelligent researches in the medical field. Most of the existing studies on temporal relation extraction remains at sentence-level tasks, however, the rich medical information and large number of specialized vocabularies in Chinese clinical medical texts lead to the fact that short clinical medical texts often contain a much larger number of medical events than conventional texts, and these events show complex inter-sentence relations. The global consistency of sentence-level temporal relation extraction results is difficult to guarantee and cannot meet the information extraction needs for clinical medical texts. Therefore, it is necessary to advance the temporal relation extraction task for medical texts from the sentence level to the chapter level. In this regard, we propose a simple and effective stepwise temporal relation extraction method. Based on the event information and the unique rules of temporal relations in medical text, the model design splits the chapter-level temporal relation extraction task into three steps, which not only can avoid the possible contradictory errors in the process of temporal relation extraction, but also can minimize the generation of redundant information to alleviate the interference of the task. Experiments show that this method can achieve better performance than the current mainstream temporal relation extraction methods.

Keywords: Natural language processing · Temporal relation extraction · Chinese clinical medical texts · Chapter level tasks

Supported by the National Natural Science Foundation of China (No. 62163033), the Talent Innovation and Entrepreneurship Project of Lanzhou, China (No. 2021-RC-49), the Natural Science Foundation of Gansu Province, China (No. 22JR5RA145, No. 21JR7RA781, No. 21JR7RA116), the Major Research Project Incubation Program of Northwest Normal University, China (No. NWNU-LKZD2021-06).

H. Xu et al. (Eds.): CHIP 2023, CCIS 1993, pp. 164–181, 2024.
https://doi.org/10.1007/978-981-99-9864-7_11

1   Introduction

Chinese clinical medical texts are key information resources for the written record of a patient's clinical case, which are not only crucial for documenting the patient's condition, but also play an important role in medical research and education [1]. However, these texts are usually written in natural language and need to be organized into structured information in order to extract the clinical medical events and relations within them [2–4]. This not only helps healthcare workers to retrieve relevant case reports more easily, but also helps to build a complete body of medical knowledge to support the handling of issues such as large global health crises.An example of a chapter-level temporal relation extraction task for a Chinese clinical medical text is shown in Fig. 1.

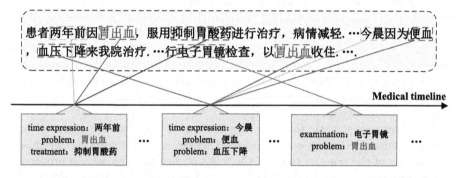

Fig. 1. Given a Chinese clinical medical text (Which means "The patient was treated with acid-suppressing medication two years ago for gastric hemorrhage, and his symptoms subsided... This morning, he came to our hospital because of blood in his stools and a drop in blood pressure, and was admitted with gastric hemorrhage after having an electronic gastroscope ..."). The text consists of multiple sentences containing a series of patient-related medical events in different temporal contexts.The dotted boxes of different colors in the figure are medical events of different event types in the text, such as "problem" events in the red box, "treatment" events in the green box, "examination" events in the blue box, and "time expression" events in the yellow box(The "time expression" type of event is a special type of event that can be subdivided into nine time expression types, as described in Sect. 4.1). "These medical events will be distributed on the timeline in a first-to-last order of occurrence based on their temporal relation to each other. In the figure below the medical timeline, the events and time expressions belonging to the same box have an "equal" temporal relation, which means that the related medical events occurred within the same time frame.Our goal is to construct a timeline of medical events without temporal conflicts for each medical text through a greedy check-and-add process. (Color figure online)

In terms of chapter-level temporal relation extraction task, by studying a large number of Chinese clinical medical texts, we found that there are important differences between the temporal relation extraction task between medical events and the common relation extraction task. In Chinese clinical medical texts, the same event expressions in different sentences do not necessarily refer to the same event. For example, in Fig. 1, there are two "problem" events expressed as "gastric hemorrhage", but these two "gastric hemorrhages" are distributed in different locations on the medical timeline, which means that they occurred at different times and and are different events with the same mention. To address this finding, we stipulated that each event in the medical text be treated as unique and independent, and extracted the temporal relations between them to construct a timeline of the patient's medical care.

2   Related Work

The task of temporal relation extraction has existed for a long time, and early research used traditional machine learning methods [5–10], as well as neural network-based approaches [11–14] to solve this problem. There are also some approaches that attempt to formulate this task as a structured prediction problem to model the temporal dependencies of events [15–17]. However, these approaches either require complex feature engineering or ignore the dependencies between temporal relations in documents, and most of them focus on extracting intra-sentence relations [18–22], which cannot effectively deal with inter-sentence relations in texts with long paragraphs.

In recent years, with the wide application of Chinese electronic medical records, temporal relation extraction for Chinese medical events has gradually become one of the popular tasks in the fields of medical information processing and natural language processing in China. A Chinese clinical medical text usually contains multiple medical events, which exhibit complex inter-sentence relations. Therefore, temporal relation extraction for medical texts focuses on chapter-level tasks. Unlike the intra-sentence relation extraction task, the chapter-level task needs to focus on the information of the whole text, which is a very challenging and difficult task.

For chapter-level relational extraction tasks, related research has focused on the overlap problem of relation triples and the interference of co-referential mentions of entities on the task. As a result, many previous researchers have centered on solving these two problems to improve chapter-level relationship classification For example, some researchers have used edge-oriented graph neural models that combine different types of nodes and edges to create chapter-level graphs, modeling the co-referential mention information of entities and dealing with the overlapping triples problem [23]. While some other researchers constructed two graphs in the model, one at the mention level and the other at the entity level, which are capable of aggregating text-aware contextual information and inferring logical relationships between texts for better extraction of chapter-level relations [24]. Other researchers have incorporated unique dependencies between co-referential mentions into the standard self-attention mechanism and throughout the encoding phase, utilizing entity structure to enhance inference of chapter-level relations [25]. As for the chapter-level temporal relation extraction task, we have learned through the example in Fig. 1 that we cannot simply rely on identical mentions of events to enhance event information. Doing so not only adds nothing to this task, but also causes loss of information and confusion, bringing noise to the model.

Dealing with temporal information in clinical medical texts has always been a challenging field. Past studies have attempted to construct medical timelines, and have even proposed the bright idea of integrating medical knowledge into temporal reasoning systems [26]. Clinical medical texts are linguistically concise and, despite their short length, contain a huge number of medical events and a correspondingly inflated number of relation triples. Therefore, the traditional temporal relation extraction method is computationally expensive. At the same time, according to the properties of temporal relations such as transmissibility and self-reversibility, a considerable portion of temporal relations can be inferred from the temporal relations related to them, so the extraction process of traditional methods produces a large amount of redundant information, which interferes with the training of the model. To solve this problem, this paper proposes an innovative step-by-step temporal relation extraction model, which can process the events in the text in batches through time intervals divided by time expressions, which not only effectively reduces the number of pairs of temporal relation events that need to be categorized, and at the same time excludes the redundant triples that do not help the construction of the timeline, but also distinguishes between different events of the same mention by the natural barriers of the time intervals and effectively reduces the likelihood of confusions or contradictions.

In conclusion, this paper proposes a stepwise temporal relation extraction method based on the characteristics of Chinese medical texts to address the main difficulties of the chapter-level temporal relation extraction task. This approach is an important inspiration in solving the temporal relation extraction problem in chapter-level Chinese clinical medical texts.

3   Method

This chapter describes the task description and the definition of our model in turn. Figure 2 illustrates our model and we will describe the different components of the model in detail in the following sections.

3.1   Task Description

Given a medical text D, consisting of n characters, ($D = \{c_i\}_{i=1}^n$. The text contains p medical events(the set of events is denoted as: $E = \{e_i\}_{i=1}^p$), and q time expressions(the set of time expressions is denoted as: $T = \{t_i\}_{i=1}^q$). The task of this paper aims to extract the temporal relations between the events and time expressions contained in medical text D in order to construct a patient-related medical timeline. The model needs to obtain a set of relations denoted as $A(A = \{R_{(e-e)} \cup R_{(e-t)} \cup R_{(t-t)}\})$, which includes the temporal relations between events in the text $R_{(e-e)}$, the temporal relations between events and time expressions $R_{(e-t)}$, and the temporal relations between time expressions $R_{(t-t)}$. In the definition,R denotes the predefined set of temporal relation types (R = { "After", "Before", "Equal", "Vague" }).

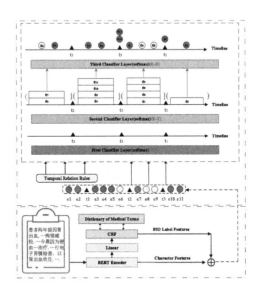

Fig. 2. A Chinese clinical medical text is fed into the model. First, the text is processed by BERT coding layer and linear layer to get the embedding vector of each token. Then, the text is processed through linear and conditional random field layers to get the named entity recognition labels of the text. Then, the model splices the token embedding vectors with the label embedding vectors to get the final representation of the event. The event representation is fed into the stepwise temporal relation classification module together with the temporal relation rule features for temporal relation classification. Eventually, the full text temporal relations obtained from the model are used to construct a chapter-level medical timeline. The triangular patterns in the figure represent the time expressions in the text, while the circular patterns of different colors represent the different types of medical events in the text.

3.2   Temporal Relation Feature Construction

Encoder. We first encode the whole text by feeding it into a pre-trained language model, BERT [27]. The emergence of BERT has greatly advanced the development of sentence-level, inter-sentence-level, and token-level tasks. Instead of relying on recurrent neural networks, it uses a transformer architecture to better capture long-distance dependencies, and is able to make predictions that go beyond natural sentence boundaries, as it is typically trained on continuous text fragments spanning multiple sentences. We chose BERT over other transformer-based models because it takes bi-directionality into account during training, a feature that we hypothesize is important for effectively capturing temporal relation interactions of events. Using BERT without the additional task of capturing information about the order of events in the text would significantly reduce model complexity. In addition, the length of our chapter-level medical text corpus is much smaller than the length of real document-level medical text, satisfying the input length limit of BERT, which is a prerequisite for us to be able to use BERT for coding in order to obtain decent performance.

In Fig. 2, our model feeds the entire medical text $D = \{c_1, c_2, ..., c_n\}$ into the BERT encoder to obtain an encoded representation of each token: $H = BERT(c_1, c_2, ..., c_n) = \{h_{cls}, h_1, h_2, ..., h_n, h_{sep}\}$, $H \in R^{l \times d}$, where l denotes the layer width, i.e., the sentence length (including the two special start and end tokens of [CLS] and [SEP]), and d denotes the hidden layer dimension of BERT. Next, with one linear layer, we obtain the label prediction vector matrix W for each token:

$$W = \lambda(w_{ner}H + b_{ner}) \tag{1}$$

where, $W \in R^{l \times m}, w_{ner} \in R^{d \times m}, b_{ner} \in R^m$, m is the number of BIO labels, m = 27, w_{ner} and b_{ner} are the learnable weight matrix and bias of the linear layer, and λ is the activation function.

After the BERT and Linear layers, we employ Conditional Random Fields (CRF) [28] to obtain the most likely BIO labels in the token sequence. We define the entity recognition task as a sequence labeling problem, referring to previous research on named entity recognition [29,30], and adopt the BIO (Beginning, Inside, Outside) encoding scheme. Since each event or time expression consists of multiple consecutive tokens in a sentence, we need to assign a tag to each token in the sentence. In this way, we can identify the start and end positions of events and time expressions, as well as their types (e.g., B_problem). With the CRF layer, we end up with a sequence of labels for the entire text token. To learn the BIO labels for each token, we compute the cross-entropy loss function L_{ner}:

$$L_{ner} = -\sum_{i=1}^{n} \log P(H'|H, \theta) \tag{2}$$

In order to improve the accuracy of the named entity recognition part of the model, we combined the relevant information in the medical field and the annotation results of medical events in our dataset, and compiled a dictionary of medical terms, which is used to correct the model for any errors or incomplete recognition that may occur when recognizing the medical events, in order to improve the accuracy of the model.

In addition, we believe that the type information of the events will be helpful for the task of extracting the temporal relations among the events. Therefore, we splice the context embedding vectors obtained through BERT encoding with the embedding vectors of the corresponding BIO label sequences to obtain the final representation of each token: $H' = \{h_{cls}', h_1', h_2', ..., h_n', h_{sep}'\}$, $H' \in R^{l \times d}$.

Event and time expressions in text usually consist of multiple consecutive characters. We use the method of averaging character sequence vectors to obtain the final representation of them. Assume that event ei consists of the ath token to the bth token and time expression tj consists of the cth token to the dth token. Then, event ei and time expression tj are represented as:

$$h_{ei} = \frac{1}{b-a+1} \sum_{i=a}^{b} h_i{}' \tag{3}$$

$$h_{tj} = \frac{1}{d-c+1} \sum_{i=c}^{d} h_i{}' \tag{4}$$

Temporal Relation Rules of Medical Event. By reading a large number of Chinese clinical medical texts and combining the annotation experience of Chinese medical event temporal relation datasets, we summarize four temporal relation rule features of medical event in Chinese medical texts, as shown below:

(1) Event type rule: Event type refers to the type of event. Statistically, we found that in our experimental corpus, when two events have the same type of event type, the probability that the temporal relation between them is "Equal" is around 50%, and the proportion of "Equal" relation between "examination" events even reaches 69%, far exceeding the proportion of the other three temporal relations. Therefore, if the first and last events of the temporal relation to be extracted have the same event type, it is specified that the feature value will be taken as 1, otherwise the feature value will be taken as 0.

(2) Event distance rule: Event distance refers to the relative distance between two events in the text, i.e., how many characters are separated between them. We believe that the relative distance between two events can help us better determine the temporal relation between them. Statistically, in our experimental corpus, the proportion of two events with the number of characters between them in the interval of [0,10] whose temporal relation is "Equal" reaches 50%. Therefore, if the number of characters separating the events of the temporal relation to be extracted is within this interval, it is specified that the feature value will be taken as 1, otherwise the feature value will be taken as 0.

(3) Medical event combination rule: There is a unique pattern of temporal relationships between different types of medical events in medical text. For example, we observed that patient-related events in the category of "problem" mostly preceded events in the category of "treatment". In our experimental corpus, two-by-two combinations involving 13 types of events yielded a total of 169 different event combinations. We counted the percentage of these event combinations with the temporal relation "Before", and the results are shown in Fig. 3. In the figure, the darker color indicates that the temporal relation of these event combinations tends to be "Before". We select the event combinations with the proportion of "Before" relation

greater than or equal to 55%, and if the head and tail events of the temporal relation to be extracted meet any of these combinations, We define this feature value to be 1; otherwise the feature value is taken to be 0. It is worth noting that the temporal relation is self-reversing, i.e., if R(A, B) = Before, then R(B, A) = After; therefore, we take the feature value of this item to be 1 if the event categories of the head and tail events of the temporal relation to be extracted correspond to one of these opposing combinations; otherwise the value of the feature is taken to be 0. Above, the rule of medical event combination needs to be captured using two feature values.

(4) Writing order rule: The writing order of events refers to the order in which the events appear in the text. Chinese medical texts usually follow the human writing habit of recording events in the objective order of their development. Therefore, in most cases, events written earlier in a medical text tend to occur earlier. Statistically, in our experimental corpus, the proportion of event pairs in which the head event appears earlier than the tail event in the text and whose temporal relation is "Before" reaches 60%. Therefore, if the head event of the event pairs to be extracted has appeared earlier than the tail event in the text, it is stipulated that the feature value will be taken as 1, otherwise the feature value will be taken as 0.

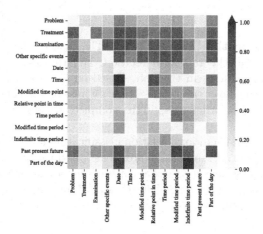

Fig. 3. Temporal relation statistics for various combinations of events

For any pair of events (e_i, e_j), extract their temporal relation rule feature vector (a five-dimensional vector) and get the temporal relation rule feature embedding of this pair of events, denoted as symbol r^*. The extraction of this feature will help to determine more accurately the temporal relation between events.

Characteristic Representation of Event Pairs. Given the vector representations corresponding to event e1 and event e1 in the text: h_{e1}, h_{e2}. Splice them
with the embedding vectors of the temporal relation rules features of this pair
of events to obtain the event pair characteristic representation of the temporal
relation to be extracted as follows:

$$f^{ee} = h_{e1} \oplus h_{e2} \oplus r^*$$

(5)

$f^{ee} \in R^{3d}$, The same reasoning leads to a characteristic representation of the pair
of event and time expressions of the temporal relation to be extracted $f^{et} \in R^{3d}$,
and the characteristic representation of a pair of time expressions $f^{tt} \in R^{3d}$.

3.3   Stepwise Temporal Relation Extraction

The chapter-level event temporal relation extraction task, in essence, is to judge
the order of occurrence of events in the text, therefore, the time information in
the text is crucial, they connect the development of all the events in the text,
which is essential for the recognition of event temporal relations. In addition,
according to the real experience, the temporal relations between time expressions
are easier to judge compared to the temporal relations between events. As a
result, this paper designs a three-layer stepwise temporal relation extraction
module.

The First Classification Layer (T-T). The task of the first classification
layer is to determine the temporal relation, i.e., the T-T temporal relation,
among all time expressions in the text. Based on the temporal order between
time expressions, this layer treats these time expressions as time anchors hitting
the relative timeline in order to split the complete timeline into multiple time
intervals.

Specifically, the first temporal relation classification layer receives the feature
vector, f^{tt}, of the pair of temporal expressions for which temporal relations are
to be extracted (these feature vectors capture the connection and information
between the two time expressions). The f^{tt} are fed into the fully connected layer,
and finally the temporal relation between them is computed by the softmax
function:

$$P(r_{ij}^{tt}, f^{tt}) = soft\max[f(w_1^{tt} \cdot f^{tt} + b_1^{tt}) \cdot w_2^{tt} + b_2^{tt}]$$

(6)

where $w_1^{tt} \in R^{h \times (3d)}$ is the learnable parameter matrix for the first fully connected layer, $b_1^{tt} \in R^h$ is the bias vector, and h is the hidden dimension of the
fully connected layer; $w_2^{tt} \in R^{c \times h}$ is the learnable parameter matrix for the second fully connected layer, $b_2^{tt} \in R^c$ is the bias vector, and c is the number of
temporal relation types, c = 4. $f(\cdot)$ is the Relu activation function.

The cross-entropy loss function for computing this layer is defined as:

$$L_{cls}^{tt} = - \sum_{t_i, t_j \in T, i \neq j} \log P(r_{ij}^{tt} | t_i, t_j), r_{ij}^{tt} \in R$$

(7)

The Second Classification Layer (E-T). The task of the second classification layer is to determine the temporal relation between the events and the time expressions in the text, i.e., the E-T temporal relation. Through this layer, we can categorize the events in the text into corresponding time intervals according to their temporal relations with the time expressions.

The second temporal relation classification layer feeds the feature vector f^{et} of the pair of event and time expressions of the temporal relation to be extracted into the fully connected layer, and finally the temporal relation between them is computed by the softmax function:

$$P(r_{ij}^{et}, f^{et}) = soft \max[f(w_1^{et} \cdot f^{et} + b_1^{et}) \cdot w_2^{et} + b_2^{et}] \qquad (8)$$

where $w_1^{et} \in R^{h \times 3d}$ is the learnable parameter matrix for the first fully connected layer, $b_1^{et} \in R^h$ is the bias vector; and h is the hidden dimension of the fully connected layer; $w_2^{et} \in R^{c \times h}$ is the learnable parameter matrix for the second fully connected layer, $b_2^{et} \in R^c$ is the bias vector. $f(\cdot)$ is the Relu activation function.

The cross-entropy loss function for computing this layer is defined as:

$$L_{cls}^{et} = - \sum_{e_i \in E, t_j \in T} \log P(r_{ij}^{et} | e_i, t_j), r_{ij}^{et} \in R \qquad (9)$$

The Third Classification Layer (E-E). The task of the third classification layer is to extract the temporal relations of the events in the time intervals obtained from the second classification layer, in order to arrange these events on the medical timeline according to their temporal relations.

The third temporal relation classification layer sends the feature vector f^{ee} of event pairs with temporal relations to be extracted in each time interval to the fully connected layer, and finally the temporal relation between them is computed by the softmax function:

$$P(r_{ij}^{ee}, f^{ee}) = soft \max[f(w_1^{ee} \cdot f^{ee} + b_1^{ee}) \cdot w_2^{ee} + b_2^{ee}] \qquad (10)$$

where $w_1^{ee} \in R^{h \times 3d}$ is the learnable parameter matrix for the first fully connected layer, $b_1^{ee} \in R^h$ is the bias vector; and h is the hidden dimension of the fully connected layer; $w_2^{ee} \in R^{c \times h}$ is the learnable parameter matrix for the second fully connected layer, $b_2^{ee} \in R^c$ is the bias vector. $f(\cdot)$ is the Relu activation function.

The cross-entropy loss function for computing this layer is defined as:

$$L_{cls}^{ee} = - \sum_{e_i, e_j \in E, i \neq j} \log P(r_{ij}^{ee} | e_i, e_j), r_{ij}^{ee} \in R \qquad (11)$$

In summary, the loss function of the stepwise temporal relation classification module is defined as:

$$L_{cls} = L_{cls}^{tt} + L_{cls}^{et} + L_{cls}^{ee} \qquad (12)$$

Once an event has been clustered into a time interval, its temporal relations with events in other time intervals have already been determined, so our approach minimizes the redundant relations generated by the model and the temporal contradiction errors that may arise during the prediction process. The efficiency of the model is also improved since the model only needs to focus on the temporal relations necessary to construct the timeline. This module provides a simple yet effective solution to the task of chapter-level temporal relation extraction.

3.4   Joint Learning

In order to synchronize the learning of the event extraction module and the temporal relation classification module so that they improve each other, we combine the loss functions of both modules to form the entire loss objective of our model:

$$L = L_{ner} + L_{\text{cls}} \qquad (13)$$

3.5   Construction of the Medical Timeline

Once our stepwise temporal relation extraction module accomplishes its task, our next critical step is to construct a complete timeline of patient care using the resulting temporal relations. This process aims to deal with any possible conflicts between the predicted outcomes of the temporal relations, which requires global reasoning. Our ultimate goal is to construct a conflict-free medical timeline through an iterative, greedy process that ensures the consistency of the temporal relations contained throughout the text. Briefly, we first sort the temporal relations in descending order according to their predicted probabilities. Then, one by one, we checked whether each predicted temporal relation, if added to the current timeline, would trigger a conflict within the timeline; if so, we removed it; if it did not trigger a conflict, we added it to the timeline. Ultimately, this process allows us to construct a complete patient medical timeline that reflects the temporal relations of the entire Chinese medical text. This approach helps ensure that our model maintains the global consistency of the extracted temporal relations over chapter-level texts.

4   Experiment

4.1   Introduction to the Dataset

Due to the scarcity of chapter-level Chinese medical event temporal relation datasets, we constructed a medical event temporal relation dataset based on Chinese electronic medical records by ourselves. We collected real patient medical data from local tertiary hospitals, covering Chinese electronic medical records of internal medicine, pediatrics, obstetrics and gynecology, oncology, and many other departments. After a simple data cleaning to remove task-irrelevant and patient privacy-related information, we finally obtained 1000 valid clinical medical texts. During the construction of the dataset, we mainly relied on manual annotation, while incorporating some automatic annotation methods to obtain reliable annotation results of the temporal relations of medical events.

In order to ensure the standardization of the dataset's annotation, we have taken into account the features related to the patient's medical timeline in the Chinese electronic medical record text, and referred to the annotation experience of Chinese CED [31], English i2b2-2012 [32], and TimeML [33], etc., to specify a set of annotation specifications applicable to our dataset.We annotate four types of events in our dataset that best reflect the patient's condition and medical treatment, including "problem", "treatment", "examination", and "other specific events". as well as nine types of time expressions, such as "date", "time", "modified time point ", "relative point in time", and so on. The definition of temporal relations includes four types: "Before", "After", "Equal" and "Vague".

The dataset contains 1,000 medical texts, a total of 12,373 events and time expressions, and 153,022 temporal relation triples. For model training and evaluation, we divided the training set, validation set, and test set in the ratio of 7.0:1.5:1.5. The statistics of various events and time expressions and temporal relation triples in the three datasets are shown in Fig. 4.

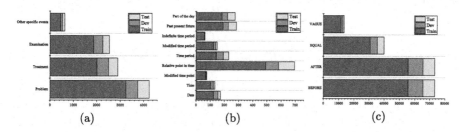

Fig. 4. Number counts of medical events (a), time expressions (b), temporal relation triples (b)

We divide all temporal relation triples into three main types, i.e., (time expression - time expression) type temporal relations (T-T), (event - time expression) type temporal relations (E-T), and (event - event) type temporal relations (E-E). Table 1 demonstrates the number of data samples in the dataset where

Table 1. Statistics on data samples

Dataset	Num of samples	T-T num (ave)/num of samples	E-T num (ave)/num of samples	E-E num (ave)/num of samples	Text length (max/min/ave)
Train	700	3.8/440	40.6/667	104.3/700	260/44/127.9
Val	150	3.0/89	39.1/139	117.4/150	253/41/132.5
Test	150	4.1/88	44.0/142	118.5/150	244/59/135.3

these three types of temporal relations exist, as well as the average number of such temporal relations contained in each data sample, and the sentence length (longest/shortest/average length) of the medical texts.

The statistics show that the number of T-T type temporal relations is the lowest, the number of E-T type temporal relations is slightly higher, and the number of E-E type temporal relations is the highest. It is worth noting that not every piece of data contains either T-T type or E-T type temporal relations.

4.2 Evaluation Indicators

In this paper, we use a strict evaluation criterion to report model performance, i.e., temporal relation extraction results are considered correct only if head and tail event representations (with complete overlap with annotations) as well as temporal relations and event types are correctly extracted. When the validation set achieves optimal results, we report the corresponding results for the test set. Since there are few similar works on Chinese related corpus available for our task, in order to be consistent with previous relation extraction methods for fair comparison, we use three different evaluation metrics including precision, recall, and F1 score to evaluate our model, which are computed using the following formulas.

$$P = \frac{TP}{TP + FP} \tag{14}$$

$$R = \frac{TP}{TP + FN} \tag{15}$$

$$F_1 = \frac{2 \times P \times R}{P + R} \tag{16}$$

where TP indicates the number of positive cases predicted correctly; FP indicates the number of negative cases predicted incorrectly; TN indicates the number of negative cases predicted correctly; and FN indicates the number of positive cases predicted incorrectly.

4.3 Baseline Models

Our approach is a BERT-based pipeline method, and in order to evaluate the performance more convincingly, we performed multiple comparisons. First, we compare it with two neural network-based joint extraction methods, namely the BERT-based BERT-CRF-joint model and the BERT-BILSTM-CRF-joint model. In addition, we also selected two current mainstream relation extraction models: CasRel [34] and the TPLinker [35]. The advantage of the CasRel model is to solve the overlapping problem of the relation triples, which embeds the relation categorization into a network of multiple pointers, and predicts the object entities and the relation categories simultaneously through multiple categorizations, in order to better deal with the complex relation situations. The TPLinker model adopts a unified joint extraction annotation framework to unify the extraction problem into a character pair linking problem, i.e., the Token Pair

Linking problem, in order to achieve a single-stage joint extraction and to solve the problem of burst bias and overlapping relation extraction in relation extraction. By comparing with these several different relational extraction models, we can more comprehensively evaluate the performance of our approach on the chapter-level temporal relation extraction task.

4.4   Experimental Results

Comparing the performance of our model with other models is shown in Table 2. From the experimental results, we find that the model that performs well in the relation extraction task does not perform well in the chapter-level temporal relation extraction task for Chinese medical events. This may be due to the fact that Chinese clinical medical record texts contain a large number of events and temporal relations far beyond ordinary texts, which increases the difficulty of temporal relation extraction. Therefore, the performance of CasRel and TPLinker models in the chapter-level temporal relation extraction task is much lower than that of the sentence-level relation extraction task.

Table 2. Comparison with other models

Model	NER			Relation Prediction		
	Precision	Recall	F1-score	Precision	Recall	F1-score
BERT-CRF-joint	0.75	0.74	0.74	0.18	0.46	0.25
BERT-BILSTM-CRF-joint	0.73	0.76	0.74	0.18	0.51	0.26
CasRel	0.83	0.80	0.81	0.39	0.32	0.35
TPLinker	0.84	0.78	0.80	0.35	0.31	0.33
Our Model	0.83	0.77	0.79	0.42	0.39	0.40

In addition, the issue of temporal granularity of time expressions is an important factor. Except for definite time expressions such as "date" and "time", most time expressions are usually fuzzy or modified time points or time periods, which naturally have different temporal granularities. However, in our Chinese temporal relation dataset, the temporal granularity features with time expressions are only roughly labeled, defining the whole time expression only based on its start time, and for the temporal relations between time expressions, comparing the sequence of their occurrences only based on their start times, without considering the time span they last. This leads to the first layer in our model, i.e., the T-T type of temporal relation extraction is not as effective as expected, and since our stepwise temporal relation extraction module is a pipelined design, the errors in the T-T layer will lead to inaccurate segmentation of the most important time intervals of the model, which in turn will lead to errors in predicting the time intervals in which the medical events are located, and the errors will keep on accumulating, which will affect the temporal relation prediction results of the whole text of the accuracy decreases, pulling down the overall performance of the model.

The comparison of the number of predicted relations to the total number of Gold relations for each model compared to our model is shown in Table 3. Traditional relation extraction models generate a large number of redundant temporal relations. In contrast, our model groups events by time intervals, and most of the relations generated can be used for timeline construction, effectively reducing redundant temporal relation generation and improving the efficiency of the task.

Table 3. Statistics on the number of temporal relations predicted by each model

Model	DEV	TEST	Number of GOLD relations
BERT-CRF-joint	18330	14128	36256
BERT-BILSTM-CRF-joint	19210	14898	36256
CasRel	14585	12978	36256
TPLinker	14912	12896	36256
Our Model	12461	9873	36256

4.5 Ablation Study

We conducted ablation experiments to analyze the validity of each part of our model. The results of performing ablation experiments are shown in Table 4.

Table 4. Result of ablation study

Model	P	R	F1	Lift ($\downarrow$)
-Fine tuning	0.19	0.20	0.19	0.21
-Dictionary of medical terms	0.35	0.40	0.37	0.03
-BIO labels embedding	0.32	0.37	0.35	0.05
-Temporal relation rules of medical events	0.40	0.39	0.39	0.01
-Stepwise temporal relation extraction	0.24	0.34	0.28	0.12
Our Model	0.42	0.39	0.40	

Based on the experimental results, we find that fine-tuning the pre-trained encoder has a significant impact on the performance. An un-fine-tuned pre-trained language model leads to a performance degradation of about 21%. Removing the information enhancement of the dictionary of medical terms decreases the entity recognition performance, which in turn affects the BIO labels embedding, resulting in a decrease in model performance of about 3%. Removing the embedding of BIO labels features and using only the contextual embedding generated by BERT as the final representation of the event and time expressions showed a decrease in model performance of about 5%, suggesting that the BIO tags provide valuable information for temporal relation classification as we expected. The temporal relation rules of medical events had a very limited improvement on the model; removing this component only decreased the model performance by about 1%, and the application of this rule may need to be explored further. Finally, we employed a simple fully-connected classification layer in place of the stepwise temporal relation extraction module, no longer distinguishing which of T-T, E-T, or E-E the combination of events of the temporal relations to be extracted belonged to, an approach that resulted in a 12% decrease in model performance. It is verified that our stepwise temporal relation extraction design improves the performance of this task significantly.

5   Conclusion

In this paper, we perform chapter-level event temporal relation extraction in a Chinese corpus of clinical medical texts to construct a patient-related medical timeline. We propose a simple pipeline method that combines the features and patterns of medical texts, and design a stepwise temporal relation extraction operation that simply and effectively removes a large number of redundant relations that may be predicted by ordinary relation extraction methods, and effectively avoids contradictory conflicts in the corpus features. On our annotated dataset, we compared our model to several pipeline-based and joint extraction models, achieving performance that outperforms these approaches. Since the effect of our model is very dependent on the extraction results of T-T class temporal relations, we will continue to explore how to improve the effect of temporal relation extraction between time expressions. In addition, due to the input limitation of BERT, we can only perform chapter-level text temporal relation extraction within a limited length now, and in future work, we would like to extend our approach to medical texts of longer length, or even to document-level medical texts in the true sense of the word.

References

1. Caufield, J.H., et al.: A reference set of curated biomedical data and metadata from clinical case reports. Sci. Data **5**(1), 1–18 (2018)
2. Soysal, E., et al.: Clamp-a toolkit for efficiently building customized clinical natural language processing pipelines. J. Am. Med. Inform. Assoc. **25**(3), 331–336 (2018)
3. Caufield, J.H., et al.: A comprehensive typing system for information extraction from clinical narratives. medRxiv, p. 19009118 (2019)
4. Alfattni, G., Peek, N., Nenadic, G.: Extraction of temporal relations from clinical free text: a systematic review of current approaches. J. Biomed. Inform. **108**, 103488 (2020)

5. Xu, Y., Wang, Y., Liu, T., Tsujii, J., Chang, E.I.C.: An end-to-end system to identify temporal relation in discharge summaries: 2012 I2B2 challenge. J. Am. Med. Inform. Assoc. **20**(5), 849–858 (2013)
6. Tang, B., Wu, Y., Jiang, M., Chen, Y., Denny, J.C., Xu, H.: A hybrid system for temporal information extraction from clinical text. J. Am. Med. Inform. Assoc. **20**(5), 828–835 (2013)
7. Khalifa, A., Velupillai, S., Meystre, S.: UtahBMI at SemEval-2016 task 12: extracting temporal information from clinical text. In: Proceedings of the 10th International Workshop on Semantic Evaluation (SemEval-2016), pp. 1256–1262 (2016)
8. Lee, H.J., et al.: UTHealth at SemEval-2016 task 12: an end-to-end system for temporal information extraction from clinical notes. In: Proceedings of the 10th International Workshop on Semantic Evaluation (SemEval-2016), pp. 1292–1297 (2016)
9. Nikfarjam, A., Emadzadeh, E., Gonzalez, G.: Towards generating a patient's timeline: extracting temporal relationships from clinical notes. J. Biomed. Inform. **46**, S40–S47 (2013)
10. MacAvaney, S., Cohan, A., Goharian, N.: GUIR at SemEval-2017 task 12: a framework for cross-domain clinical temporal information extraction. In: Proceedings of the 11th International Workshop on Semantic Evaluation (SemEval-2017), pp. 1024–1029 (2017)
11. Dligach, D., Miller, T., Lin, C., Bethard, S., Savova, G.: Neural temporal relation extraction. In: Proceedings of the 15th Conference of the European Chapter of the Association for Computational Linguistics: Volume 2, Short Papers, pp. 746–751 (2017)
12. Guan, H., Li, J., Xu, H., Devarakonda, M.: Robustly pre-trained neural model for direct temporal relation extraction. In: 2021 IEEE 9th International Conference on Healthcare Informatics (ICHI), pp. 501–502. IEEE (2021)
13. Galvan-Sosa, D., Matsuda, K., Okazaki, N., Inui, K.: Empirical exploration of the challenges in temporal relation extraction from clinical text. J. Nat. Lang. Process. **27**(2), 383–409 (2020)
14. Lin, C., Miller, T., Dligach, D., Sadeque, F., Bethard, S., Savova, G.: A BERT-based one-pass multi-task model for clinical temporal relation extraction (2020)
15. Ning, Q., Feng, Z., Roth, D.: A structured learning approach to temporal relation extraction. arXiv preprint arXiv:1906.04943 (2019)
16. Han, R., et al.: Deep structured neural network for event temporal relation extraction. arXiv preprint arXiv:1909.10094 (2019)
17. Han, R., Ning, Q., Peng, N.: Joint event and temporal relation extraction with shared representations and structured prediction. arXiv preprint arXiv:1909.05360 (2019)
18. Luan, Y., He, L., Ostendorf, M., Hajishirzi, H.: Multi-task identification of entities, relations, and coreference for scientific knowledge graph construction. arXiv preprint arXiv:1808.09602 (2018)
19. Bekoulis, G., Deleu, J., Demeester, T., Develder, C.: Joint entity recognition and relation extraction as a multi-head selection problem. Expert Syst. Appl. **114**, 34–45 (2018)
20. Wadden, D., Wennberg, U., Luan, Y., Hajishirzi, H.: Entity, relation, and event extraction with contextualized span representations. arXiv preprint arXiv:1909.03546 (2019)
21. Giorgi, J., Wang, X., Sahar, N., Shin, W.Y., Bader, G.D., Wang, B.: End-to-end named entity recognition and relation extraction using pre-trained language models. arXiv preprint arXiv:1912.13415 (2019)

22. Nguyen, D.Q., Verspoor, K.: End-to-end neural relation extraction using deep biaffine attention. In: Azzopardi, L., Stein, B., Fuhr, N., Mayr, P., Hauff, C., Hiemstra, D. (eds.) ECIR 2019, Part I. LNCS, vol. 11437, pp. 729–738. Springer, Cham (2019). https://doi.org/10.1007/978-3-030-15712-8_47
23. Christopoulou, F., Miwa, M., Ananiadou, S.: Connecting the dots: document-level neural relation extraction with edge-oriented graphs. arXiv preprint arXiv:1909.00228 (2019)
24. Zeng, S., Xu, R., Chang, B., Li, L.: Double graph based reasoning for document-level relation extraction. arXiv preprint arXiv:2009.13752 (2020)
25. Xu, B., Wang, Q., Lyu, Y., Zhu, Y., Mao, Z.: Entity structure within and throughout: modeling mention dependencies for document-level relation extraction. In: Proceedings of the AAAI Conference on Artificial Intelligence, vol. 35, pp. 14149–14157 (2021)
26. Zhou, L., Hripcsak, G.: Temporal reasoning with medical data-a review with emphasis on medical natural language processing. J. Biomed. Inform. **40**(2), 183–202 (2007)
27. Devlin, J., Chang, M.W., Lee, K., Toutanova, K.: BERT: pre-training of deep bidirectional transformers for language understanding. arXiv preprint arXiv:1810.04805 (2018)
28. Lafferty, J., McCallum, A., Pereira, F.C.: Conditional random fields: probabilistic models for segmenting and labeling sequence data (2001)
29. Lample, G., Ballesteros, M., Subramanian, S., Kawakami, K., Dyer, C.: Neural architectures for named entity recognition. arXiv preprint arXiv:1603.01360 (2016)
30. Ma, X., Hovy, E.: End-to-end sequence labeling via bi-directional LSTM-CNNs-CRF. arXiv preprint arXiv:1603.01354 (2016)
31. Zhang, Z.C., Zhang, M.Y., Zhou, T., Qiu, Y.L.: Pre-trained language model augmented adversarial training network for Chinese clinical event detection. Math. Biosci. Eng. **17**, 2825–2841 (2020)
32. Sun, W., Rumshisky, A., Uzuner, O., Szolovits, P., Pustejovsky, J.: The 2012 I2B2 temporal relations challenge annotation guidelines. Manuscript (2012). https://www.i2b2.org/NLP/TemporalRelations/Call.php
33. Saurí, R., Littman, J., Knippen, B., Gaizauskas, R., Setzer, A., Pustejovsky, J.: TimeML annotation guidelines. Version **1**(1), 31 (2006)
34. Wei, Z., Su, J., Wang, Y., Tian, Y., Chang, Y.: A novel cascade binary tagging framework for relational triple extraction. arXiv preprint arXiv:1909.03227 (2019)
35. Wang, Y., Yu, B., Zhang, Y., Liu, T., Zhu, H., Sun, L.: TPLinker: single-stage joint extraction of entities and relations through token pair linking. arXiv preprint arXiv:2010.13415 (2020)

Combining Biaffine Model and Constraints Inference for Chinese Clinical Temporal Relation Extraction

DeYue Yin[ID], ZhiChang Zhang[(✉)][ID], Hao Wei[ID], and WenJun Xiang[ID]

College of Computer Science and Engineering, Northwest Normal University, Lanzhou, Gansu, China
zzc@nwnu.edu.cn

Abstract. The extraction of clinical events and their temporal relation from electronic medical records (EMRs) is crucial and plays a significant role in the development of various intelligent clinical applications. Nevertheless, achieving precise extraction of such information from Chinese electronic medical records (CEMRs) presents a formidable challenge due to the limited availability of Chinese language resources in this field. To address this challenge, we create a dataset comprising clinical events and their temporal relations extracted from CEMRs. Previous methods for extracting clinical events and temporal relations typically relied on sequential pipeline models, which involve initially identifying events and then training classifiers to recognize temporal relations between them. However, this step-by-step approach can result in the accumulation of errors at each stage. Therefore, we propose a joint extraction model utilizing a biaffine architecture to simultaneously extract clinical events and temporal relations. To enhance the model's performance, we incorporate constraints related to relatedness and irreversibility, resulting in an efficient approach for extracting temporal relations from CEMRs. Our joint extraction model performs admirably on the Chinese dataset we constructed.

Keywords: Chinese Electronic Medical Records · Clinical Temporal Relation Extraction · Biaffine Model · Constraint Inference

1 Introduction

In recent years, the development and popularization of medical information technology has seen Chinese electronic medical records (CEMRs) gradually

Supported by the National Natural Science Foundation of China (No. 62163033), the Talent Innovation and Entrepreneurship Project of Lanzhou, China (No. 2021-RC-49), the Natural Science Foundation of Gansu Province, China (No. 22JR5RA145, No. 21JR7RA781, No. 21JR7RA116), the Major Research Project Incubation Program of Northwest Normal University, China (No. NWNU-LKZD2021-06). The funding body had no role in study design, data collection and analysis, decision to publish, or preparation of the manuscript.

H. Xu et al. (Eds.): CHIP 2023, CCIS 1993, pp. 182–194, 2024.
https://doi.org/10.1007/978-981-99-9864-7_12

replace traditional paper medical records as the primary form of medical records. CEMRs provide enhanced clinical decision-making support and medical quality management for medical personnel due to their efficient and reliable characteristics. However, the vast amount of vital clinical event and temporal relation information [1–3] contained in CEMRs, such as disease diagnosis, treatment processes, and medication history, holds significant value for medical research and clinical practice. Owing to the limitations of available data resources, fully leveraging this value is currently challenging.

We have developed a dataset based on CEMRs to identify clinical events and temporal relations. Specifically, we obtained CEMR text from a first-class hospital in China and processed it manually. Furthermore, we processed the raw data into an independent medical text and removed any patient privacy information, including names and addresses. Next, we utilized the TimeML [4] and I2B2 [5] annotation guidelines and established a unified annotation standard based on CEMR's characteristics. We manually annotated clinical events (CEvent) and time expressions (Timex3) and temporal links (TLink) [6–8] on each event pair, including CEvent-CEvent, CEvent-Timex3, Timex3-Timex3, where the temporal relation includes Before, After, Equal, and Vague.

In recent years, temporal relation extraction have been mainly implemented using pipeline models [2,9] and joint extraction models [10]. While the pipeline model involves detecting clinical events before extracting temporal relations, errors in event extraction can lead to lower accuracy in temporal relation identification. Therefore, we used a joint extraction model to concurrently extract clinical event and temporal relation. Specifically, we employed a biaffine model [10–13] to construct a unified table structure for extracting clinical events and temporal relations. In the table, events are represented as squares distributed diagonally, while temporal relations are represented as rectangles distributed non-diagonally.

Figure 1 illustrates a clinical narrative that states *"The patient had been suffering from uremia for over a year and had completed the relevant examinations..."*, where the clinical event *"E1: uremia"* is a disease labeled as *problem-label* (PRO), the time expression *"E2: over a year"* is labeled as *modified duration-label* (MDUR), and the clinical event *"E3: relevant examinations"* belongs to laboratory examination and is labeled as *examination-label* (EXA). The temporal relation between events satisfies irreversibility, meaning that the order of events cannot be changed. The relation between *"E1: uremia"* and *"E2: over a year"* is **Equal**. If *"E1: uremia"* is the head event and *"E3: relevant examinations"* is the tail event, their temporal relation is **Before**. On the contrary, if *"E3: relevant examinations"* is the head event and *"E1: uremia"* is the tail event, their temporal relation is **After**. Similarly, when *"E2: over a year"* is the head event and *"E3: relevant examinations"* is the tail event, the temporal relation is **Before**, while when *"E2: over a year"* is the head event and *"E3: relevant examinations"* is the tail event, the temporal relation is **After**.

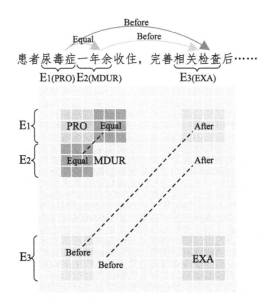

Fig. 1. Example of a table for joint extraction model.

Previous research [6,9] have treated temporal relation extraction as a multi-classification problem, thereby making it challenging to maintain logical constraints between temporal relations. To tackle this issue, [6–9,14] introduced a constraint inference method that enforces logical coherence by incorporating supplementary losses. Inspired by this, this study incorporated constraints relate to relatedness and irreversibility, resulting in an efficient approach for extracting temporal relations from CEMRs. To ensure relatedness, we aimed to maximize the probability of events in the table while minimizing the probability of temporal relations in the same row and column. An example is illustrated in Fig. 1, the probability of "*E1: uremia*" and "*E2: over a year*" should exceed the probability of (E1, Equal, E2) in the table. The irreversibility constraint conditions, including (E1, Equal, E2) and (E2, Equal, E1), must be satisfied by the rectangle representing temporal relation with diagonal symmetry.

We have developed a dataset of events and temporal relations from CEMRs, which aims to facilitate the development of Chinese medical information extraction. We proposed a novel joint extraction model that employs a biaffine architecture to concurrently extract clinical events and temporal relations. By incorporating constraints related to relatedness and irreversibility, we developed an efficient approach for extracting temporal relations from CEMRs. Our contributions to this work are listed as follows:

– We have constructed a dataset consisting of clinical events and temporal relations extracted from Chinese electronic medical records, which has the potential to advance the field of medical information extraction in the Chinese language.

- We proposed a joint extraction model utilizing a biaffine architecture to concurrently extract clinical events and temporal relations.
- The use of biaffine architecture and constraint inference techniques to extract clinical events and their temporal relations shows a practical and innovative approach.

2   Related Work

2.1   Relation Extraction

In recent years, research on relation extraction has primarily focused on entity relation extraction (ERE) [15–17]. ERE is a process of extracting entity and their related relation from text, ultimately producing a set of triples in the format (*head entity, relation, tail entity*). Experiments in ERE tasks often involve overlapping modes, including single entity overlap (SEO) [15–17], entity pair overlap (EPO) [15–17], and subject object overlap (SOO) [17]. SEO refers to the scenario where an entity has relations with two or more other entities, while EPO indicates the possibility of a pair of entities having multiple relation types. Furthermore, SOO describes a triplet where the head and tail entities share common elements.

Researchers have proposed various research strategies for different tasks. For instance, [15] proposed a cascade binary tagging framework that is a joint ERE method that leverages parameter sharing. In [16], the authors proposed a one-stage joint extraction model that addresses three overlap issues. After continuous attempts, [17] designed a component that predicts potential relation and constrains the subset of relation extracted by entities. They then constructed corresponding global components to align relation triplets. Moreover, [10,12] used one-pass to classify relation among all entity mention while locating relation from all entity mention. These methods involve filling out tables.

2.2   Temporal Relation Extraction

Temporal relation extraction is a specialized field within event relation extraction. Unlike entity relation extraction, temporal relation extraction focuses on identifying the temporal order of events in natural language texts. This involves utilizing common sense [18] and constraint inference [2,6,9]. For instance, in the clinical domain, it is common knowledge that a patient is diagnosed with a disease before being admitted for treatment.

Previous research aimed to extract temporal relations between events in a large corpus [19,20] for the first time, with the goal of applying this knowledge to the news domain [8]. In [6], constraints of symmetry and transitivity were utilized to optimize event temporal relations model. [21] represented events using hyper-rectangles and identified their order of based on whether the rectangles overlapped or contained each other. Meanwhile, [22] proposed an end-to-end hyperbolic neural structure to model events and their temporal relations in hyperbolic space. To better model the constraints between temporal relations, [2,3] proposed a global constraint inference pipeline model, which has made significant contributions.

3   Method

This section presents our joint extraction model, which is depicted in Fig. 2. Specifically, we fine-tuned a pre-trained language model (PLM) [23–26] to learn contextual vector representations. Two multi-layer perceptrons (MLPs) are employed to predict the vector representations of the head and tail events, enabling the prediction of the table structure (Sect. 3.2). The model is further optimized through constraint inference (Sect. 3.3).

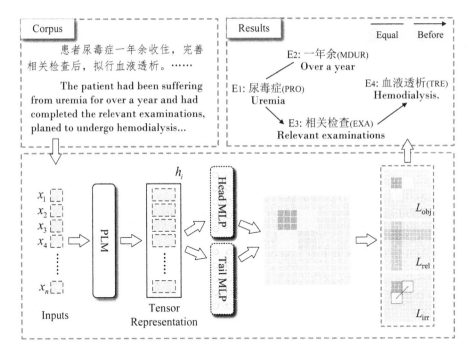

Fig. 2. Overall framework of our model.

3.1   Task Definition

We set the input sequence $x = \{x_1, x_2, \ldots, x_n\}$ to have a length of n. The objective is to detect events e and temporal relations r. Each event e is assigned a distinct label $\varepsilon \in \gamma_\varepsilon$, such as PRO or DUR. Each event pair is linked by a temporal relation $r \in \gamma_R$ represented as a triplet of (e_1, r, e_2), where e_1 and e_2 are events and r represents a temporal relation. For any given text, we constructed a table T of size $|n| \times |n|$, where each cell (i, j) is assigned a label $s(i, j) \in \gamma$. Each cell (i, j) represent a head x_i and tail x_j, and should be filled ε or r. Note that cells (i, j) in any square on the diagonal of the table can only be labeled with $s(i, j) \in \gamma_\varepsilon \cup \oslash$, whereas cells (i, j) in non-diagonal rectangles can only be labeled with $s(i, j) \in \gamma_R \cup \oslash$. The symbol $\oslash$ represents no filling.

3.2   Biaffine Model

We formulated the joint extraction model as a table structure prediction via a biaffine model. We fed the input sequence x into a PLM as an encoder context representation $h_i \in \mathbb{R}^d$. The output of the PLM is:

$$h_i = \mathsf{PLM}(x_i) \tag{1}$$

Next, we used a biaffine model to represent each token in the table T, which is effective for dependency parsing tasks [10–13]. Specifically, we used two MLPs, head event h^{head} and tail event h^{tail} to learn the projection representations, which are calculated using the learned representations as follows:

$$h_i^{head} = W_2^{head}(ReLU(W_1^{head}h_i^{enc})), h_j^{tail} = W_2^{tail}(ReLU(W_1^{tail}h_j^{enc})) \tag{2}$$

where $h_i^{head} \in \mathbb{R}^d$ and $h_j^{tail} \in \mathbb{R}^d$, and d is the hidden state. Finally, we realized the biaffine model to attain $s_{i,j}$, which is a scoring tensor. We calculated the scoring vector by:

$$s_{i,j} = \mathsf{Biaffine}(h_i, h_j) \tag{3}$$
$$= (h_i^{head})^T U_1 h_j^{tail} + U_2(h_i^{head} \oplus h_j^{tail}) + b \tag{4}$$

where $U_1 \in \mathbb{R}^{n \times n \times \mathbb{Z}}$ and $U_2 \in \mathbb{R}^{2n \times \mathbb{Z}}$ are learnable weight parameters, b is the bias, $\oplus$ denotes vector concatenation.

The obtained scoring vector $s_{i,j}$ is fed into a softmax function to predict the probability distribution, where $s_{i,j} \in \gamma_\varepsilon \cup \gamma_R \cup \oslash$. We trained our model using the following objective function to calculate the loss:

$$p(y_{i,j}|x) = Softmax(s_{i,j}) \tag{5}$$

$$L_{obj} = -\frac{1}{|n|^2} \sum_{i=1}^{|n|} \sum_{j=1}^{|n|} \log p(y_{i,j}|x) \tag{6}$$

3.3   Constraints Inference

To improve the performance of our model, we incorporated additional constraints. Specifically, we merged the structural characteristics of the biaffine model with constraints that ensure relatedness and irreversibility. The relatedness constraint, which is based on the biaffine model, states that cells on the diagonal of the table should have a higher probability of being identified as events than as relations in the same row or column. Additionally, temporal relations must be irreversible, which means that they must be symmetrical about the diagonal in the table T. We designated the predicted probability $\mathbb{S}_{i,j,k}$ for each cell (i, j) in the table T, where $\mathbb{S} \in \mathbb{R}^{|n| \times |n| \times |\gamma|}$.

Relatedness. Due to the fact that event existence is a prerequisite for relation existence, the probability of relation existence should be lower than that of event existence. To ensure this constraint, we set the maximum probability of event type $\mathbb{S}_{i,i,k}$ for each cell (i, i) on the diagonal should not be lower than that of other cells in the same row $\mathbb{S}_{i,:,k}$ or column $\mathbb{S}_{:,i,k}$ of relation type.

$$L_{rel} = \frac{1}{|n|} \sum_{i=1}^{|n|} \left[\max_{k \in \gamma_R} \{\mathbb{S}_{:,i,k}, \mathbb{S}_{i,:,k}\} - \max_{k \in \gamma_\varepsilon} \{\mathbb{S}_{i,i,k}\} \right]_* \tag{7}$$

where $[u]_* = max(u, 0)$ is a hinge function.

Irreversibility. Temporal relations between events are irreversible, meaning that the temporal order of events cannot be changed. The square corresponding to an event must be symmetrical about the diagonal. When a pair of events is treated as a head and tail event, the corresponding temporal relation in the table is distributed on both sides of the diagonal. For example, the relations $(e_1, \text{Before}, e_2)$ and (e_2, After, e_1) are equivalent.

$$L_{irr} = \frac{1}{|n|^2} \sum_{i=1}^{|n|} \sum_{j=1}^{|n|} |\mathbb{S}_{i,j,k} - \mathbb{S}_{j,i,k}| \tag{8}$$

Finally, we optimized all three loss functions jointly during training using the combined loss function $L_{obj} + L_{rel} + L_{irr}$.

4   Experiments

In this section, we presented an overview of the dataset and experimental results from multiple perspectives.

4.1   Dataset

We obtained raw data from a first-class hospital in China, which required manual processing and developed annotation guidelines before annotation. This involve first course records, ward rounds, and examination records. During the manual processing stage, the raw data was transformed into a single medical text and was removed any privacy information including names and addresses. The annotation guidelines were developed based on the unique characteristics of CEMRs. As shown in Fig. 3, the annotation process mainly involves five steps to ensure the quality of the data: event annotation, event checking, relation annotation, relation checking, and relation generation. The dataset consists of 6 CEvent, 12 Timex3, and 4 TempRel, as presented in Table 1, 2, and 3. According to Table 3, we calculated the distribution of the four temporal relations and found that the number of **Before** and **After** is equal, which satisfies the irreversibility constraint. However, the **Vague** nature of certain events in clinical narratives makes it challenging to identify them with complete accuracy at the time of occurrence. We divided the dataset into training, validation, and test sets in a 6:3:1 ratio (Table 4).

Table 1. Clinical Event Statistics.

CEVENT label	Acronyms	Count	Ratio (%)
Problem	PRO	4,397	27.84
Examination	EXA	3,502	22.18
Treatment	TRE	2,863	18.13
Clinical Department	CD	309	1.96
Evidence	EVI	1,124	7.12
Occurrence	OCC	799	5.06

Table 2. Time Expressive Statistics.

TIMEX3 label	Acronyms	Count	Ratio (%)	TIMEX3 label	Acronyms	Count	Ratio (%)
Season	–	11	0.07	Duration	DUR	271	1.72
Age	–	105	0.66	Modified Duration	MDUR	166	1.05
Date	–	183	1.16	Unspecified Duration	UDUR	62	0.39
Time	–	133	0.84	Past, Now, Future	PNF	215	1.36
Relative Time	RTime	937	5.93	Part of Day	POD	358	2.27
Modified Time	MTime	91	0.58	Set	–	266	1.68

Table 3. Temporal Relation Statistics.

TempRel Type	Count	Ratio (%)
Before	76,714	38.6
After	76,714	38.6
Equal	38,802	19.5
Vague	6,478	3.3

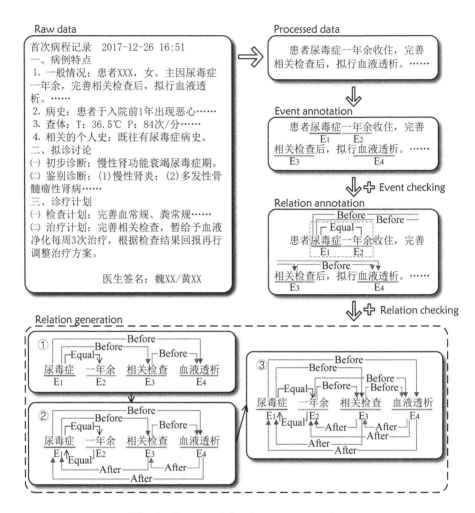

Fig. 3. Process of the dataset annotation.

Table 4. Number of Dataset Allocation.

	Text	Event	Relation
Train	1,200	10,163	92,194
validation	600	4,260	30,422
test	200	1,369	9,362
all	2,000	15,792	131,978

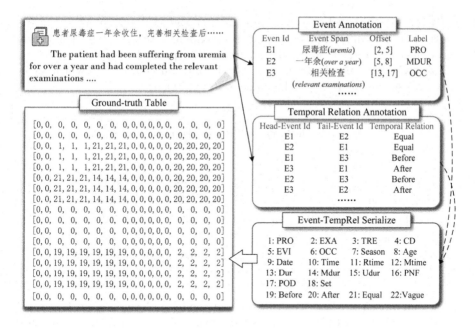

Fig. 4. Example of model input data.

4.2 Implementation Details and Hyperparameter Settings

We realized the joint extraction model through designed a table structure. As illustrated in Fig. 4, the input data for this model consists of annotated events and temporal relations. Since each event can have multiple tokens, accurately identifying event boundaries is crucial. Therefore, all event labels and relation types are serialized, and a ground-truth table is generated. During training, we aimed for the learned content close to the rows and columns corresponding to any event in the table.

The batch size of each data input into the model during training is 16, and the maximum length of the text is 256. We used four Chinese pre-trained language models, such as BERT [23], RoBERTa [24], AlBERT [25], and MacBERT [26]. Furthermore, we set the hidden state size of 768, the learning rate is 5e-5, and the dropout rate is 0.3. Based on this, we trained 200 epochs to train our model.

4.3 Performance Comparison

Table 5 summarizes our experimental results and a comparative baseline analysis. We evaluated the performance of our model using [27] and Precision (P), Recall (R), and F1 score (F1) throughout the experiment. Our comparison baseline includes three methods:

1. **BERT+softmax:** A pipeline approach that aims to detect clinical events and classify temporal relations using BERT and softmax.

2. **BERT+LSTM+MAP:** We adopted BERT and LSTM to detect events and extract temporal relations and used the maximum posterior (MAP) optimization method to train our model, following the approach proposed by [2].
3. **Joint Constraints Learning** (JCL): [14] introduced the JCL, which incorporates logic constraints and commonsense knowledge.

Table 5. Overall Results Display.

Model	Events			TempRel		
	P (%)	R (%)	F1 (%)	P (%)	R (%)	F1 (%)
BERT + softmax	82.4	81.1	81.7	42.2	41.6	41.8
BERT + LSTM + MAP	83.5	82.9	83.2	48.6	47.9	48.2
Joint Constrained Learning	83.6	85.8	84.7	54.6	52.6	53.8
Ours	**85.7**	**86.1**	**85.9**	**54.9**	**53.7**	**54.3**

In comparison to these experiments, our model performs better. Given the reliance of NLP on PLMs, we conducted experiments to verify the pre-trained ability of our model. Specifically, we fine-tuned four PLMs to encode medical record text (Table 6).

Table 6. The comparison (F1 score) of different PLM.

Encoder	Events (%)	TempRel (%)
BERT-base [23]	84.5	53.6
RoBERTa-large [24]	85.1	53.8
ALBERT-xxlarge [25]	85.5	54.1
MacBERT-base [26]	**85.9**	**54.3**

4.4   Ablation Study

The results presented in Table 7 demonstrate the effectiveness of our model, including a biaffine model and constraint inference. The '-relatedness inference' and '-irreversibility inference' techniques remove part of constraints, while '-constraint inference' removes both relatedness and irreversibility constraints and is only applicable to experiments using the biaffine model. However, identified temporal relations results were significantly lower when using '-constraint inference' due to its impact on temporal information. We removed the PLM and now use only embeddings to learn token-level context representations, and the comparison results showed that our model based on the PLM is effective in identifying events and temporal relations.

Table 7. The comparison (F1 score) with different setting.

	Events (%)	TempRel (%)
Ours	85.2	53.9
- relatedness inference	83.4	49.2
- irreversibility inference	83.7	47.6
- constraint inference	83.1	44.5
- MLP→embedding	80.1	36.8

5 Conclusions

We have developed a Chinese clinical events and temporal relations dataset composed of authentic medical records from various hospitals, encompassing various diseases and clinical scenarios. To conduct experiments, we employed natural language processing techniques and deep learning models. Specifically, we used a joint extraction model through a biaffine model, optimizing it using relatedness and irreversibility constraints. The experimental results demonstrate that our model, incorporating the biaffine model and constraint inference, is effective in handling temporal relation extraction tasks.

References

1. Leeuwenberg, A., Moens, M.F.: Structured learning for temporal relation extraction from clinical records. In: Proceedings of the 15th Conference of the European Chapter of the Association for Computational Linguistics: Volume 1, Long Papers, pp. 1150–1158 (2017)
2. Han, R., Zhou, Y., Peng, N.: Domain knowledge empowered structured neural net for end-to-end event temporal relation extraction. arXiv preprint arXiv:2009.07373 (2020)
3. Zhou, Y., et al.: Clinical temporal relation extraction with probabilistic soft logic regularization and global inference. In: Proceedings of the AAAI Conference on Artificial Intelligence, vol. 35, pp. 14647–14655 (2021)
4. Saurí, R., Littman, J., Knippen, B., Gaizauskas, R., Setzer, A., Pustejovsky, J.: TimeML annotation guidelines. Version 1(1), 31 (2006)
5. Sun, W., Rumshisky, A., Uzuner, O.: Evaluating temporal relations in clinical text: 2012 I2B2 challenge. J. Am. Med. Inform. Assoc. 20(5), 806–813 (2013)
6. Ning, Q., Feng, Z., Roth, D.: A structured learning approach to temporal relation extraction. arXiv preprint arXiv:1906.04943 (2019)
7. Meng, Y., Rumshisky, A.: Context-aware neural model for temporal information extraction. In: Proceedings of the 56th Annual Meeting of the Association for Computational Linguistics (Volume 1: Long Papers), pp. 527–536 (2018)
8. Ning, Q., Subramanian, S., Roth, D.: An improved neural baseline for temporal relation extraction. arXiv preprint arXiv:1909.00429 (2019)
9. Han, R., Ning, Q., Peng, N.: Joint event and temporal relation extraction with shared representations and structured prediction. arXiv preprint arXiv:1909.05360 (2019)

10. Wang, Y., Sun, C., Wu, Y., Zhou, H., Li, L., Yan, J.: UniRE: a unified label space for entity relation extraction. arXiv preprint arXiv:2107.04292 (2021)
11. Yu, J., Bohnet, B., Poesio, M.: Named entity recognition as dependency parsing. arXiv preprint arXiv:2005.07150 (2020)
12. Verga, P., Strubell, E., McCallum, A.: Simultaneously self-attending to all mentions for full-abstract biological relation extraction. arXiv preprint arXiv:1802.10569 (2018)
13. Dozat, T., Manning, C.D.: Deep biaffine attention for neural dependency parsing. arXiv preprint arXiv:1611.01734 (2016)
14. Wang, H., Chen, M., Zhang, H., Roth, D.: Joint constrained learning for event-event relation extraction. arXiv preprint arXiv:2010.06727 (2020)
15. Wei, Z., Su, J., Wang, Y., Tian, Y., Chang, Y.: A novel cascade binary tagging framework for relational triple extraction. In: Proceedings of the 58th Annual Meeting of the Association for Computational Linguistics, pp. 1476–1488 (2020)
16. Wang, Y., Yu, B., Zhang, Y., Liu, T., Zhu, H., Sun, L.: TPLinker: single-stage joint extraction of entities and relations through token pair linking. arXiv preprint arXiv:2010.13415 (2020)
17. Zheng, H., et al.: PRGC: potential relation and global correspondence based joint relational triple extraction. arXiv preprint arXiv:2106.09895 (2021)
18. Zhou, B., Ning, Q., Khashabi, D., Roth, D.: Temporal common sense acquisition with minimal supervision. arXiv preprint arXiv:2005.04304 (2020)
19. Chambers, N., Cassidy, T., McDowell, B., Bethard, S.: Dense event ordering with a multi-pass architecture. Trans. Assoc. Comput. Linguist. **2**, 273–284 (2014)
20. Ning, Q., Wu, H., Roth, D.: A multi-axis annotation scheme for event temporal relations. arXiv preprint arXiv:1804.07828 (2018)
21. Hwang, E., Lee, J.Y., Yang, T., Patel, D., Zhang, D., McCallum, A.: Event-event relation extraction using probabilistic box embedding. In: Proceedings of the 60th Annual Meeting of the Association for Computational Linguistics (Volume 2: Short Papers), pp. 235–244 (2022)
22. Tan, X., Pergola, G., He, Y.: Extracting event temporal relations via hyperbolic geometry. arXiv preprint arXiv:2109.05527 (2021)
23. Devlin, J., Chang, M.W., Lee, K., Toutanova, K.: BERT: pre-training of deep bidirectional transformers for language understanding. arXiv preprint arXiv:1810.04805 (2018)
24. Liu, Z., Lin, W., Shi, Y., Zhao, J.: A robustly optimized BERT pre-training approach with post-training. In: Li, S., Sun, M., Liu, Y., Wu, H., Kang, L., Che, W., He, S., Rao, G. (eds.) CCL 2021. LNCS (LNAI), vol. 12869, pp. 471–484. Springer, Cham (2021). https://doi.org/10.1007/978-3-030-84186-7_31
25. Lan, Z., Chen, M., Goodman, S., Gimpel, K., Sharma, P., Soricut, R.: ALBERT: a lite BERT for self-supervised learning of language representations. arXiv preprint arXiv:1909.11942 (2019)
26. Cui, Y., Che, W., Liu, T., Qin, B., Wang, S., Hu, G.: Revisiting pre-trained models for Chinese natural language processing. arXiv preprint arXiv:2004.13922 (2020)
27. Taillé, B., Guigue, V., Scoutheeten, G., Gallinari, P.: Let's stop incorrect comparisons in end-to-end relation extraction! arXiv preprint arXiv:2009.10684 (2020)

Healthcare Natural Language Processing

Biomedical Event Detection Based on Dependency Analysis and Graph Convolution Network

Xinyu He[✉], Yujie Tang, Xue Han, and Yonggong Ren

School of Computer and Artificial Intelligence, Liaoning Normal University, Dalian, China
hexinyu@lnnu.edu.cn

Abstract. Biomedical event detection is one of the most important tasks in biomedical event extraction, providing an important basis for disease prevention and drug development. The existing methods treat event detection tasks as multi-classification or sequence annotation tasks, only considering the sequence representation of sentences and striving to obtain more contextual information in sequence models. However, they overlook the shortcomings of sequence modeling methods in capturing long-distance dependency problems and the impact of syntactic structure dependencies on event detection performance. Therefore, the paper proposes a biomedical event detection model based on dependency analysis and graph convolutional neural networks. Firstly, we constructed a feature extraction framework based on BioBERT word embedding combined with entity type embedding and dependency parsing, effectively extracting sentence level features from natural language texts. In addition, dependency analysis is used to perform syntactic analysis on sentences, identify the grammatical dependencies between words in the sentence, and construct a dependency syntactic structure graph. Finally, a graph convolutional neural network is used to perform convolution operations on the dependency syntax graph, and the dependency relationships between various nodes in the dependency structure graph are dynamically updated during the training process, more fully capturing long-distance dependency relationships in sentences, effectively identifying and classifying the event trigger words in the sentences. The experimental results show that the proposed method achieves better performance on the MLEE dataset.

Keywords: BioBERT · BiLSTM · Dependency analysis · Graph convolutional network · Event detection

1 Introduction

In recent years, the biomedical field has grown continuously, and the number of biomedical literature has grown exponentially. Biomedical information plays an important role in biomedical research, and how to efficiently extract the biomedical information needed by researchers in massive data becomes a major challenge. For biomedical researchers, it is one of the main tasks of biomedical information extraction to extract the structured information from the unstructured data, which can greatly improve the research efficiency

© The Author(s), under exclusive license to Springer Nature Singapore Pte Ltd. 2024
H. Xu et al. (Eds.): CHIP 2023, CCIS 1993, pp. 197–211, 2024.
https://doi.org/10.1007/978-981-99-9864-7_13

and quickly detect the effective biomedical events from the biomedical information. A biomedical event consists of a trigger word and multiple elements. The trigger word is a word or phrase that triggers the whole event. The type of the trigger word determines the type of the event; the element is the participant of the event, which can be an entity or another event. As shown in Fig. 1, it is an example of a biomedical event in a sentence containing two events "Development" and "Negative Regulation" in the sentence "Thalidomide inhibited the formation of capillary tubes.", and the event structure is as follows:

E1 (Type: Development, Trigger: formation, Theme: capillary tubes);

E2 (Type: Negative Regulation, Trigger: inhibited, Theme: E1 Cause: Thalidomide);

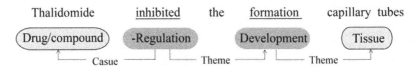

Fig. 1. Examples of the biomedical events

A complete biomedical event detection task includes biomedical named entity identification, biomedical trigger word recognition, and trigger word classification. For most event detection tasks, the standard entity is given in the relevant text corpus, so as a subtask of biomedical event extraction, biomedical event detection only needs to identify the biomedical event trigger word from the text and detect its type. Therefore, the event detection task can be regarded as a trigger word recognition task, and the identified trigger words can be classified into pre-defined event types. How to correctly identify the event trigger word and determine the event type is pretty important for the event extraction.

Most of the previous methods used for biomedical event detection are rule-based or traditional machine learning based. The rule-based method relies on manual rule making, which takes a lot of time; While the methods based on traditional machine learning, such as SVM (Support Vector Machine) and CRF (Conditional Random Field), have better performance in event detection compared with the methods based on rules, but they rely on a large number of manually designed complex features, have poor generalization ability. At present, the deep learning method based on neural network has gradually become the mainstream method. Using word vectors to represent words can not only improve the data sparse problem caused by high-dimensional vector space, but also contain more semantic feature information [1]. Using neural network model can automatically learn text features and achieve good results in many natural language processing tasks. At present, in biomedical event detection tasks, many researchers treat biomedical event detection tasks as multi-classification tasks or sequence annotation tasks, and are committed to obtaining more context information in the sequence model. However, sentence level sequence modeling methods are still insufficient in capturing long-distance dependency, which ignore the impact of syntactic structure dependencies in sentences on the performance of event detection tasks. And because syntactic structure dependency can determine the relationship between different words and phrases in a sentence, the semantic differences in different syntactic dependency structures and the types of dependency labels in dependency structures are often ignored, and text features cannot be well extracted. To solve the above problems, this paper presents a model for biomedical event detection, combining BioBERT (Biomedical Bidirectional Encoder Representation from Transformers) [2] word embedding and entity type word embedding to encode sentences, obtaining the vector representation of the entire input sentence, and then combines the bidirectional long short term memory neural network BiLSTM (Bidirectional Long Term Memory) to obtain sufficient context information, the syntactic dependency graph is obtained by dependency parsing to represent syntactic dependency, which effectively shortens the distance from one trigger word to another in a sentence. The GCN (Graph Convolutional Neural) [3] is used to process the dependency syntactic structure data, and dynamically update the dependency relationships between the nodes in the dependency structure graph during the training process, so as to more fully capture the long-distance dependency in sentences and the semantic differences in different syntactic structures. In addition, this paper introduces multi head attention perception MUH (Multi Head Attention) [4] after GCN to enhance biomedical event information. The performance of the model and its advantages in the experiment were evaluated on MLEE (Multi Level Event Extraction) [5], a general data set in the biomedical field. The experimental results show the effectiveness of the model in the event detection task. To sum up, the main contributions of this paper are as follows:

- A feature extraction framework based on BioBERT word embedding combined with entity type embedding and dependency analysis is proposed to effectively extract sentence-level features in natural language texts.
- Design a biomedical event detection model based on dependency analysis and graph convolutional network, through the sentence syntactic analysis, identify the grammar dependence between the words in the sentence, build dependent syntactic structure, using graph convolution neural network dependent graph convolution operation, and the dependency relationships between nodes in the dependency syntax graph are dynamically updated, effectively identify and classify the event trigger words in the sentence.
- Experiments are conducted on MLEE, a general dataset in the biomedical field, and the experimental results show that the proposed event detection model performs better than other models.

2   Related Work

The biomedical event detection examined in this paper is mainly about identifying the trigger word from the text and detecting its type. The existing biomedical event detection methods still have some difficulties, which require researchers to continuously explore and innovate. At present, the biomedical trigger word recognition methods mainly include: rule-based methods, traditional machine learning-based methods and deep learning-based methods. Rule-based methods mainly rely on manually formulated rules, which do not need the dataset to be labeled with labels, but their rules are generally defined for specific data sets, and have poor generalization ability. Methods based on traditional machine learning mainly rely on artificial design features to train traditional machine learning algorithms. Pyysalo et al. [5] input manually designed context-dependent features into the support vector machine SVM to complete biomedical event extraction. Zhou et al. [6] used the learned expertise in the external corpus as a feature embedding to train a multi-core classifier. He et al. [7] used SVM to combine complex features to enable two-stage biomedical event trigger word detection. Traditional machine learning methods require a lot of labor, are more complex, and have poor generalization ability. With the continuous development of deep learning technology, in order to solve the problems of complex artificial design rules and features and the lack of semantic information and features, deep learning methods based on word vector and neural network in traditional machine learning methods, and gradually become the mainstream method. Nie et al. [8] proposed based on the PubMed corpus training word vector-assisted neural network prediction model for biomedical event detection. Liu et al. [9] embedded the pre-trained words based on the NYT corpus into the auxiliary neural network prediction model for event detection. The above method is based on the specific field corpus training word embedding, and different from many fields general corpus, biomedical corpus has a large number of professional terms nouns (such as resistance, transcription), and these professional terms are easy to be understood by professional biomedical researchers, but not universal, so in the biomedical text mining task has no good training effect. Massive biomedical information contains a large amount of biomedical information of great scientific research value, and the performance of biomedical event detection model is very important in the task of biomedical event detection. Lee et al. [10] proposed that based on the study of biomedical events, they found that BERT (Bidirectional Encoder Representation from Transformers) pre-trained language model can be further optimized in biomedical events, and proposed that using BERT model for word vector training has achieved good results. The BioBERT model trained by the biomedical corpus PubMed (PubMed Abstracts) and PMC (PMC full-text articles) has a better effect on biomedical events than the BERT model. In this paper, we use the pre-trained word vector of BioBERT model based on training. Rahul et al. [11] proposed to extract complex features in sentences based on the recurrent neural network model, used for biomedical event detection. Li et al. [12] proposed a parallel multi-pooling convolutional neural network model for biomedical event extraction. Wang et al. [13] proposed a word embedding and deep learning model based on dependency analysis to improve the performance of the event detection task. Li et al. [14] proposed to use CNN (Convolutional Neural Networks) training character-level vector and word vector combination with large-scale background corpus training as input, and build BLSTM-CRF deep neural network model for biomedical event detection. Chen et al. [15] proposed the DMCNN model to using the improved convolutional neural network and improved the pooling layer to achieve two-stage event detection. Fei et al. [16] proposed a RecurNN-CRF model, which combined the dependency-tree based RNN with CRF layer using a recurrent neural network to globally represent the entire dependency tree to better integrate dependency-based syntax letters. Wei et al. [17] introduced a language model to dynamically calculate the word representation of the context, and proposed a multi-layer residual bidirectional long and short-time memory structure to detect biomedical events for the problem of labeled ambiguity in the biomedical corpus. All of the above research methods have important references, but the influence of dependence and long-distance dependence on event detection performance is not considered. This paper proposes to rely on dependency analytical and graph convolutional neural network modeling, it effectively solves the problem that recurrent neural network and convolutional network cannot obtain distant word information, further improves the detection performance in the biomedical event detection tasks.

3   Methods

This paper presents a biomedical event detection model based on dependent analytic and graph convolutional networks, integrate dependency syntactic information into a graph convolutional network, dynamic update dependency edge in graph convolution network, using the multi head attention perception enhance event information, strengthen the connection between events to complete biomedical event detection. As shown in Fig. 2, the event detection model proposed in this paper, the whole model is divided into five layers: sentence coding layer, BiLSTM layer, graph convolutional network layer based on dependency analysis, multi head attention layer and event classification layer.

3.1   Sentence Coding Layer

The sentence coding layer converts each word in a sentence into a real valued vector, which contains sentence semantic information and entity information. The sentence coding layer in this paper consists of pre-trained word embedding and entity type word embedding. First, each sentence is truncated to a fixed length L, and the blank part of the shorter sentence is filled by specific special characters. Then, the pre-trained word embedding corresponding to each word in the sentence is spliced with the entity type word embedding to obtain the representation of each word x_i. Therefore, a sentence will be represented as $\{x_1, x_2, \ldots, x_L\}$. In the sentence coding layer, in order to improve the expression ability of initial features, each word in the sentence is converted into a real value vector by splicing word embedding and entity type word embedding:

Word Embedding
At present, the most typical pre-trained language model is BERT [10], which uses bidirectional transformer for coding, and comprehensively considers context features when predicting words. BERT has achieved good optimization results on some general domain corpora, but cannot achieve higher performance for specific specialized words in the biomedical field. This paper uses the pre-trained language model BioBERT for the biomedical field, which assigns trigger word labels to each word in the sentence using the BIO label method. In the sentence encoding layer, the BioBERT pre-trained model is used to convert the input sentence into a fixed length embedding representation e_i.

Entity Type Embedding
Event trigger words are verbs or gerund connecting entities in text. In biomedical text, a word is a trigger word in a specific sentence, and may be part of an entity in another sentence. The presence of entities and their corresponding entity types in sentences may affect the detection of trigger words. Therefore, this paper introduces entity type embedding in the sentence encoding layer, annotates the entities mentioned in the sentence

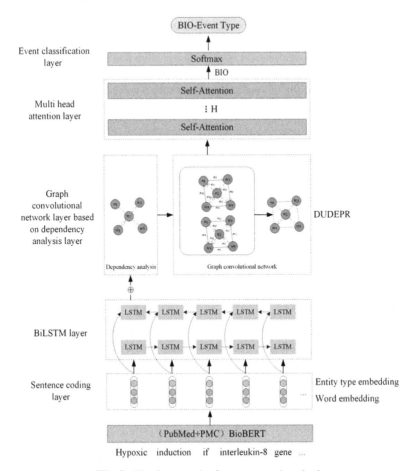

Fig. 2. The framework of our proposed method

using BIO label method, and maps the type information of each word (such as PER (person name), LOC (location), ORG (organization)) to a low dimensional vector matrix to obtain an oriented quantization representation. As the model is trained and updated, we define it as the entity vector representation of the word v_i.

3.2 BiLSTM Layer

Long short-term memory is a special structured recurrent neural network. By controlling the long-term information in the recording sequence through input gates, forgetting gates, and output gates, the problem of long-term dependence in RNN is solved. In order to capture the long distance context information of a sentence, this paper uses bidirectional long short term memory neural network to extract sentence level features. Specifically, it involves encoding and analyzing the word features x_t obtained from the sentence encoding layer at time t, concatenating the forward LSTM hidden layer vector representation $\overrightarrow{h_t}$ with the reverse LSTM hidden layer vector representation

$\overleftarrow{h_t}$ to obtain the final output h_t, and then obtaining the hidden state representation of sequences incorporating context information, as shown in (1–3):

$$\overrightarrow{h_t} = \overrightarrow{LSTM}(x_t) \tag{1}$$

$$\overleftarrow{h_t} = \overleftarrow{LSTM}(x_t) \tag{2}$$

$$h_t = [\overrightarrow{h_t}, \overleftarrow{h_t}] \tag{3}$$

3.3 Graph Convolutional Network Layer Based on Dependency Analysis

Construction of the Dependency Analysis Graph
Dependency syntactic parsing, also known as dependency analysis, can identify and determine the interdependence between various components in a sentence, analyze the grammatical structure of the sentence. Different dependency structures may have significant semantic differences. Therefore, dependency syntax can better understand sentences and improve the precision of tasks such as event detection. The dependency syntactic structure graph represents the syntactic dependency relation of a sentence as a directed graph, where the directed arc represents the grammatical dependency relation between words. The graph convolution operation of the word can focus on the word most related to the current word, avoiding the modeling of unrelated sequences.

This paper uses the Stanford-CoreNLP dependency parser to obtain the dependency syntactic structure of each sentence, and then takes the word representation obtained from the upper layer as the node, and represents the dependency as the connection between each node. For example, the dependency syntactic structure of sentence w can be obtained as shown in Fig. 3. Where, the word "mediated" is the root word (root) the root word does not depend on other words, other words are directly dependent on one word or more words in the sentence. The sentence W contains "Positive_regulation" events triggered by "induction", "Gene_expression" events triggered by "expression", and "Regulation" events triggered by "mediated".

W: Hypoxic induction of HIF-1alpha and VEGF expression in head and neck squamous cell carcinoma lines is mediated by stress activated protein kinases.

Let graph $G = \{V, E\}$ be the syntactic dependency structure of sentence w, where V is the node set $V = \{w_1, w_2, \ldots, w_n\}$ of graph G, w_i represents the ith node in set V, E represents the edge set of graph G, and each directed edge (w_i, w_j) in set E represents a directed edge from the head node $(head)w_i$ to the dependent node $dep(w_j)$, and the attribute of the edge is $L(w_i, w_j)$, and the attribute of the edge is the dependency label. For example, in the syntactic dependency structure diagram of sentence W, there is a directed edge from the initial node w_i = "induction" to the dependent node w_j = "Hypoxic", the directed edge attribute $L(w_i, w_j) = L("induction", "Hypoxic") = $ amod, and amod represents adjective modifier. The trigger word "induction" and trigger word "mediated" are associated through syntactic dependency structure to form a event "Regulation", and the dependency type of trigger word "induction" and trigger word "mediated" is

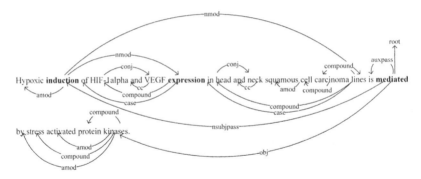

Fig. 3. Dependency syntactic structure graph example

L("induction", "mediated") = nsubjpass. Therefore, dependency syntactic structures and dependency types can provide important information for event detection.

Graph Convolutional Neural Network Updated by Syntactic Edges
Graph convolution network [3] is a method that can directly perform convolution operation on graph data. Graph convolutional neural network updated by syntactic edges first convolutes node feature vectors according to the attribute feature information of neighbor nodes, and aggregates the information from the neighbor nodes together. In each layer, each node transmits information to its neighbor nodes along the edges in the graph. Dependency parsing can explain the relation between different words and phrases in a sentence. The different dependency structures may have large semantic differences. The dependency label information of this type is merged into the feature aggregation process to obtain a better representation. Then, according to the context representation of each node in the sentence, this paper dynamically updates the dependency representation between nodes in the syntactic dependency structure graph, combines the semantic information of the context and the syntactic structure relation, so as to obtain the dynamic syntactic dependency edge. For each node u in the graph, the calculation equation at the $k + 1(k \geq 0)$ level is:

$$(H^{k+1}, E^{k+1}) = \text{DUDEPR\_GCN}(H^k, E^k) \tag{4}$$

$$E_{i,j}^{k+1} = \text{DUDEPR}(E_{i,j}^k, H_i^k, H_j^k) = W_u(E_{i,j}^k \oplus H_i^k \oplus H_j^k), i, j \in [1, n] \tag{5}$$

$$H_u^{k+1} = \text{ReLU}(\sum_{v \in N(u)} W_{L(u,v)}^k H_v^k + b_{L(u,v)}^k) \tag{6}$$

where ReLU is a non-linear activation function; $E^k \in R^{n \times d}$ is the node representation output for the layer k. DUDEPR is a dynamic update node dependency module, H_i^k represents the node representation of the node i in layer k, H_j^k represents the node representation of the node j in layer k, Wu is a learnable transfer matrix, $L(u, v)$ is the dependency type passing between DUDEPR module node u and node v, dependency type updates with the dependent edge, $W_{L(u,v)}^k$ and $b_{L(u,v)}^k$ are the weight matrix and the deviation, respectively.

3.4 Multi Head Attention Perception Layer

In order to fully mine the context information in sentences, this paper uses multi head attention perception. The input of multi head attention is three same vector matrices: *Q(Query)*, *K(Key)* and *V(Value)*. First, perform linear transformation on *Q*, *K*, and *V* respectively, and then calculate the scaled dot product attention. The calculation equation is as follows:

$$\text{Attention}(Q, K, V) = \text{softmax}(\frac{QK^T}{\sqrt{d_w}})V \tag{7}$$

where, d_w represents the dimension of the key, which is the sequence of word vectors of the input sentence. Scaling the point product attention combined with the linear transformation needs to be calculated h times, one head at a time, and is calculated in parallel, so that the model can learn relevant information in different subspaces. Multi-head attention is calculated as shown in (8) and (9):

$$head_i = \text{Attention}(QW_i^Q, KW_i^K, VW_i^V) \tag{8}$$

$$\text{MUH}(Q, K, V) = (head_1 \oplus head_2 \oplus \cdots \oplus head_h)W^o \tag{9}$$

where $W_i^Q \in R^{d_w/h \times d_w}$, $W_i^K \in R^{d_w/h \times d_w}$, and $W_i^V \in R^{d_w/h \times d_w}$ are respectively the weight parameter matrix of different parameters to be trained, $W^o \in R^{d_w \times d_w}$ is the linear transformation matrix. The *h* head corresponds to the *h* dimensions, and each dimension is an embedding.

3.5 Event Classification Layer

The output of the multi head attention perception layer is input to a full connection layer, and then the softmax network is used to complete the classification prediction of the last event, and the credibility of each event type is output. The BIO lable method is used to label each trigger word in the sentence. "B-" indicates the starting position of the trigger word, "I-" indicates the middle or rear position of the trigger word of this type, and "O" indicates that it is not a trigger word.

$$y_{t_i} = \text{softmax}(W_t M_i + b_t) \tag{10}$$

where, y_{t_i} is the final prediction output of the ith token, softmax function often used for multiple classification tasks, represent the probability that a certain element is taken, $M_i \in R^d$ represents the probability of an element being taken, represents the output representation of the ith token in the multi head attention layer, *d* represents the node dimension, and the loss function of the model is the cross entropy loss function.

4 Experiment

4.1 Dataset

In this paper, we use Pyysalo [5] to organize the labeled dataset MLEE to study the whole trigger word recognition task. The MLEE dataset contains medical noun events from the molecular level to all levels of biological individuals, and its annotation method is also based on the BioNLP Shared Task. The overview of MLEE corpus data is shown in Table 1.

Table 1. Data overview of the MLEE corpus

Type	Train+Dev	Test	Toal
Document	175	87	262
Sentences	1749	878	2627
Event	4471	2206	6677

4.2 Experimental Parameter Setting and Evaluation Indicators

In the experiment, the deep learning framework was used as pytorch [18], and the Stanford-CoreNLP toolkit was used to preprocess the experimental data for dependency resolution and entity type annotation. The hidden dimension of BioBERT pre-trained word embedding was 768 dimensions, and the dimension of entity type word vector was 25 dimensions. One layer of BiLSTM, hidden dimension was 100 dimensions, two layers of GCN, output dimension was 150 dimensions. The model optimizer was Adam [19] optimization algorithm, we set the dropout of BiLSTM and GCN to 0.5 and the learning rate is set to 1e−3 from {0.1, 0.01, 1e−3, 1e−4, 1e−5}. The specific experimental parameter settings are shown in Table 2.

In this paper, $P(Precision)$, $R(Recall)$, and $F1$ score are used as model performance evaluation indicators, calculated as (11).

$$P = \frac{TP}{TP + FP} \times 100\% \quad R = \frac{TP}{TP + FN} \times 100\% \quad F1 = \frac{2 \times P \times R}{P + R} \times 100\%$$

$$(11)$$

4.3 Experimental Results and Analysis

Biomedical Events Detection Results

The performance of the biomedical event detection method based on dependency analysis and graph convolution neural network proposed in this paper is compared with other advanced event detection methods. The performance of each method on the event detection task is shown in Table 3.

Table 2. Experimental parameter setting

Parameter	Value
BioBERT word embedding	768 dim
Entity type embedding	25 dim
BiLSTM	$(2\times)100$ dim
GCN	$(2\times)150$ dim
Dropout	0.5
Learning Rate	1e$-$3
Batch size	16
Optimizer	Adam
Label Schema	BIO

- Pyysalo et al. [5] proposed an SVM model connecting context and dependency features.
- Zhou et al. [6] proposed an SVM classifier model with word embedding and hand-made features.
- Rahul et al. [11] proposed an embedded biomedical event detection model that excludes dependent information and considers only words and entity types.
- Wei et al. [17] introduced a language model for dynamically calculating the expression of upper and lower cultural words, and proposed a multi-layer residual bidirectional long-term and short-term memory architecture.
- Li et al. [20] proposed that the gating polarity attention mechanism explicitly applies dependent representation learning and triple context representation learning to biomedical event detection tasks.
- Wang et al. [21] introduced an attention mechanism into Child-Sum Tree-LSTMs for the detection of biomedical event triggers.

Table 3. Performance comparison of event detection methods

Method	P (%)	R (%)	F1 (%)
Pyysalo et al. [5]	70.79	81.69	75.84
Zhou et al. [6]	75.35	81.60	78.32
Nie et al. [8]	71.04	84.60	77.23
Rahul et al. [11]	79.78	78.45	79.11
Wei et al. [17]	79.89	81.61	80.74
Li et al. [20]	81.95	81.31	81.63
Wang et al. [21]	**83.24**	80.90	82.05
Proposed	81.67	**85.09**	**83.35**

As shown in Table 3, it can be seen that the model in this paper achieved a competitive performance of 83.35% of $F1$ score under the architecture based on dependency analysis and graph convolutional network. Compared with Pyysalo et al. [5] and Zhou et al. [6] manual feature extraction methods, our model avoids any manual participation in Feature Engineering, which saves the time and labor costs associated with data processing and feature selection. Compared with Nie et al. [8] who used skip gram to generate word embedding to optimize the performance of neural network, we used BioBERT pre-trained word embedding to effectively extract biomedical event features and obtain more sufficient context information. In this paper, the Stanford-CoreNLP toolkit is used to build dependencies. Compared with Rahul et al. [11], considering word embedding in the event detection task, $F1$ score is improved by 5.14%. Compared with literature [20], which also adopts dependency relation, this paper uses a combination of bidirectional long short term memory network to obtain context information, graph convolution network to model the syntactic dependency relation of sentences, capture the long-distance dependency relation in sentences, and achieve better performance. $F1$ scores are increased 1.72%, dependency analysis has a good impact on the precision of the detection of event triggered words in sentences. Compared with the residual bidirectional long short term memory sequence modeling method proposed by Wei et al. [17] and the an attention mechanism into Child-Sum Tree-LSTMs method proposed by Wang et al. [21], the graph convolution network model has achieved better performance in capturing long-distance dependence, and the $F1$ score has increased by 2.61% and 1.30% respectively. The experimental results show that the performance of the model can be better improved by using the graph convolutional network and dependency syntax structure based on BioBERT word embedding combined with entity type embedding and BiLSTM combined with dynamic updating dependency.

4.4 Ablation Experiments

In this paper, ablation experiments were carried out on MLEE dataset to verify the effectiveness of each method. In this paper, Embedding+BiLSTM+GCN was used as the baseline model, and dependency label (DEPL) module, dynamic update dependency relation(DUDEPR) module and multi head attention perception (MUH) module were added on the basis of the baseline model. The experimental results are shown in Table 4. Compared with the baseline model, adding dependency label increased $F1$ score by 0.83%; Dependency syntactic information expresses the hierarchical syntactic relation between words in a sentence. Dependency labels can provide sufficient information for event detection. Graph convolutional neural network can effectively model sentences. The dependency label module and the dynamic update dependency module were introduced, and the $F1$ score increased by 1.77%, indicating that the dynamic update dependency representation can dynamically integrate contextual semantic information and syntactic information effectively. Adding the dependency label (DEPL) module, the dynamic update dependency relation (DUDEPR) module and the multi head attention perception (MUH) module, the $F1$ score increased by 2.33%, indicating that the multi head attention perception can more fully capture the connection between trigger words in sentences, enhance the event information, and obtain a more focused event representation after the graph convolutional network modeling.

Table 4. Performance comparison for each method

Method	$F1$ (%)
Embedding+BiLSTM+GCN	81.02
Embedding+BiLSTM+DEPL+GCN	81.85
Embedding+BiLSTM+DEPL+GCN+DUDEPR	82.79
Embedding+BiLSTM+DEPL+GCN+DUDEPR+MUH	**83.35**

5 Conclusion

In this paper, a biomedical event detection model based on dependency analysis and graph convolution network is proposed. Firstly, we splice BioBERT word embedding and entity type embeddings to encode the text sentence. The BiLSTM is used to obtain a more sufficient context representation, and then the syntactic dependency structure graph is obtained through dependency analysis, the GCN is modeled on this basis by incorporating the dependency label information into the feature aggregation process. During the training process, the syntactic dependency edges are dynamically updated to effectively enrich the extracted feature information and overcome the long-distance dependency problem in the trigger word detection process. After that, multi head attention perception is used to strengthen the connection between events for each word in the sentence. Finally, the event detection is carried out through the fully connected classification network. The proposed method has achieved excellent performance on the generic biomedical event detection corpus MLEE.

Although our proposed model has achieved good results in biomedical event tasks, research has found that the performance of the model depends on the understanding of context semantics. In future research, we will focus on the direct use of dependencies, rely on syntactic relationships to directly train dependency word embedding, and the sparsity of dependency labels also affects the performance of the model.

Acknowledgement. This work is supported by the National Natural Science Foundation of China (No. 62006108, 61976109), Postdoctoral Research Foundation of China (No. 2022M710593), Liaoning Province General Higher Education Undergraduate Teaching Reform Research Project (Liaoning Education Office [2022] No. 160), The Ministry of Education's Industry School Cooperation Collaborative Education Project (220802755304633), Liaoning Normal University Undergraduate Teaching Reform Research and Practice Project (No. LSJG202210).

References

1. Mikolov, T., Sutskever, I., Chen, K., Corrado, G., Dean, J.: Distributed representations of words and phrases and their compositionality. In: Proceedings of the 26th International Conference on Neural Information Processing Systems - Volume 2 (NIPS 2013), pp. 3111–3119. Curran Associates Inc. Red Hook (2013)
2. Lee, J., et al.: BioBERT: a pre-trained biomedical language representation model for biomedical text mining. Bioinformatics **36**(4), 1234–1240 (2020)

3. Kipf, T.N., Welling, M.: Semi-Supervised classification with graph convolutional networks. Neural. Process. Lett. **54**(4), 2645–2656 (2022)

4. Vaswani, A., et al.: Attention is all you need. In: Proceedings of the 31st International Conference on Neural Information Processing Systems (NIPS 2017), pp. 6000–6010. Curran Associates Inc., Red Hook (2017)

5. Pyysalo, S., Ohta, T., Miwa, M., Cho, H.-C., Tsujii, J., Ananiadou, S.: Event extraction across multiple levels of biological organization. Bioinformatics **28**(18), 575–581 (2012). https://doi.org/10.1093/bioinformatics/bts407

6. Zhou, D., Zhong, D., He, Y.: Event trigger identification for biomedical events extraction using domain knowledge. Bioinformatics **30**(11), 1587–1594 (2014). https://doi.org/10.1093/bioinformatics/btu061

7. He, X., Li, L., Liu, Y., Yu, X., Meng, J.: A two-stage biomedical event trigger detection method integrating feature selection and word embeddings. J. IEEE/ACM Trans. Comput. Biol. Bioinform. **15**(4), 1325–1332 (2017)

8. Nie, Y., Rong, W., Zhang, Y., Ouyang, Y., Zhang, X.: Embedding assisted prediction architecture for event trigger identification. J. Bioinform. Comput. Biol. **13**(03), 575–577 (2015)

9. Liu, S., Chen, Y., He, S., Liu, K., Zhao, J.: Leveraging framenet to improve automatic event detection. In: Proceedings of the 54th Annual Meeting of the Association for Computational Linguistics (Volume 1: Long Papers), pp. 2134–2143. Association for Computational Linguistics, Berlin (2016). https://doi.org/10.18653/v1/P16-1201

10. Devlin, J., Chang, M.-W., Lee, K., Toutanova, K.: BERT: pre-training of deep bidirectional transformers for language understanding. In: Proceedings of the 2019 Conference of the North American Chapter of the Association for Computational Linguistics: Human Language Technologies, Volume 1 (Long and Short Papers), pp. 4171–4186. Association for Computational Linguistics, Minneapolis (2019)

11. Rahul, P.V.S.S.S., Sahu, K., Ashish, A.: Biomedical event trigger identification using bidirectional recurrent neural network based models. In: BioNLP 2017, pp. 316–321. Association for Computational Linguistics, Vancouver (2017)

12. Li, L., Liu, Y.: Exploiting argument information to improve biomedical event trigger identification via recurrent neural networks and supervised attention mechanisms. In: 2017 IEEE International Conference on Bioinformatics and Biomedicine (BIBM), Kansas City, MO, USA, pp. 565–568 (2017). https://doi.org/10.1109/BIBM.2017.8217711

13. Wang, J., et al.: Biomedical event trigger detection by dependency-based word embedding. In: 2015 IEEE International Conference on Bioinformatics and Biomedicine (BIBM), Washington, DC, pp. 429–432 (2015). https://doi.org/10.1109/BIBM.2015.7359721

14. Li, L., Yang, L., Qin, M.: Extracting biomedical events with parallel multi-pooling convolutional neural networks. IEEE/ACM Trans. Comput. Biol. Bioinformatics **17**(2), 599–607 (2020). https://doi.org/10.1109/TCBB.2018.2868078

15. Chen, Y., Xu, L., Liu, K., Zeng, D., Zhao, J.: Event extraction via dynamic multi-pooling convolutional neural networks. In: Proceedings of the 53rd Annual Meeting of the Association for Computational Linguistics and the 7th International Joint Conference on Natural Language Processing (Volume 1: Long Papers), pp. 167–176 (2015)

16. Fei, H., Ren, Y., Ji, D.: A tree-based neural network model for biomedical event trigger detection. Inf. Sci. **512**, 175–185 (2020)

17. Wei, H., Zhou, A., Zhang, Y., Chen, F., Lu, M.: Biomedical event trigger extraction based on multi-layer residual BiLSTM and contextualized word representations. Int. J. Mach. Learn. Cyber. **13**, 721–733 (2022). https://doi.org/10.1007/s13042-021-01315-7

18. Ketkar, N.: Introduction to pytorch. In: Deep Learning with Python, pp. 195–208. Apress, Berkeley (2017)

19. Kingma, D., Ba, J.: Adam: a method for stochastic optimization. In: Computer Science (2014)
20. Li, L., Zhang, B.: Exploiting dependency information to improve biomedical event detection via gated polar attention mechanism. Neurocomputing **421**(7), 210–221 (2021)
21. Wang, L., Cao, H., Yuan, L., Yuan, L., Guo, X., Cui, Y.: Child-sum EATree-LSTMs: enhanced attentive child-sum tree-LSTMs for biomedical event extraction. BMC Bioinform. **24**, 253 (2023). https://doi.org/10.1186/s12859-023-05336-7

Research on the Structuring of Electronic Medical Records Based on Joint Extraction Using BART

Yu Song[1], Pengcheng Wu[1], Chenxin Hu[2], Kunli Zhang[1(✉)], Dongming Dai[1], Hongyang Chang[3], and Chenkang Zhu[1]

[1] College of Computer and Artificial Intelligence, Zhengzhou University, Zhengzhou, China
{ieysong,ieklzhang}@zzu.edu.cn, pcwu2022@gs.zzu.edu.cn
[2] Henan Cancer Hospital/Affiliated Cancer Hospital of Zhengzhou University, Zhengzhou 450003, China
[3] Unit 63893 of the People's Liberation Army, Luoyang 471000, China

Abstract. Medical institutions commonly utilize electronic medical records (EMRs) to document patients' medical conditions, which contain invaluable medical information. However, EMRs often consist of semi-structured or unstructured data, posing significant challenges in processing and analysis. In this paper, addressing the requirements for subsequent tasks such as clinical decision-making, we present the process of structuring EMRs, focusing on lung cancer EMRs. This process encompasses EMR structure analysis, data preprocessing, information extraction, and data integration. Notably, entity and entity relationship extraction are pivotal steps in this workflow. To accomplish this, we employ a joint extraction model using BART for information extraction tasks in lung cancer EMRs. When compared to existing models, our model achieves an F1 score of 64.86%. Furthermore, we validate the model's generalization capability by conducting experiments on a pediatric epilepsy dataset, ultimately achieving the structuring of EMRs tailored to the requirements of subsequent tasks.

Keywords: Electronic Medical Records · Lung Cancer · Structured · Entity Relationship Extraction

1 Introduction

Lung cancer is one of the most prevalent and deadliest malignancies worldwide, with an overall five-year survival rate relatively lower than many other major cancers. Early diagnosis and prognosis of lung cancer are crucial for improving patient survival rates. Although artificial intelligence has found wide applications in clinical assistance for lung cancer, the complete process, from medical record documentation to diagnostic support, still presents numerous challenges. Efficiently organizing and utilizing existing information related to lung cancer, rapidly and accurately extracting valuable information from these vast datasets, and uncovering new knowledge will greatly advance medical research and lead to significant breakthroughs.

H. Xu et al. (Eds.): CHIP 2023, CCIS 1993, pp. 212–226, 2024.
https://doi.org/10.1007/978-981-99-9864-7_14

EMRs document detailed patient medical histories and professional diagnoses by healthcare providers, making them a vital and primary source of reference in clinical diagnostics. This has positioned EMRs as a crucial resource for the analysis of large-scale health data. Within these records, the quantity of semi-structured and unstructured data significantly outweighs structured data, yet they contain a wealth of valuable medical knowledge. The challenge lies in processing and making use of this semi-structured or unstructured data, as it presents a more complex task but holds great potential for improving diagnostic accuracy. Therefore, the importance of the task of structuring EMRs is becoming increasingly urgent.

In this study, we use lung cancer EMRs as a case study to illustrate the process of structuring EMRs. The primary steps encompass data collection, data preprocessing, data annotation, joint extraction of entities and entity relationships, and data integration. In the entity and entity relationship extraction segment, we validate the method's generalizability using a pediatric epilepsy EMRs dataset.

2 Related Work

2.1 BART

BERT [1] has demonstrated exceptional performance in natural language understanding tasks by providing bidirectional context representation. However, it is not directly applicable to generative tasks. On the other hand, GPT [2] has showcased the effectiveness of attention mechanisms within an autoregressive structure for sequence generation tasks. Nevertheless, due to differences between its pre-training objective and discriminative task objectives, along with its autoregressive nature, GPT exhibits limited performance in discriminative tasks.

BART (Bidirectional and Auto-Regressive Transformers) is a generative pre-trained model based on the Transformer architecture, introduced by Facebook AI in 2019 [3]. BART amalgamates the characteristics of autoregressive and bidirectional encoding, endowing it with robust text generation and comprehension capabilities. Unlike traditional autoregressive models, BART employs a Masked Language Model for pre-training. During the pre-training phase, it masks and perturbs input text, enabling the model to acquire more generalized representations, while simultaneously facilitating bidirectional text generation (Fig. 1).

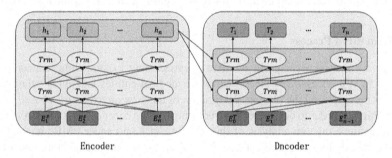

Encoder   Dncoder

Fig. 1. BART model structure diagram

2.2 Electronic Medical Record Structuring

EMR structuring currently has two mainstream solutions: pre-structuring and post-structuring. The pre-structuring method, initially employed in the medical field, rigorously constrains data format during the data collection process. However, its drawback lies in the requirement for healthcare professionals to input data in prescribed formats, which may not align with their habitual clinical note-taking practices. As a result, post-structuring methods have gradually become the focus of contemporary research. These methods predominantly entail the post-collection structuring of data in the background, employing machine learning and deep learning techniques.

Zeng et al. [4] introduced a named entity recognition approach that integrates an attention mechanism with BiLSTM-CRF, which achieved promising results on the CCKS2018 dataset. With the widespread adoption of pre-trained models, Zhang et al. [5] successfully applied BERT-BiLSTM-CRF to Chinese EMRs for named entity recognition, outperforming baseline models on the CCKS2017 dataset.Huang et al. [6] proposed a representation method for medical text based on XLNet, effectively harnessing sequential information within EMR texts, thereby accomplishing modeling within the medical text domain. Chang et al. [7] conducted comprehensive research and improvements based on the existing CasREL framework. They specifically addressed two prominent issues in Chinese medical texts, namely, entity overlap and the relatively higher average triplet count in single-sentence corpora. This endeavor resulted in significant performance enhancements.

3 Analysis and Construction of a Lung Cancer Electronic Medical Record Dataset

The acquisition of EMRs for lung cancer typically encompasses a wide range of data types, with semi-structured data comprising the majority, and also includes some structured information. These structured data effectively enhance the accuracy of information extraction. In addition to structured data, EMRs contain a substantial amount of unstructured data, such as free text. However, this unstructured data inevitably contains errors and redundant information. Therefore, for existing EMR documents, conducting structured analysis and data organization becomes of paramount importance. This process aims to clearly define data elements, thereby improving data usability and quality, providing a more reliable foundation for subsequent research and clinical practice.

3.1 Structured Process

The primary task in structuring involves preprocessing existing lung cancer EMRs. Subsequently, it necessitates the extraction of medical entities and entity relationships from these records and the ultimate integration of these extracted entities based on their relationships, in order to complete the structuring of lung cancer electronic health record data. To achieve this, an analysis of the structure of lung cancer EMRs is conducted, and specific labeling standards are devised. Both automatic pre-labeling and manual labeling are employed, involving the participation of specialized medical professionals and graduate students. These individuals carried out three rounds of labeling and quality reviews for 200 lung cancer cases. Following the labeling, the data is subjected to joint extraction experiments and then applied to unlabeled data before being integrated. The specific workflow of this entire process is illustrated in the diagram below (Fig. 2).

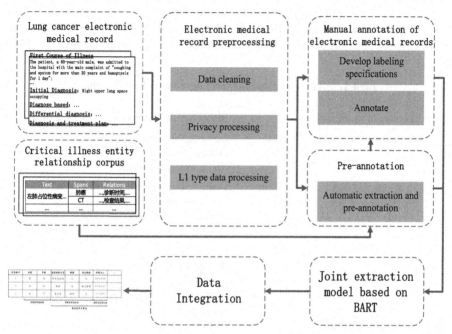

Fig. 2. Lung cancer electronic medical record structured flow chart

3.2   Structural Analysis of Lung Cancer Electronic Medical Records

Presently, the documentation of EMRs in China primarily adheres to the "Basic Standards for Electronic Health Records (Trial)" [8], which were issued in 2010, serving as the fundamental guiding principles. The documentation centers around the patient and is typically presented in the form of free text. In this section, we aim to analyze and describe the basic structure and characteristics of real lung cancer EMRs, which have been collected for the purpose of this research. Specifically, we will delve into the writing features and data organization methods of lung cancer EMRs using the key elements outlined in Table 1.

Given the research objective for downstream clinical tasks, and following surveys and consultations with expert physicians, four semi-structured and structured sections of lung cancer EMRs have been selected. These primarily include admission records, initial course records, and discharge records. In this section, the data from these EMRs will undergo structural analysis, attribute delineation, and data preprocessing.

The purpose of attribute delineation is to clarify the data hierarchy and employ different medical record text structuring strategies based on these hierarchies. Data hierarchies are categorized into two levels: L1 and L2. L1 refers to original information that is structured and can be accurately extracted through mapping or filtering of specific fields. L2 denotes original information embedded in extensive text and cannot be accurately extracted using rule-based methods; instead, deep learning methods are needed for field extraction.

Through an in-depth analysis of the existing EMR data, we have summarized the primary structure and attribute delineation of lung cancer EMRs. These filtered datasets will facilitate more precise subsequent research in clinical decision support.

Table 1. Analysis and description of lung cancer EMR structure

Main structure of medical records		Main content description	Attribute division
admission record	Allergy history	Describe the patient's history of drug, food, or environmental allergies	L1
	Chief complaint	Describe the patient's self-reported reason for admission and description of symptoms	L2
	History of present illness	A detailed narrative describing the patient's current condition and progression of symptoms	L2
	Past history	Describe the patient's past illness, examination, and treatment history	L1, L2
	Personal history	Describe the patient's personal information such as lifestyle, diet, and hobbies	L1
	Marriage and childbearing history	Records describing marital status and parenthood	L1
	Family history	Describe the genetic and disease history associated with family members	L1
	Physical examination	Describe a doctor's detailed examination of a patient's physical condition	L1

(*continued*)

Table 1. (*continued*)

Main structure of medical records		Main content description	Attribute division
	Specialist examination	Describes a professional examination and evaluation by a physician in a specific field	L1
	Auxiliary inspection	Describe laboratory, imaging and other auxiliary diagnostic results	L2
	Initial diagnosis	Describe the doctor's tentative diagnosis based on the patient's information	L1
first course of illness	Admission status	Describe the description of the patient's symptoms and signs on admission	L2
	Discussion of proposed diagnosis	The medical team initially discusses the patient's possible diagnosis	L2
	Diagnosis and treatment plan	Treatment plans and plans developed by your doctor	L1
Discharge records	Admission status	Describe the description of the patient's symptoms and signs on admission	L2
	Admission diagnosis	Describe the doctor's tentative diagnosis based on the patient's information	L1
	Diagnosis and treatment process	A detailed description of the treatment and care the patient received in the hospital	L2
	Discharge diagnosis	The patient's final diagnosis or physician's assessment at discharge	L1
	Discharge status	The patient's general health status and recommendations at discharge	L1

(*continued*)

Table 1. (continued)

Main structure of medical records		Main content description	Attribute division
	Discharge Instructions	Treatment and life advice provided by doctors to patients after discharge	L1

The above table provides a brief overview of the primary structure and content of the studied lung cancer EMRs. Through our analysis, it has become evident that the crucial aspects in need of structuring within lung cancer EMRs include disease and symptoms, examination events, treatment events, and diagnostic events:

Disease and Symptoms. "Disease" refers to disruptions in the patient's physiological regulation, resulting in abnormal states or disturbances in essential life processes. "Symptoms" encompass the discomfort or abnormal reactions observed within the patient's body, as well as unusual conditions detected through examinations. Notably, ICD-11 lacks a specific classification for symptoms, thus necessitating the utilization of the Chinese symptom knowledge base [9] and "Diagnostics" to ascertain symptom entities during the annotation process. These symptom entities primarily encompass statements made by the patient, family members, or other proxies regarding abnormal conditions. Additionally, they encompass abnormal physiological conditions identified by medical practitioners through observations, inquiries, palpations, and medical imaging procedures. Specific examples are provided below:

- **Chest and back pain** for more than 1 year, and **lung cancer** diagnosed for more than 1 year.
- Two months ago, the patient suddenly developed **cough** and **sputum** without obvious inducement.

Check Event. Examinations encompass specific procedural investigations or the utilization of pertinent instruments to identify or confirm diseases and symptoms, aiding physicians in diagnosing the patient's condition. Within the realm of EMRs concerning lung cancer, commonly encountered examination entities comprise radiological examinations, pathological examinations, immunohistochemical examinations, tumor marker examinations, and routine blood examinations. In the process of record structuring, examinations manifest frequently within both the present medical history and past medical history, carrying significant implications for the physician's diagnostic process. Consequently, the accurate extraction of examination events stands as a pressing concern in medical record structuring. Specific examples are elaborated below:

- A cervical and **chest CT** performed on *** on July 10, 2020 showed: 1. **Multiple enlarged lymph nodes on the left side of the neck** 2. **Massive soft tissue shadows in the basal segment of the lower lobe of the right lung.** Enhanced scanning is recommended for further examination 3. **Multiple nodules in both lungs section**, short-term follow-up is recommended 4. **Multiple enlarged lymph nodes in the**

mediastinum 5. Calcification of the aortic wall and coronary artery, mitral valve calcification 6. **Multiple enlarged lymph nodes in the left armpit** 7. **Cystic low-density lesions in the left lobe of the liver**, please combine Ultrasonography.

Treatment Event. Treatment encompasses therapeutic procedures, medication administration, and intervention measures aimed at improving physiological regulation, addressing underlying causes, or alleviating symptoms. It is typically classified into pharmacological treatment, surgical treatment, and other modalities based on the mode of therapy. In the course of treating lung cancer patients, the primary modalities revolve around medication and chemotherapy, involving treatment cycles and precise timing for initiation and cessation of treatment. Consequently, within the ambit of structuring tasks, the accurate extraction of treatment entities and delineation of treatment cycles hold paramount significance.

– **One cycle** of chemotherapy with the "**pemetrexed + carboplatin**" regimen was given on July 25, 2020.
– The "**nab-paclitaxel + carboplatin + tislelizumab**" regimen was used for **4 cycles** of chemotherapy.

Diagnostic Event. Diagnosis encompasses a comprehensive process involving the collection and analysis of diverse patient information, such as clinical manifestations, medical history, laboratory tests, and imaging examinations, among others. This process aims to determine the disease type, disease status, etiology, prognosis, and subsequently formulate appropriate treatment plans. Within tumor diagnosis, the TNM staging of cancer stands as a critical diagnostic outcome significantly emphasized by physicians. In accordance with the TNM staging method advocated by the Union for International Cancer Control (UICC), the **T** parameter delineates the size and extent of the primary tumor, the **N** parameter evaluates whether the tumor has spread to lymph nodes, providing insights into the extent of lymph node involvement, while the **M** parameter ascertains whether the cancer has metastasized to other parts of the body, indicating distant metastasis. The TNM staging within the diagnostic section holds pivotal clinical significance in lung cancer diagnosis, assisting physicians in crafting treatment strategies, predicting patient prognosis, and establishing a foundational framework for clinical research.

- Preliminary diagnosis: 1. Primary right lung squamous cell carcinoma cT4N2M0 stage IIIB PD-L1 (22C3 positive 1%) (SP263 positive 1%) EGFR gene (-), ALK (-).

3.3 Lung Cancer Electronic Medical Record Data Preprocessing

In general, data retrieved from hospital EMRs databases display characteristics such as diversity, incompleteness, and redundancy. These attributes notably influence the final application performance and represent a vital aspect of EMRs structuring. Hence, preprocessing of EMR data is imperative to guarantee accuracy, completeness, consistency, and the preservation of patient privacy. The data preprocessing process involves procedures such as data cleansing, privacy protection, and handling of L1-type data to elevate data quality and enhance usability.

Data Cleaning. Due to the templated and repetitive nature of EMR documentation, the data concerning physical examinations, specialized examinations, auxiliary examinations, etc., recorded in the patient's admission record, are also presented in the discharge record when the patient is discharged. This redundancy in data is not beneficial for named entity recognition and subsequent structuring tasks in EMR; instead, it adds to the annotation workload. Therefore, it is essential to eliminate redundant information before efficient structuring to avoid unnecessary extraction efforts. In this paper, initially, using the cosine similarity measurement algorithm, the text similarity between the initial course text and the specialized examination section of the admission record was calculated to be 93.06%, as seen in Formula (1).

$$\cos\alpha = \frac{\sum_{i=1}^{k} f_{A_i} \cdot f_{B_i}}{\sqrt{\sum_{i=1}^{k} \left(f_{A_i}\right)^2} \cdot \sqrt{\sum_{i=1}^{k} \left(f_{B_i}\right)^2}} \tag{1}$$

where $F(A) = \left[f_{A_1}, f_{A_2}, \cdots, f_{A_k}\right]$ and $F(B) = \left[f_{B_1}, f_{B_2}, \cdots, f_{B_k}\right]$ employ word frequencies extracted from the text as feature values. These values are then vectorized to derive vectors $\overrightarrow{A} = \left(f_{A_1}, f_{A_2}, \cdots, f_{A_k}\right)$ and $\overrightarrow{B} = \left(f_{B_1}, f_{B_2}, \cdots, f_{B_k}\right)$. These vectors are utilized to compute the cosine similarity between the texts. In consideration of the logical consistency and comprehensiveness of the text, we choose to retain the "auxiliary examinations" and "physical examinations" sections from the admission record.

By employing regular expressions and tokenization methods, we identify keywords such as "specialized examination", "physical examination", and "auxiliary examination". This enables the removal of a substantial amount of redundant content pertaining to specialized and auxiliary examinations. The remaining text is then concatenated, and annotations are included to denote the deduplication process. Ultimately, the original medical record text, following deduplication processing, aligns with the standards necessary for subsequent data processing tasks.

Privacy Processing. In both patient and parental datasets, a significant volume of sensitive information is present. Ensuring proper de-identification of this private data is an essential step in processing EMRs data. EMRs data is primarily characterized by non-continuous text, often organized within a record-based framework. To address this, the TS-GRU model [10] has been introduced to effectively integrate contextual information extracted from EMRs. This integration streamlines the de-identification process for sensitive data elements such as age, name, address, and more.

L1 Type Data Processing. L1-type data refers to the templated and structured data within EMRs, allowing for precise field extraction using rule-based methods. Taking the physical examination section in the EMRs as an example, upon observing the original EMR text, it becomes evident that the data in the physical examination section is largely structured, allowing for direct data extraction. Utilizing rule-based regular expressions for data extraction, patient vital signs such as body temperature by matching the character 'T' and heart rate information by matching the character 'P' can be accurately extracted. This process primarily extracts patient information related to body temperature, heart rate, blood pressure, weight, height, and general condition.

4 Joint Extraction of Entity Relationships Based on BART

In the process of structuring EMRs pertinent to lung cancer, a pipeline approach is commonly adopted following data preprocessing. This approach aims to identify medically significant entities and entity relationships relevant to the diagnosis. These entities encompass diseases, symptoms, pertinent examinations, and other relevant information documented in the patient's medical history. Moreover, lung cancer EMR texts often involve single entity overlap (SEO) and entity pair overlap (EPO). In comparison to general domain datasets, the relationships between entities in lung cancer EMRs are notably more intricate. This complexity gives rise to challenges such as a higher number of triplets within a single corpus and a prevalent overlap of entities among triplets. The presence of multiple triplets and overlapping entities within a single piece of text poses a significant challenge in the task of entity relationship extraction.

Considering these practical challenges, this study employed the generative model BART for a joint extraction approach. Experimental analysis was conducted on lung cancer EMRs to successfully accomplish the task of structuring medical records.

4.1 Model Architecture

The BART model, utilizing a standard Transformer structure, was introduced to address the prevalence of triplet data and the substantial issue of entity overlap within triplets in lung cancer EMRs [11]. This selection was based on its remarkable adaptability to pretraining objectives and downstream tasks, resulting in enhanced generation outcomes. BART operates as a denoising autoencoder for pretraining seq2seq models. Leveraging BART's generative decoding approach enables the model to repeatedly decode candidate words from the candidate word list, proving advantageous in addressing the challenge of overlapping entities in triplets, thus eliminating the necessity for intricate sequence labeling strategies.

In the training phase of the model, the encoder initially learns the encoded representation of the source sentence denoted as S. Subsequently, the encoded sentence representation is fed into the decoder of the model. The decoder is provided with the input of the target triplet sequence T, marked with a <sos> token. Throughout the training process, the decoder is trained to predict the next word based on the subsequence from <sos> to the current word in the target sequence, inferring the shifted sequence of the target sequence. The optimization of the model is achieved by minimizing the negative log-likelihood estimation loss using an optimizer. The specific definition of the loss function is presented in Formula (2).

$$loss = -\log P_{t_n}^{\text{gold}} (S, T_{i<n}; \theta) \tag{2}$$

where $P_{t_n}^{\text{gold}}$ represents the probability that the model infers correctly at the nth position; θ represents the model parameters.

The BART encoder encodes the source sentence S into a feature vector H^E of dimensions $s \times h$. The decoder utilizes the previously generated sequence $T_{i<n}$ and H^E to generate the representation $H_{t_n}^D$ for the next target word t_n within the decoder. Subsequently,

an internal classifier in the decoder transforms $H_{t_n}^D$ into a probability distribution over the various vocabulary words in the word table.

$$H^E = Encoder(S; \theta_E) \tag{3}$$

$$H_{t_0}^D = Embedding(<sos>) \tag{4}$$

$$H_{t_n}^D = Decoder\left(H^E, T_{i<n}; \theta_D\right) \tag{5}$$

$$P_{t_n} = Softmax\left(WH_{t_n}^D + b\right) \tag{6}$$

In this context, θ_E and θ_D represent the encoder and decoder weights, respectively, while W signifies the trainable weights of the internal decoder classifier. The BART model appends the generated target word t_n to the sequence $T_{i<n}$ in an autoregressive manner, which becomes the input for the next decoding round. This process iterates continuously until it generates the designated end character <eos>, completing the iterative generation of the source sentence. The specific iterative formula is outlined in Formula (7).

$$P(T \mid S) = \prod_{i=1}^{m} P(t_i \mid S, T_{<i}; \theta) \tag{7}$$

where m is the length of the sequence generated by the decoder. The model architecture is shown in Fig. 3.

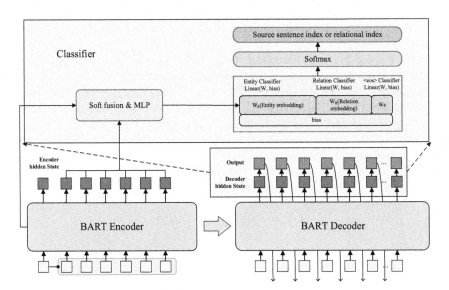

Fig. 3. The model architecture

Encoder. The encoder section encodes the input text S, and the encoding process is depicted in Formulas (8) and (9). The encoded representation of the extracted sentences, in the form of a hidden layer vector H_l^E, is passed on to the decoder section of the model. In this model, the encoder is constructed using the BART encoder, which comprises multiple layers of Transformer modules [12]. The BART-base model consists of 6 layers, while the BART-large model consists of 12 layers.

$$H_0^E = Embedding(S) + Embedding(S_{pos}) \tag{8}$$

$$H_l^E = Trans(H_{l-1}^E), l \in [1, L] \tag{9}$$

where, H_0^E represents the embedding layer weights of the BART encoder, $Embedding()$ denotes the word embedding applied to the current sentence, and S_{pos} represents the positional sequence of words in the input sentence. $Trans()$ signifies the Transformer module within the encoder, and l indicates the number of hidden layers.

Decoder. The BART model integrates the decoder portion of the GPT model, utilizing a decoder architecture based on the self-attention mechanism of Transformers. The encoder learns the overall contextual information of the input text through the self-attention mechanism, while the decoder's task is to predict the next word based on the current input and the model's previous state [13]. Subsequently, the predicted word is appended to the input sequence for the next step, iterating continuously until a complete sequence is generated. Unlike the GPT model, which is a left-to-right unidirectional autoregressive model, the BART model introduces an encoder. This addition enables the BART model to utilize contextual information from the source sentence on the encoder side during inference. This strengthens the relationship between the source sentence and the generated sequence, enhancing decoding effectiveness [14].

4.2 Dataset

The experiment involved annotating EMRs related to lung cancer collected from a tertiary hospital. After data analysis, the EMR texts from patient admission records, ward rounds, and discharge records were retained. Additionally, it was observed during the analysis that complete files for every patient were not available (some patients were not discharged). In the end, 1,497 EMRs were curated, and a subset of 200 records was chosen for annotation. With guidance from specialized physicians and training provided to 22 annotators, the process included the formulation of annotation guidelines, trial annotations, guideline refinement, and three rounds of annotation.

The document-level lung cancer EMR annotation corpus underwent sentence segmentation, resulting in 6,189 annotated sentences. This corpus comprises 26,594 triplets. After eliminating duplicates in the dataset, there were a total of 6,641 unique entities and modifiers, constituting 12,956 triplets. The specific statistical information is detailed in the table below (Table 2).

The lung cancer EMRs dataset was divided based on an 8:1:1 ratio for training, validation, and testing sets. This division resulted in 4,951, 618, and 620 sentences in the respective sets. Analysis of the corpus revealed that in over 70% of sentences,

Table 2. Statistics on the number of entities and entity relationships in the dataset

Entities and modifications	Quantity		Entities and modifications	Quantity	
	Remove duplicates	Total		Remove duplicates	Total
Disease	495	7,596	Examine - result	1,671	5,612
Symptom	2,009	18,587	Examine - Symptoms	1,845	8,213
Examine	386	5,981	Time - Symptoms	1,368	4,356
Treatment	478	3,560	Body - Disease	245	968
Modify	265	9,145	Time - Disease	698	1,735
Time	469	845	Disease - Symptoms	1,567	3,576
Body	680	5,479	Modify - Disease	274	2,259
Examine result	1859	3,017	Examine - Disease	544	1,092
–	–	–	Treatment - Symptom	156	945
Sum	6,641	54,210	Sum	8,368	28,756

there were 2 or more triplets present. Additionally, approximately 30% of the sentences contained 5 or more triplets. There were instances where a single sentence contained both SEO and EPO scenarios. Notably, in most examination-related sentences, the SEO situation was prevalent due to the necessity of establishing relationships between the examination name and symptoms or diseases from the examination results.

4.3 Experimental Results and Analysis

In the entity and entity relationship extraction steps of EMR structuring, experiments were conducted using carefully partitioned lung cancer records to validate the effectiveness of the BART joint extraction model in structuring lung cancer EMRs. In this experiment, we employed the BART-Large model with both encoder and decoder set to 12 layers to maintain consistency in the number of layers with BERT-Large and RoBERTa-Large models. Accuracy (Pre), recall (Rec), and F1 score were utilized as evaluation metrics to assess the model's performance. The specific results are shown in Table 3.

Table 3. Main experimental results

Dataset	Model	P (%)	R (%)	F1 (%)
Lung cancer EMR	ERNIE	58.74	61.35	59.63
	BERT-Large	60.56	64.83	63.49
	RoBERTa-Large	60.95	65.41	63.86
	BART-Large	**63.41**	**66.37**	**64.86**

5 Conclusion

In this paper, we present the core process and key techniques for structuring EMRs based on lung cancer EMRs, with a focus on addressing subsequent tasks such as clinical decision-making. The data preprocessing stage employs data cleaning to handle characters and redundant data, optimizing the annotation process. The TS-GRU model is utilized to de-identify patient information and extract structured data (L1 data). In the information extraction phase, we employ a BART-based joint extraction approach to accomplish the crucial steps in structuring lung cancer EMRs. This model takes input sentences, encodes them using an encoder to obtain sentence encoding information, and then employs a soft fusion strategy to obtain encoding representations at different depths of the sentences. Using a specific starting token <sos> as input for the decoder, the decoder utilizes the encoding representation of the source sentence and embedded representation of relationships as weights for entity and relationship classification. The softmax function is applied to obtain the probability distribution of candidate words, from which the word with the highest probability is selected and added to the sequence starting with <sos>, serving as input for the decoder to infer the next word in the sequence. This process is iterated until the decoder infers the end token <eos>. Finally, the identified medical entities are integrated to achieve the structured EMRs for subsequent tasks such as auxiliary diagnosis.

Acknowledgement. We appreciate the constructive feedback from the anonymous reviewers and the support provided for this research by the following projects: Henan Provincial Department of Science and Technology Science and Technology Research Project, research on key technologies for multi-source knowledge fusion for knowledge graph construction No. 232102211033, and the Science and Technology Innovation 2030 "New Generation of Artificial Intelligence" Major Project under Grant No. 2021ZD0111000.

References

1. Devlin, J., Chang, M.W., Lee, K., et al.: BERT: pre-training of deep bidirectional transformers for language understanding. arXiv preprint arXiv:1810.04805 (2018)
2. Radford, A., Narasimhan, K., Salimans, T., et al.: Improving language understanding by generative pre-training (2018)

3. Lewis, M., Liu, Y., Goyal, N., et al.: BART: denoising sequence-to-sequence pre-training for natural language generation, translation, and comprehension. arXiv preprint arXiv:1910. 13461 (2019)

4. Zeng, Q., Xiong, W., Du, J., et al.: Named entity recognition in electronic health records using BiLSTM-CRF with self-attention. J. Comput. Appl. Softw. **38**(03), 159–162+242 (2021)

5. Jiang, S., Zhao, S., Hou, K., et al.: A BERT-BiLSTM-CRF model for Chinese electronic medical records named entity recognition. In: 2019 12th International Conference on Intelligent Computation Technology and Automation (ICICTA), pp. 166–169. IEEE (2019)

6. Huang, K., Singh, A., Chen, S., et al.: Clinical XLNet: modeling sequential clinical notes and predicting prolonged mechanical ventilation. arXiv preprint arXiv:1912.11975 (2019)

7. Chang, H., Zan, H., Guan, T., et al.: Application of cascade binary pointer tagging in joint entity and relation extraction of Chinese medical text. Math. Biosci. Eng. **19**(10), 10656–10672 (2022)

8. Li, X.Y.: Ministry of health issues basic standards for electronic health records. Chin. Commun. Phys. **13**, 21 (2010)

9. Zan, H.Y., Han, Y.C., Fan, Y.X., et al.: Establishment and analysis of a Chinese symptom knowledge base. J. Chin. Inf. Process. **34**(4), 30–37 (2020)

10. Zhao, Y.S., Zhang, K.L., Ma, H.C., et al.: Leveraging text skeleton for de-identification of electronic medical records. BMC Med. Inform. Decis. Mak. **18**, 65–72 (2018)

11. Chang, H., Xu, H., van Genabith, J., Xiong, D., Zan, H.: JoinER-BART: joint entity and relation extraction with constrained decoding, representation reuse and fusion. IEEE/ACM Trans. Audio Speech Lang. Process. (2023). https://doi.org/10.1109/TASLP.2023.3310879

12. Das, A., Du, X., Wang, B., et al.: Automatic error analysis for document-level information extraction. In: Proceedings of the 60th Annual Meeting of the Association for Computational Linguistics (Volume 1: Long Papers), pp. 3960–3975 (2022)

13. Lee, C.Y., Li, C.L., Dozat, T., et al.: FormNet: structural encoding beyond sequential modeling in form document information extraction. In: Proceedings of the 60th Annual Meeting of the Association for Computational Linguistics (Volume 1: Long Papers), pp. 3735–3754 (2022)

14. Lu, Y., Liu, Q., Dai, D., et al.: Unified structure generation for universal information extraction. In: Proceedings of the 60th Annual Meeting of the Association for Computational Linguistics (Volume 1: Long Papers), pp. 5755–5772 (2022)

Privacy-Preserving Medical Dialogue Generation Based on Federated Learning

Bo Xu[1], Yingjie Zhou[2], Linlin Zong[3(✉)], Hongfei Lin[1], and Fang Mei[1]

[1] School of Computer Science and Technology, Dalian University of Technology, Dalian, China

[2] National University of Defense Technology, Changsha, China

[3] School of Software, Dalian University of Technology, Dalian, China
llzong@dlut.edu.cn

Abstract. Large-scale pre-trained dialogue models have shown outstanding performance across various dialogue-related natural language processing tasks. However, in privacy-sensitive domains like healthcare, concerns related to legal regulations and data security continue to pose challenges, resulting in data silos as a major barrier to building secure medical dialogue generation models. Federated learning is a distributed model training approach that allows models to be trained using data without the data leaving its local environment, making it an effective solution to address data silos in medial dialogue generation. In this paper, we focus on the task of medical dialogue generation, which utilizes medical dialogue data collected from three different Chinese short video platforms to train federated medical dialogue generation model. We employ the FedAvg algorithm to merge parameters of models trained on data from different sources. Experimental results demonstrate that in collaborative scenarios involving large organizations, federated learning effectively enhances the performance of medical dialogue models, improving the accuracy of output predictions. The effectiveness of federated learning varies among participants with different data volumes. Compared to the ideal scenario of centralized training, federated training yields an acceptable range of performance loss in the medical dialogue generation models.

Keywords: Federated Learning · Medical Dialogue Generation · Natural Language Generation

1 Introduction

Intelligent remote healthcare is gaining increasing attention due to its higher resource utilization, safety, and convenience for medical consultations [8]. Medical dialogue models thus become a cutting-edge research topic in the field of Natural Language Processing (NLP) for monitoring remote medical consultations. To build powerful medical dialogue models, the quality and quantity of dialogue data play a crucial role in model effectiveness. In recent years, Chinese short video platforms, such as Kuaishou and Douyin, accumulated rich doctor-patient dialogue data released by doctor accounts, which not only facilitates the patients to pre-diagnose their health conditions, but also provides a rich source of data for medical dialogue model training [14]. However, in medical domain, data privacy is a major concern. Strict privacy regulations limit the availability of high-quality and abundant labeled medical data. Moreover. Small datasets are prone to encountering overfitting issues during model training [11]. To overcome this problem, this work mainly seeks to build privacy-preserving medical dialogue models by employing federated learning approaches. The emergence of federated learning provides hope for collaborative data efforts among different institutions without compromising privacy, overcoming the limitations posed by data scarcity on model performance [17].

Federated learning is a decentralized solution with the main idea being to ensure that data doesn't leave the jurisdiction of the organization it belongs to. While maintaining data security, different institutions collaborate to perform efficient machine learning among multiple participants or computing nodes. This involves jointly training a global model with more refined features using data from various owners without the need for data exchange between institutions. The key distinction from distributed learning is that federated learning doesn't require centralized data. Rather than focusing primarily on efficiency, it emphasizes privacy and security. Therefore, we adopt federated learning to build privacy-preserving medical dialogue generation model.

This paper focuses on preserving user privacy in medical dialogue generation. We attempt to incorporate federated learning into the general process of training generative models, specifically in the pre-training and fine-tuning phases. The goal is to address the challenge faced by general medical dialogue models in privacy-sensitive domains where centralized collection of user data is not feasible. The design concept of federated generative models involves using local data for local training, transmitting model parameters instead of private data to ensure data security. Central servers manage model parameter updates, incorporating different participants' learned feature information to optimize model performance. The paper conducts three different experiments and arrives at the following conclusions:

(1) Federated generative models for medical dialogue generation outperform original pre-trained dialogue models, effectively extracting data features from three parties and promoting secure data collaboration among different institutions.
(2) Federated generative models perform better than models trained individually by participating parties, particularly benefiting participants with lower data proportions, offering significant improvements for all participants involved in federated training of medical dialogue models.
(3) The performance of federated generative models improve privacy-preserving performance despite some acceptable loss due to communication and non-independent distributed data. Under the experimental conditions of this paper, the decrease of performance is less than 10% compared to traditional centralized training.

2 Related Work

2.1 Medical Dialogue Generation

In the field of medical dialogue generation, researchers and practitioners have been focusing on developing natural language processing (NLP) models and techniques to facilitate communications between healthcare professionals, patients, and chatbots. Recent advances in medical dialogue systems have benefited medical applications such as psychological consultation [1], elderly care [3], and disease pre-diagnosis [10]. To build effective medical dialogue systems, related studies are focusing on optimizing medical dialogue from various aspects. Wei et al. [13] proposed a method that utilizes patient self-reports and automatically identifies symptoms from the patient's dialogue history. They generate responses using reinforcement learning and templates. Building upon this work, Lin et al. [5] extracted symptom graphs from a dataset to model the relationships between symptoms, thereby improving symptom extraction performance. Xu et al. [15] developed a dialogue system that incorporates an external knowledge graph. They combined this knowledge graph with annotated patient dialogue information to calculate the probability of symptoms and diseases. This probability is then used in decision-making through reinforcement learning, and the final responses are generated using templates. Zhang et al. [19] introduced a Medical Information Extractor (MIE) tailored for medical dialogues. MIE is designed to extract information related to symptoms, surgeries, and other medical aspects. The authors employed a sliding window approach to annotate online medical consultation dialogues, which is considered a more straightforward method compared to sequential annotation. Du et al. [2] presented a model capable of extracting symptoms and their states mentioned in clinical dialogues. The authors also created their own corpus, which includes approximately 3,000 dialogues annotated by professional medical transcriptionists. This corpus serves as a valuable resource for training and evaluating the model's performance in symptom extraction from clinical conversations. Xu et al. [14] collected and annotated a wide range of meta-data with respect to medical dialogue including doctor profiles, hospital departments, diseases and symptoms for fine-grained analysis on language usage pattern and clinical diagnosis. And evaluated the performance of medical response generation on the data set. However, the above methods did not take into account the issue of user privacy protection, which remains an open research question for future studies.

2.2 Federated Learning for Nautral Lauguage Processing

In recent years, Federated Learning (FL) has yielded numerous creative achievements in the field of NLP [4,7,16,20]. For instance, Google LLC, in 2019, was among the first to apply FL to the Google keyboard and published a series of technical papers primarily addressing word-level language modeling problems in the mobile industry. Apple Inc. is using FL for wake word detection in Siri within the realm of speech recognition tasks. In sequence tagging, Liu and Miller [6] employs federated learning to fine-tune the BERT model for named entity recognition tasks. Furthermore, as natural language processing models have evolved towards larger pre-trained models, the demand for data has become more significant. Stremmel and Singh [12] used GPT-2 as a language model but due to the very large number of parameters in GPT-2, they proposed dimensionality reduction techniques to reduce the word embedding layer dimensions of GPT-2 to smaller values. Currently, the application of federated learning in the field of medical dialogue generation still requires exploration.

3 Our Federated Medical Dialogue Generation Model

The idea of the federated medical dialogue generation model is as follows: it utilizes local data from participants for local training, transmitting model parameters instead of privacy data to ensure data security. The central server manages model parameter updates, assimilates different participant-learned feature information, and optimizes model performance. As shown in Fig. 1, the specific process includes: (1) The server-side initiates model pre-training, providing a common basic generative model GPT-2 architecture and word embedding matrix to participants in a broadcast manner, reducing local computational overhead, and improving model convergence speed. (2) Federated training participants perform model training using local data and transmit the parameters of their local training models to the central server. (3) The central model conducts model fusion using federated learning algorithm FedAvg and broadcasts the updated model back to all participants until the model's performance stabilizes. We introduce the key elements in the following.

3.1 The Generative Model

Using pretrained language models and fine-tuning on medical datasets is a common approach in the development of medical dialogue systems. The main steps involve pretraining on large public datasets and fine-tuning on task-specific datasets. In this paper, a Chinese pretrained model based on GPT-2 was chosen for the initial training phase, with adaptions made to accommodate Chinese data input and output. The overall structure of GPT-2 is depicted as shown in Fig. 2, the model comprises an input layer, self-attention learning layers, and an output prediction layer.

Input Layer. The input layer is designed to preprocess data into a standardized format that the model can work with efficiently, facilitating feature extraction and memory in this specific format. The input layer consists of two steps: word embedding and positional embedding.

Word embedding is a technique that transforms input words from variables that are unrelated to each other into low-dimensional variables that capture their relationships. This transformation is achieved using a word embedding matrix

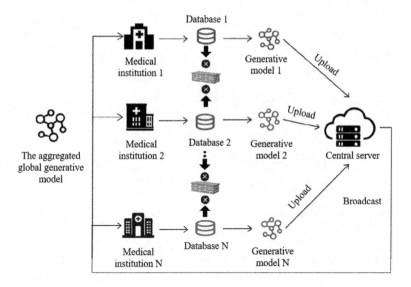

Fig. 1. Framework of Federated Medical Dialogue Generation.

$W_{n \times d} = U_{n \times m} We_{m \times d}$, where We is the initialize embedding matrix and U is the sequence of the input text.

Positional embedding involves adding positional information to the input for different positions of words. This helps the model to recognize and understand the different meanings of the same words in different positions within the input. To input position information into the model, it first need to construct a position vector PE.

After constructing the positional embedding vector, it is added to the word embedding matrix calculated in the previous step to obtain the model's input.

$$input_{n \times d} = U_{n \times m} We_{m \times d} + Wp_{n \times d} \tag{1}$$

where Wp is the position matrix.

Self-attention Learning Layers. The model's self-attention layer consists of 10 stacked transformer decoders, and the computations between these layers can be represented using the following formula:

$$h_0 = UWp + We; h_l = transformer_block(h_{l-1}); P(u) = softmax(h_n We^T) \tag{2}$$

where n is the number of layers, U is the vectors of the first k inputs, We is the word embedding matrix, Wp is the position matrix. The transformer block is shown in Fig. 2. Except for the first layer, where the input is the word embeddings and position embeddings, the input for each subsequent layer is the output of the previous layer.

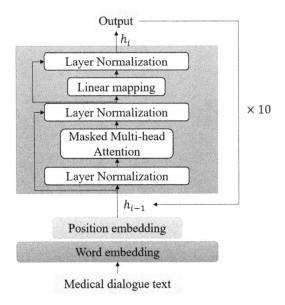

Fig. 2. Framework of GPT-2.

In the transformer block, layer normalization helps accelerate the convergence speed of the network by summarizing and calculating the mean and variance of the input data from the same layer and normalizing the input data from the previous layer. The masked multi-head attention calculates attention scores to obtain the attention matrix, where each row represents the attention of the current word position to other words. Standardization is then applied to avoid overfitting, and finally, softmax is used for normalization. The entire process can be described by the following formula:

$$Attention(Q, K, V) = softmax(\frac{Q^T K}{\sqrt{d}})V \qquad (3)$$

where Q, K, V are vectors obtained by transforming the word embedding matrix, and d represents the variance calculated during the standardization process.

Output Layer. The output layer maps the unsupervised outputs learned by the model to the vocabulary and selects output words based on a certain strategy. The performance of the output layer significantly influences aspects of the model, such as its expressive richness.

3.2   The Uploaded Parameters

The model parameters correspond to the model structure and are mainly divided into: the token embedding matrix W_{te} (weight of token embedding), the positional embedding matrix W_{pe} (weight of positional embedding), and the parameters of 10 transformer blocks. Specifically, the matrix dimensions are as follows:

W_{te} has dimensions of 13317×768, and W_{pe} has dimensions of 300×768. The 300 dimension corresponds to the standard input length $n = 300$. Each transformer block performs self-attention learning with 12 attention heads internally and optimizes the parameters recorded in the parameter matrix. Although this model has only 10 layers of transformer blocks, it has a total parameter count close to 100 million.

3.3   The Federated Updates and Aggregations

We adopt the relatively simple yet highly effective FedAvg algorithm [9]. FedAvg aims to address the privacy and security issues associated with using private data on mobile devices for model training. This algorithm has been extensively evaluated and proven to be robust against imbalanced and non-IID data distributions.

The core idea of FedAvg is as follows: There is one server and a fixed set of clients, with a total of clients, each having its own local dataset. Before each training round, C clients are randomly selected. The server sends the current global model to these C clients. These C clients then perform local training on their respective local datasets for several local epochs using the received global model. After local training, these C clients send back their updated models to the server, which synchronizes these updates into the global model. This process continues for a certain number of global epochs or until the model reaches a certain level of accuracy. The objective of this algorithm can be represented by the following equation.

$$min_w f(w) = \frac{1}{C} \sum_{i=1}^{n} f_i(W) \tag{4}$$

where $f_i(W)$ is the corresponding loss function for the task. w represents the parameters updated in each round of iteration. C represents the total number of clients randomly selected to participate in this round of iteration.

4   Experiments

4.1   Datasets and Settings

To study whether medical dialogue models can be pre-trained and fine-tuned using different data sources using federated learning methods, we designed the following experimental process: select the pre-trained GPT-2 model from a unified data source; select three fine-tuned data sources Corresponding to three clients, named as client1, client2, client3; set up a federated server, named as server, to execute the federated learning FedAvg algorithm and perform parameter fusion. The following training is performed respectively: on the server side, perform model evaluation on the model that has not been pre-trained; on client1, client2, and client3, we use local data to train separately to evaluate the performance of their respective models; perform federated fine-tuning, and perform parameter fusion on the server side.

The public large-scale MedDialog-CN dataset [18] is used for pre-training on the server side. The short video based RealMedDial dataset is used for the fine-tuning process [14]. The original RealMedDial only contains dialogue collected from the Kuaishou platform. To increase the data source for federated learning, we enrich the data by collecting short video based medical dialogue from Douyin and Xiaohongshu platforms. The final collected data are divided into three parts according to different platforms: Kuaishou data, Douyin data, and Xiaohongshu data. The statistics of the used datasets are shown in Table 1.

Table 1. Statistics of the used datasets

dataset	No. of Dialogue	No. of Disease	No. of Departments
MedDialog-CN	3,407,494	172	51
RealMedDial (Kuaishou)	2637	55	17
Xiaohongshu	240	31	9
Douyin	208	25	13

Different automatic evaluation metrics are used to evaluate the model effectiveness, including Perplexity, NIST-n (where n is the size of the n-gram and is set to 4), BLEU-n (where n is set to 2 and 4), Entropy-n (where n is set to 4), Dist-n (where n is set to 1 and 2), and Perplexity that measure whether the generated text is rich enough and of high quality. The calculated value of Perplexity can be understood as the type of reasonable words that the model can provide when predicting a certain word. The higher the Perplexity value on the same data set, the better the model performance.

4.2 The Effect of Federated Learning on Medical Dialogue Generation

This group of experiments compares the performance of the full-process federated training model with the pre-trained model without fine-tuning to verify whether the global model can effectively learn feature knowledge from dispersedly stored data. From the Table 2, we can see that

(1) The Perplexity value has decreased after federated training compared with each client, indicating that federated training comprehensively uses data from all parties and effectively enhances the model's prediction ability;
(2) The values of BLEU and NIST are slightly increased after federated training. There is a greater improvement compared to the model that does not participate in fine-tuning, which shows that the federated training method can effectively improve the prediction ability on the datasets;
(3) The value of Entrop-4 and Dist indicators shows that during the federated fine-tuning process, the model can obtaining richer word representations from the data increases the richness of the generated text;

Table 2. Experimental Results

	before fine-tuning	Client1	Client2	Client3	Federated Training
loss	0.163	0.128	0.131	0.0893	0.0832
BLEU-2	0.003	0.018	0.015	0.055	0.062
BLEU-4	0.001	0.005	0.004	0.027	0.031
Dist-1	0.007	0.005	0.005	0.004	0.006
Dist-2	0.015	0.010	0.012	0.008	0.009
Entropy-4	1.202	0.718	0.824	0.606	0.595
NIST-4	0.005	0.845	0.768	1.033	1.063
Perplexity	31647	6597	8977	309.874	288.260

(4) When there is a significant difference in the local data volume, the participants with smaller data volumes achieve significantly better results with the federated model compared to their locally trained models. In this experiment, client3's data volume represents more than 70% of the total data, which shows that while the federated model has some improvements compared to its local training, its performance is far from significant compared to the other two clients.

Overall, the results prove that the federated learning method could be used in language model training, and can keep the model performance while increasing the privacy-preserving utility.

4.3   Loss Change in Federated Learning and Centralized Training

The Table 3 below shows the results of the experiments where the federated parameters from four rounds, each consisting of 20 local training iterations, were compared to the equivalent centralized training with 80 local training iterations, where all three clients' data were aggregated at the server for centralized training.

Table 3. The comparison of loss change between federated training and centralized training

	Centralized training	Federated Training
loss	0.0775	0.0832
BLEU-2	0.105	0.062
BLEU-4	0.033	0.031
Dist-1	0.009	0.006
Dist-2	0.020	0.009
Entropy-4	1.674	0.595
NIST-4	1.494	1.063
Perplexity	220.071	288.260

The results indicate that while federated training has advantages in protecting data privacy, it suffers some performance loss. Compared to centralized training, the models trained through federated training exhibit inferior performance in certain performance metrics. This suggests that while federated learning is a powerful method for privacy protection, it may lead to a sacrifice in model performance under certain circumstances.

5   Conclusion

Due to the increase in model size, there is a growing need in the training process to aggregate more high-quality data to enhance the model's capabilities. However, in privacy-sensitive domains like healthcare, traditional methods of purchasing or collecting relevant data are subject to strict legal regulations. Faced with the "data island" problem in the medical dialogue generation field, we propose to combine the federated learning approach with pre-trained dialogue generation models, forming the architecture of federated generation models. The concept of federated learning was incorporated in the GPT-2 model. Training was distributed across different client institutions with non-independent distributed data. This approach enabled distributed training while keeping data on the clients' local institutions, ensuring privacy and data security. The experimental results indicate that federated learning methods can have a positive impact on medical dialogue generation for privacy preserving.

Acknowledgment. This work is supported by grant from the Natural Science Foundation of China (No. 62006034), the Ministry of Education Humanities and Social Science Project (No. 22YJC740110).

References

1. Das, A., et al.: Conversational bots for psychotherapy: a study of generative transformer models using domain-specific dialogues. In: Proceedings of the 21st Workshop on Biomedical Language Processing, Dublin, Ireland, pp. 285–297 (2022)
2. Du, N., Chen, K., Kannan, A., Tran, L., Chen, Y., Shafran, I.: Extracting symptoms and their status from clinical conversations. In: Proceedings of the 57th Conference of the Association for Computational Linguistics, Florence, Italy, pp. 915–925 (2019)
3. Keshmiri, S., Sumioka, H., Yamazaki, R., Ishiguro, H.: Decoding the perceived difficulty of communicated contents by older people: toward conversational robot-assistive elderly care. IEEE Robot. Autom. Lett. 4(4), 3263–3269 (2019)
4. Kim, Y., Kim, J., Mok, W., Park, J., Lee, S.: Client-customized adaptation for parameter-efficient federated learning. In: Findings of the Association for Computational Linguistics: ACL 2023, Toronto, Canada, 9–14 July 2023, pp. 1159–1172. Association for Computational Linguistics (2023)
5. Lin, X., He, X., Chen, Q., Tou, H., Wei, Z., Chen, T.: Enhancing dialogue symptom diagnosis with global attention and symptom graph. In: Proceedings of the 2019 Conference on Empirical Methods in Natural Language Processing and the 9th International Joint Conference on Natural Language Processing, Hong Kong, China, pp. 5032–5041 (2019)

6. Liu, D., Miller, T.A.: Federated pretraining and fine tuning of BERT using clinical notes from multiple silos. CoRR abs/2002.08562 (2020)
7. Liu, Y., Bi, X., Li, L., Chen, S., Yang, W., Sun, X.: Communication efficient federated learning for multilingual neural machine translation with adapter. In: Findings of the Association for Computational Linguistics: ACL 2023, Toronto, Canada, 9–14 July 2023, pp. 5315–5328. Association for Computational Linguistics (2023)
8. Mann, D.M., Chen, J., Chunara, R., Testa, P.A., Nov, O.: COVID-19 transforms health care through telemedicine: evidence from the field. J. Am. Med. Inform. Assoc. **27**(7), 1132–1135 (2020)
9. McMahan, B., Moore, E., Ramage, D., Hampson, S., y Arcas, B.A.: Communication-efficient learning of deep networks from decentralized data. In: Proceedings of the 20th International Conference on Artificial Intelligence and Statistics, Fort Lauderdale, FL, USA, vol. 54, pp. 1273–1282 (2017)
10. Nasreen, S., Hough, J., Purver, M.: Rare-class dialogue act tagging for Alzheimer's disease diagnosis. In: Proceedings of the 22nd Annual Meeting of the Special Interest Group on Discourse and Dialogue, Singapore and Online, pp. 290–300 (2021)
11. Qiu, X., Sun, T., Xu, Y., Shao, Y., Dai, N., Huang, X.: Pre-trained models for natural language processing: a survey. CoRR abs/2003.08271 (2020)
12. Stremmel, J., Singh, A.: Pretraining federated text models for next word prediction. CoRR abs/2005.04828 (2020)
13. Wei, Z., et al.: Task-oriented dialogue system for automatic diagnosis. In: Proceedings of the 56th Annual Meeting of the Association for Computational Linguistics, Melbourne, Australia, pp. 201–207 (2018)
14. Xu, B., et al.: RealMedDial: a real telemedical dialogue dataset collected from online chinese short-video clips. In: Proceedings of the 29th International Conference on Computational Linguistics, Gyeongju, Republic of Korea, pp. 3342–3352 (2022)
15. Xu, L., Zhou, Q., Gong, K., Liang, X., Tang, J., Lin, L.: End-to-end knowledge-routed relational dialogue system for automatic diagnosis. In: The Thirty-Third AAAI Conference on Artificial Intelligence, Hawaii, USA, pp. 7346–7353 (2019)
16. Xu, Z., et al.: Federated learning of gboard language models with differential privacy. In: Proceedings of the The 61st Annual Meeting of the Association for Computational Linguistics, ACL 2023, pp. 629–639. Association for Computational Linguistics (2023)
17. Yang, Q., Liu, Y., Chen, T., Tong, Y.: Federated machine learning: concept and applications. ACM Trans. Intell. Syst. Technol. **10**(2), 12:1–12:19 (2019)
18. Zeng, G., et al.: MedDialog: large-scale medical dialogue datasets. In: Proceedings of the 2020 Conference on Empirical Methods in Natural Language Processing, EMNLP 2020, Online, 16–20 November 2020, pp. 9241–9250. Association for Computational Linguistics (2020)
19. Zhang, Y., et al.: MIE: a medical information extractor towards medical dialogues. In: Proceedings of the 58th Annual Meeting of the Association for Computational Linguistics, Online, pp. 6460–6469 (2020)
20. Zhang, Z., et al.: FEDLEGAL: the first real-world federated learning benchmark for legal NLP. In: Proceedings of the 61st Annual Meeting of the Association for Computational Linguistics (Volume 1: Long Papers), ACL 2023, Toronto, Canada, 9–14 July 2023, pp. 3492–3507. Association for Computational Linguistics (2023)

FgKF: Fine-Grained Knowledge Fusion for Radiology Report Generation

Kunli Zhang, Xiyang Huang, Hongying Zan[(⊠)], Yutuan Ma, Qianxiang Gao, and Yaoxu Li

College of Computer and Artificial Intelligence, Zhengzhou University, Zhengzhou, China
{ieklzhang,iehyzan}@zzu.edu.cn

Abstract. Radiology imaging examination is an important basis for disease diagnosis and treatment. Based on existing radiology images and reports, automated generation of image-to-report can effectively relieve pressure on physicians. The generation of radiology reports utilizes the terminology and expertise inherent to the field of radiology. The integration of this specialized knowledge into automated report generation not only enhances the precision of disease findings descriptions, but also significantly elevates the quality of the reports produced. In this paper, we propose a fine-grained knowledge fusion model for radiology report generation that reduces the gap between visual and textual features by fusing image features with fine-grained radiographic knowledge. Specifically, the image-text cross-modal retrieval model, CLIP, is utilized to retrieve report from the dataset that are similar to the current image. The feature representations of the image and the fine-grained knowledge which are extracted from the similar report, are aligned by an Entities-Enhanced Multi-Head Attention mechanism. Then the fused features are decoded by a Transformer decoder with a semantic information fusion module to generate the radiology report. Experimental results on IU X-Ray and MIMIC-CXR show that the fusion of fine-grained knowledge guides the model to produce higher quality radiology reports.

Keywords: Report Generation · Radiology Images · Cross-modal Alignment

1 Introduction

In the clinic, the reading of medical images is completed by professional radiologists, and the accurate writing of radiology reports depends on the professional knowledge and clinical experience of doctors, which has high requirements for their professional level [1]. With the advancement and widespread use of radiological imaging technology, the size of imaging data in hospitals has grown by leaps and bounds. Topol [2] posited that the need for diagnosing and drafting reports for image-based examinations significantly surpasses the medical capabilities of physicians. This scarcity of specialized physicians is particularly pronounced in resource-limited nations [3]. Deep learning's swift advancements in computer vision and natural language processing have opened up promising avenues for applications within the medical sector [4]. Given the vast repository of existing radiographic images and reports, there is a compelling research interest in developing models capable of autonomously generating diagnostic reports from images. Such an innovation could significantly aid radiologists and alleviate physicians' workload.

The text of a radiology report contains rich semantic information and medical knowledge, including terminology, descriptive conventions, etc. When using only image features as input, it is difficult for the model to learn fine-grained semantic information in radiology reports. Radiologists often refer to existing reports for revision and refinement when writing radiology reports. Drawing on this process, incorporating fine-grained knowledge in the training process enables the model to learn more information and improves the quality of the reports generated by the model. In this regard, we explore Fine-grained Knowledge Fusion for radiology report generation (FgKF). Specifically, we obtain similar reports of input images through image-to-text cross-modal retrieval and extract anatomical entities and observed entities in similar reports as knowledge information. When performing knowledge fusion, an Entities-Enhanced Multi-Head Attention mechanism (EEMHA) is proposed for image features alignment with entities features. A decoder with a semantic information fusion module is used to finally decode and generate the radiology report. We have experimented and analyzed our approach on two datasets, IU X-Ray [5] and MIMIC-CXR [6].

Our contributions can be summarized as follows: (1) We propose a radiology report generation model FgKF that incorporates fine-grained knowledge, which makes full use of radiology domain knowledge and enables the model to generate radiology reports that are more in line with the requirements of the radiology domain. (2) Our model achieves alignment and fusion of visual and textual features to strengthen the connection between the current image and related descriptions through Entities-Enhanced Multi-Head Attention and semantic information fusion module. (3) A series of tests conducted on two publicly accessible datasets, namely IU X-Ray and MIMIC-CXR, substantiate the efficacy of our proposed methodology.

2 Related Work

2.1 Image Captioning

Image captioning refers to describing the visual content of an image in natural language. Early research on image description mostly used traditional machine learning methods [7–9]. The advent of deep learning, particularly the popularity of encoder-decoder architectures [10–12], has led to an exponential surge in the evolution of image captioning models [13–15]. Based on the good performance of Transformer [16] in the field of natural language processing and computer vision, a large number of Transformer-based methods have been applied to the field of image caption. Fang [17] et al. proposed a purely visual Transformer-based image captioning model called ViTCAP, which uses a grid representation without extracting regional features. To improve the performance, a novel Concept Token Network (CTN) is introduced to predict the semantic concepts, which are then incorporated into the end-to-end description generation. The rich semantic information contained in the semantic concepts effectively improves the performance of the model. Li et al. [18] introduced COS-Net (Comprehending and Ordering Semantics Networks), an image captioning model designed to comprehend and order semantic information. This model integrates rich semantic information and a learnable semantic ordering process into a unified structure. The system procures sentences related to the image via cross-modal retrieval, fetches corresponding words through the same process, and refines and supplements semantic words through tasks of both single and multi-classification. In recent years, contrastive learning-based visual-language pre-training models have made significant strides in representation learning. A prime example of this is Microsoft's CLIP [19] (Contrastive Language-Image Pre-training) model. Leveraging CLIP, text is processed through data augmentation to construct negative samples with grammatical errors. A classifier is then employed to predict positive and negative samples from these examples. This process is combined with reinforcement learning, which is rewarded with natural language generation metrics to jointly enhance the performance of the text encoder. This approach effectively improves both the relevance of the generated descriptions to the image and their grammatical correctness.

2.2 Radiology Report Generation

The automatic generation of radiology reports, which uses radiological images as input and generates report text describing the content of the images, is an application of image captioning in the medical field. Therefore, some methods in image captioning have reference significance for radiology report generation. Similar to image captioning, early research on radiology report generation was based on CNN-RNN structures. Jing et al. [20] proposed a multi-task learning model that uses CNN to extract image features from various sub-regions of the image and calculates the interaction between image features and semantic features through joint attention to strengthen the correspondence between images and reports. In reality, doctors often follow a certain template to write reports, and then modify them according to specific findings. Based on this observation, Li et al. [21] proposed a reinforcement learning model that integrates retrieval and generation, attempting to combine human prior knowledge and learning-based generation methods to automatically generate diagnostic reports. With the advent of the Transformer encoder-decoder structure, Chen et al. [22] introduced a memory-driven, Transformer-based structure for generating radiology reports, achieving state-of-the-art results at the time. Unlike the image captioning model where each word carries equal weight, the mention of disease keywords in radiology reports is of paramount importance. Therefore, greater emphasis should be placed on disease keywords and their attributes when assessing the quality of the generated report. In response to this, Zhang et al. [23] proposed a graph structure model equipped with a priori knowledge of chest findings. They constructed a chest abnormality graph for common diseases and their attributes in the report and introduced a novel evaluation mechanism, MIRQI (Medical Report Quality Index). This mechanism provides a more accurate measure of the generated report's accuracy in the medical domain compared to traditional generation metrics. You et al. [24] predicted disease labels on input images and employed a multi-layer stacked attention module to align image features and disease labels at multiple levels of granularity. This approach not only heightened the model's focus on disease keywords but also effectively mitigated data bias issues. Wang et al. [25] propose a cross-modal prototype driven network to promote cross-modal pattern learning and exploit it to improve the task of radiology report generation. Current research on radiology report generation is predominantly data-driven, with relatively little focus on incorporating knowledge. However, domain knowledge can significantly enhance the medical expertise of generated reports. In light of this, our work will concentrate on studying the automatic generation of radiology reports with fine-grained knowledge fusion.

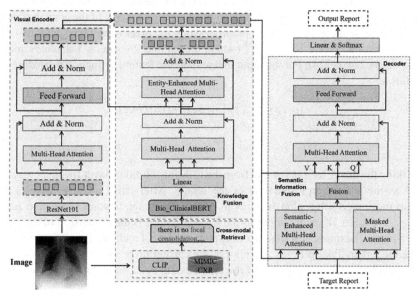

Fig. 1. Overview of our proposed FgKF which consists of four modules, namely visual encoder, knowledge fusion, cross-modal retrieval and decoder with a semantic information fusion module.

3 Proposed Methodology

3.1 Model Architecture

As shown in Fig. 1, the visual encoder mainly preprocesses the input images and uses the pre-trained ResNet101 [26] as the image features extraction model to extract image features from the pre-processed images, after which the image features are encoded by the Transformer encoder. Based on the image-text cross-modal pre-training model CLIP [19] and the training set of MIMIC-CXR, an offline process of retrieving reports from images is pre-constructed, so that the retrieval results can be used directly during model training. The retrieved similar reports are used as a source of knowledge, which is combined with the entity types defined in the Knowledge Graph RadGraph [27] to extract fine-grained knowledge. In the process of knowledge fusion, fine-grained knowledge is first encoded by a pre-trained Bio_ClinicalBERT [28]. When performing entities information fusion, an Entities-Enhanced Multi-Head Attention is designed to facilitate interaction and alignment between different features. Finally, image features fused with fine-grained knowledge are decoded by a decoder with a semantic information fusion module to generate the report.

3.2 Visual Content Encoding

In this work, ResNet101 [26] is used as an image feature extraction model. Before feature extraction, the images are first normalized to remove the photometric and color differences in the images to better fit the training of the network. The images are also scaled to a fixed size to accommodate the input size requirements of the convolution and pooling layers in the network. After preprocessing, the pixel value representation of the image is obtained $Img \in \mathbb{R}^{3 \times 224 \times 224}$ (which means that it contains 3 channels and the image size is 224×224). For the input image Img, the feature extraction procedures are as follows:

$$\{p_1, p_2, \ldots, p_n\} = ResNet101(Img) \tag{1}$$

$$\{x_1, x_2, \ldots, x_n\} = Linear(p_1, p_2, \ldots, p_n) \tag{2}$$

Taking the image features output from the fifth convolutional layer $\{p_1, p_2, \ldots, p_n\} \in \mathbb{R}^{2048}$ as the feature representation of the image. Afterwards, a linear layer is used to map the image sub-region features to obtain the image features extraction results $\{x_1, x_2, \ldots, x_n\} \in \mathbb{R}^d$ as the input to the encoder and d is the dimension of the model hidden layer. The image features encoding part consists of multiple Transformer encoder stacked together. Taking H^l as the input of the current layer and H^{l+1} as the output of the current layer, the computation of the image features encoding are as follows:

$$H_1^l = LayerNorm\left(MHSA\left(H^l, H^l, H^l\right) + H^l\right) \tag{3}$$

$$H^{l+1} = LayerNorm\left(FeedForward\left(H_1^l\right) + H_1^l\right) \tag{4}$$

where MHSA denotes Multi-Head Self-Attention Mechanism, *FeedForward* denotes Feedforward Neural Network, *LayerNorm* denotes Layer Normalization and H_1^l denotes intermediate state. The first layer input is the image features representation $\{x_1, x_2, \ldots, x_n\}$, the input of subsequent layers is the output of the previous layer, and finally the hidden layer state of the image representation is $H_i = \{i_1, i_2, \ldots, i_n\} \in \mathbb{R}^d$.

3.3 Cross-Modal Retrieval

To obtain the text of the radiology reports associated with the input images, a large-scale image-text cross-modal pre-trained model CLIP [19] is used as a retrieval engine based on its fine-tuning on the radiology image dataset. The fine-tuning of the CLIP is performed on the training set of the MIMIC-CXR. A retrieved sample is shown in Fig. 2, where it can be seen that the retrieved report contains a correct description of the heart and lungs (underlined and italicized sections).

For the current input image, the fine-grained entities information contained in the similarity report is obtained as knowledge based on the retrieval of the similarity report. Two types of entities, Anatomy and Observation, are defined in the knowledge graph Rad-Graph [27]. And three attributes, positive, negative and uncertain, are defined for Observation. This fine-grained information can provide more accurate and specific anatomical and imaging knowledge for radiology report generation models. For example, in the report text "Increased right lower lobe opacity, concerning for infection. No evidence of pneumothorax.", which contains the Anatomy entities "right", "lower" and "lobe", as well as the Observation entities "Increased", "opacity", "infection" and "pneumothorax". The attribute information contained within an Observation entity is appended to the entity word. This is done by "present", "absent", or "uncertain", depending on the label type. The entities information corresponding to the aforementioned report will ultimately be "increased, opacity present, right, lower, lobe, infection present, pneumothorax absent". This information accurately encapsulates the medical features associated with the current input image and the interconnections among these features. In this work, we utilize this information as the fine-grained knowledge corresponding to the input image.

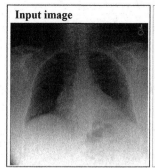

Input image	Ground truth : *The lungs remain clear without focal consolidation, effusion, or edema.* Moderate cardiomegaly is similar compared to prior. No acute osseous abnormalities. **Retrieval** : frontal and lateral views of the chest are obtained. enlargement of the cardiac silhouette persists. the mediastinum and hilar contours are stable. *no focal consolidation pleural effusion or evidence of pneumothorax is seen. no overt pulmonary edema is seen.* degenerative changes are seen along the spine.

Fig. 2. A retrieved sample of the CLIP

3.4 Fine-Grained Knowledge Fusion

Prior to the fusion of fine-grained knowledge, the Bio_ClinicalBERT [28] is employed to obtain a superior feature representation for the fine-grained entities in the retrieved similarity report. Bio_ClinicalBERT has been pre-trained on the BioBERT [29], which is specifically optimized for the biomedical domain. The procedure can be formulated as follows:

$$Emb(e) = T(e) + P(e) \tag{5}$$

$$\{he_1, he_2, \ldots, he_k\} = Bio\_ClinicalBERT(e_1, e_2, \ldots, e_k) \tag{6}$$

$$\{e_1, e_2, \ldots, e_k\} = Linear(he_1, he_2, \ldots, he_k) \tag{7}$$

where $T \in \mathbb{R}^{|v| \times d_b}$ represents the word embedding, $P \in \mathbb{R}^{512 \times d_b}$ represents the positional embedding, $|v|$ and d_b denote the size of the word list and the dimension of the hidden layer of the Bio_ClinicalBERT, respectively. Obtain the last hidden layer state of the Bio_ClinicalBERT model and map it to $H_e = \{e_1, e_2, \ldots, e_k\} \in \mathbb{R}^d$ to keep the dimensions consistent and k denotes the length of the entities.

There may be some discrepancies between the retrieved similarity reports and the true reports corresponding to the current image. As shown in Fig. 2, among the retrieved similar reports, "Enlargement of the cardiac silhouette persists", "No focal consolidation pleural effusion", "No focal consolidation pleural" and "No overt pulmonary edema is seen" are relevant descriptions that are consistent with the current image features, while the rest of them belong to the noise information introduced during the knowledge acquisition process. In order to make the model pay more attention to the relevant descriptions, the Entities-Enhanced Multi-Head Attention (EEMHA) is proposed, which calculates the interaction between image features and entities features to strengthen the connection between the current image and the relevant descriptions. The process for fine-grained knowledge fusion can be formulated as follows:

$$\left\{\widetilde{e_1}, \widetilde{e_2}, ..., \widetilde{e_k}\right\} = MHA(H_e, H_e, H_e) \tag{8}$$

$$\{i_1', i_2', \ldots, i_n'\} = MHA\left(H_i, \widetilde{H_e}, \widetilde{H_e}\right) \tag{9}$$

$$\{e_1', e_2', \ldots, e_l'\} = EEMHA\left(\widetilde{H_e}, H_i', H_i'\right) \tag{10}$$

$$EEMHA\left(\widetilde{H_e}, H_i', H_i'\right) = MHA\left(\widetilde{H_e}, MHA\left(H_i', \widetilde{H_e}, \widetilde{H_e}\right), MHA\left(H_i', \widetilde{H_e}, \widetilde{H_e}\right)\right) \tag{11}$$

$$H_{ie} = Concat\left(i_1, \ldots, i_n, e_1', \ldots, e_l'\right) \tag{12}$$

where MHA denotes Multi-Head Attention Mechanism, $\widetilde{H_e} = \left\{\widetilde{e_1}, \widetilde{e_2}, \ldots, \widetilde{e_k}\right\}$ is the updated entities features representation. $H_i' = \{i_1', i_2', \ldots, i_n'\}$ is the image representation after incorporating shallow entity information. The computation of EEMHA is divided into two parts. Firstly, H_i' is used as the query matrix Q and $\widetilde{H_e}$ is used as the K, V for computation of the multi-head attention. Then $\widetilde{H_e}$ is used as the query matrix Q and the result of the previous step as K and V for one more computation of the multi-head attention to get the updated feature representation $H_e' = \{e_1', e_2', \ldots, e_l'\}$. Finally, H_i and H_e' are concatenated to obtain the output of the fine-grained knowledge fusion layer. $H_{ie} = \{h_1, h_2, \ldots, h_{n+l}\} \in \mathbb{R}^d$, denotes concatenation along the sequence dimension.

3.5 Sentence Decoding

The decoder consists of multiple stacked Transformer blocks, each of which includes multi-head attention mechanism, semantic information fusion module, feed-forward neural network layers, residual connectivity and layer normalization. Segment the reference report by word to get the input sequence $Y = \{y_1, \ldots, y_L\}$, the word embedding and positional embedding of the reference report are obtained by word embedding matrix and position embedding matrix, which are summed up as the embedding representation of the reference report $Emb(Y)$. Take H^l as the input of the current layer, H^{l+1} as the output of the current layer, $H_1^{(*)l}$, H_2^l and H_3^l as the intermediate states. The masked multi-head attention is first computed on H^l to obtain the semantic context $H_1^{(s)l}$. Then H^l as query Q, the output of the visual encoder H_{ie}, which incorporates fine-grained knowledge as key-value pair K, V, is subjected to the computation of Semantic-Enhanced Multi-Head Attention (SEMHA) to obtain the overall visual context $H_1^{(c)l}$:

$$H_1^{(s)l} = MMHA\left(H^l, H^l, H^l\right) \tag{13}$$

$$H_1^{(c)l} = SEMHA\left(H^l, H_{ie}, H_{ie}\right) \tag{14}$$

The overall visual context and semantic context are fused by a sigmoid gate function [18]. And the learnt hidden layer state H_2^l is used as the query Q for the next multi-head attention:

$$H_2^l = LayerNorm\left(\left(g*H_1^{(s)l} + (1-g)*H_1^{(c)l}\right) + H^l\right) \tag{15}$$

$$g = Sigmoid\left(W_g\left[H_1^{(s)l}, H_1^{(c)l}\right]\right) \tag{16}$$

The output of the encoding layer H_{ie} is then used as the key-value pair K, V for multi-head attention computation. Finally a feedforward neural network layer is connected, adding residual connections and layer normalization after all three layers:

$$H_3^l = LayerNorm\left(MHA\left(H_2^l, H_{ie}, H_{ie}\right) + H_2^l\right) \tag{17}$$

$$H^{l+1} = LayerNorm\left(FeedForward\left(H_3^l\right) + H_3^l\right) \tag{18}$$

After obtaining the output H of the last layer of the decoder, a linear layer and a *Softmax* activation function is used to map the feature dimension to the size of the list of words reported by the diagnostic and compute the predicted probability distribution for each word:

$$p_i = Softmax(Linear(H))\# \tag{19}$$

Building on the aforementioned structure, the process of radiology report generation unfolds in an aggressive manner. At each time step, reports are generated word-by-word, based on the encoder state and the current sequence, until either the predetermined maximum sequence length is reached or a terminator is generated. The model's training process can be conceptualized as a recursive application of chain rules given the radiological images and fine-grained knowledge E:

$$p(Y|Img) = \prod_{t=1}^{T} p(y_t|y_1, \ldots, y_{t-1}, Img; E) \tag{20}$$

The model is optimized by a cross-entropy loss function and θ denotes the parameters of the model:

$$\mathcal{L} = -\sum_{t=1}^{N} log(P_\theta(y_t|y_{<t}, Img; E)) \tag{21}$$

4 Experiments and Results

4.1 Datasets and Metrics

Datasets. We conduct experiments to evaluate the effectiveness of the proposed FgKF on two widely used radiology report generation benchmarks, i.e., IU-Xray [5] and MIMIC-CXR [6]. The IU X-Ray is a chest X-ray collection that includes 7,470 X-ray images and 3,955 corresponding reports. MIMIC-CXR is the largest publicly available chest X-ray dataset containing radiology reports. The dataset contains 227,827 studies involving 377,110 X-ray images, where one study corresponds to one or more exams of a single patient, and one radiology report corresponds to images from single or multiple views. In the course of the experiments, samples with missing image findings were omitted from both datasets. In other words, images corresponding to different views of the same report were treated as distinct samples. The statistics of the filtered datasets are shown in Table 1.

Table 1. Statistical information on IU X-Ray and MIMIC-CXR

Datasets	IU X-Ray			MIMIC-CXR		
	TRAIN	VAL	TEST	TRAIN	VAL	TEST
IMAGE	4,138	592	1,108	270,790	2,130	3,858
REPORT	2,069	292	590	138,267	1,158	2,344
AVG. LEN	36.44	35.71	32.50	53.00	53.05	66.40

Metrics. To gauge the performance, we employ the widely-used natural language generation (NLG) metrics. We utilize the most widely used BLEU [30] as the main evaluation metric. At the same time, evaluation based solely on N-tuples easily ignores the grammatical soundness of the generated text, as well as synonyms and near-synonyms. To address the aforementioned problems, we incorporate the METEOR [31] and ROUGE-L [32] metrics, which provide a more comprehensive evaluation.

4.2 Implementation Details

ViT-B/32 [33] and ResNet101 [26] are utilized as the visual encoder for the fine-tuning of the CLIP. For ViT-B/32, experiments are conducted with learning rates of $1e-6$ and $5e-6$, respectively. For ResNet101, experiments are conducted with learning rates of $5e-5$ and $5e-6$, respectively. The weight decay is set to a relatively large 0.2. The number of training rounds is set to 15 and the batch size is set to 64. The experimental parameter settings are consistent with [22]. For the IU X-Ray dataset, samples that included both frontal and lateral frontal views were retained. The image features from both views were amalgamated to serve as input for a single sample. On the other hand, for the MIMIC-CXR dataset, images were utilized as base units. In other words, images corresponding to different views of the same report were treated as distinct samples.

4.3 Results and Analysis

Main Results. In order to validate the effectiveness, we compare the performances of our model with a wide range of state-of-the-art models on the IU-Xray and MIMIC-CXR, which include image captioning models [14, 34, 35] and radiology report generation models [22, 36, 37]. The BLEU-4 score is used as a measure of model performance during training. The experimental results are presented in Table 2, where FgKF denotes the model proposed in this work. The models used for comparison include ST [34], ATT2IN [35], R2Gen [22], PPKED [37], and others [14, 36].

Table 2. Comparison on IU-Xray (upper part) and MIMIC-CXR datasets (lower part)

Dataset	Methods	B-1	B-2	B-3	B-4	M	R-L
IU X-Ray	ST	0.216	0.124	0.087	0.066	-	0.306
	ATT2IN	0.224	0.129	0.089	0.068	-	0.308
	ADAATT	0.220	0.127	0.089	0.068	-	0.308
	R2Gen	0.470	0.304	0.219	0.165	0.187	0.371
	R2GenCMN	0.475	0.309	0.222	0.170	0.191	0.375
	PPKED	**0.483**	**0.315**	0.224	0.162	0.190	**0.376**
	FgKF	0.470	0.306	**0.225**	**0.177**	**0.193**	0.364
MIMIC-CXR	ST	0.299	0.184	0.121	0.084	0.124	0.263
	ATT2IN	0.325	0.203	0.136	0.096	0.134	0.276
	ADAATT	0.299	0.185	0.124	0.088	0.118	0.266
	R2Gen	0.353	0.218	0.145	0.103	0.142	0.277
	R2GenCMN	0.353	0.218	0.148	0.106	0.142	0.278
	PPKED	**0.360**	**0.224**	**0.149**	0.106	**0.149**	**0.284**
	FgKF	0.347	0.215	0.146	**0.106**	0.138	0.278

As shown in Table 2, our proposed FgKF model outperforms all the compared models on the BLEU-3, BLEU-4 and METEOR on the IU X-Ray dataset. Compared to the models that are not optimized for the healthcare domain [14, 34, 35], our model shows significant improvement in all the metrics. The BLEU-3 and BLEU-4 scores of our FgKF outperform those of the models designed for radiology report generation [22, 36, 37], which illustrates the effectiveness of our introduction of fine-grained knowledge and fusion in the decoding process. However, we notice that on the MIMIC-CXR dataset, there is still a performance gap between our model and the best baseline (i.e., PPKED [37]). The reason may be that after integrating fine-grained knowledge information, the model's ability to model long-term dependencies in the text is improved, resulting in slightly lower scores on BLEU-1 to BLEU-3.

Ablation Studies. In order to explore the impact of fine-grained knowledge fusion on model performance, we perform ablation tests, and the ablation results are listed in Table 3. "Base" refers to the foundational Transformer model. There are two variants: (1) wo/EEMHA, which does not consider EEMHA but directly concatenates the visual embedding with the entities embedding, (2) wo/KF, which only considers the Transformer-base decoder but not the semantic information fusion decoder. As shown in Table 3, compared to the full model, the performance of wo/EEMHA drops significantly on both datasets. This illustrates the importance of introducing fine-grained entity information. However, for wo/KF, the performance of various metrics remains nearly the same as the full model. This could be due to the fact that during the fusion process of the overall visual context and semantic context, the fine-grained entity information integrated in the overall visual context duplicates with the semantic information in the semantic context. Then, the sigmoid gate filters out the unique information from each and retains the duplicated information. Therefore, during the knowledge fusion process, some good methods for fusing and filtering the two parts of knowledge may have a positive impact on the results. Moreover, the improved performance of the model on the IU X-Ray dataset suggests that using the MIMIC-CXR training set as a knowledge base is feasible when spanning datasets. Since RadGraph was developed based on the MIMIC-CXR dataset, the use of RadGraph will not affect the portability of the model.

Table 3. Ablation studies

		B-1	B-2	B-3	B-4	M	R-L
IU X-Ray	Base	0.396	0.254	0.179	0.135	0.164	0.342
	wo/EEMHA	0.411	0.269	0.196	0.151	0.175	0.347
	wo/KF	0.467	0.301	0.222	0.172	0.184	0.364
	FgKF	0.470	0.306	0.225	0.177	0.193	0.364
MIMIC CXR	Base	0.314	0.192	0.127	0.090	0.125	0.265
	wo/EEMHA	0.328	0.201	0.135	0.097	0.131	0.271
	wo/KF	0.337	0.210	0.142	0.103	0.138	0.277
	FgKF	0.347	0.215	0.146	0.106	0.138	0.278

Qualitative Analysis. To further investigate the effectiveness of the proposed method, reports generated by different models are compared and analyzed. As depicted in Fig. 3, for a randomly chosen sample from the IU X-Ray dataset, both the R2Gen, R2GenCMN and FgKF models correctly describe imaging manifestations such as "no pleural effusion or pneumothorax" and "osseous structures of the thorax are without acute abnormality" in their generated reports. However, the R2Gen inaccurately describes "the heart and mediastinum are within normal limits" as "cardiomediastinal silhouette is unremarkable" and the report generated by the R2GenCMN model lacks the observation of "lungs are clears". In contrast, the FgKF model, which incorporates fine-grained knowledge, provides a more accurate description of the heart and generates reports that align closely with the actual reports. This indicates that the integration of fine-grained knowledge enhances the model's ability to generate more precise radiology reports. To better observe the impact of incorporating fine-grained knowledge on the model, we obtained and mapped the attentional weights of the cross-attention module in the last hidden layer in the decoder (i.e., the attentional weights between the report text and the image) to the original image.

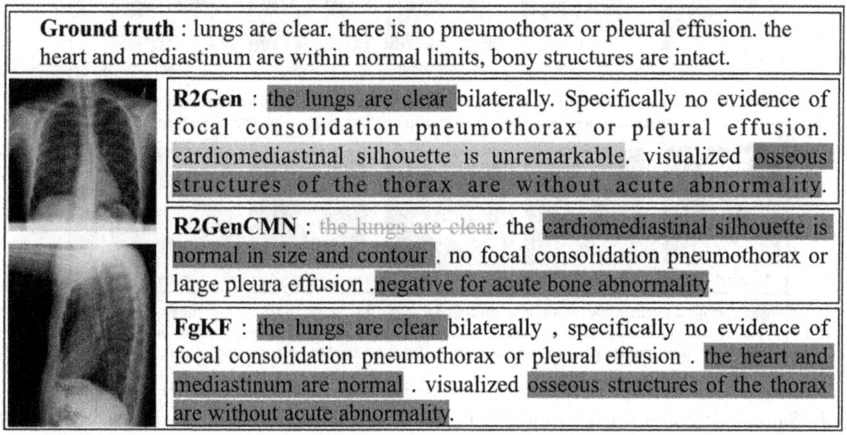

Ground truth : lungs are clear. there is no pneumothorax or pleural effusion. the heart and mediastinum are within normal limits, bony structures are intact.

R2Gen : the lungs are clear bilaterally. Specifically no evidence of focal consolidation pneumothorax or pleural effusion. cardiomediastinal silhouette is unremarkable. visualized osseous structures of the thorax are without acute abnormality.

R2GenCMN : the lungs are clear. the cardiomediastinal silhouette is normal in size and contour. no focal consolidation pneumothorax or large pleura effusion .negative for acute bone abnormality.

FgKF : the lungs are clear bilaterally , specifically no evidence of focal consolidation pneumothorax or pleural effusion . the heart and mediastinum are normal . visualized osseous structures of the thorax are without acute abnormality.

Fig. 3. Sample report generated by FgKF, "Ground truth" stands for the real report. Correct and incorrect descriptions in the generated report are marked with different colors.

As illustrated in Fig. 4, after incorporating fine-grained knowledge, the model not only correctly describes "no pleural effusion" and "cardiomediastinal silhouette appears grossly unchanged", but also identifies and describes surgically implanted devices. Moreover, the transition from "coarsened lung markings" to "underlying emphysema" aligns with the logic of the true report "compared to prior study in the background of emphysema". The attention distribution map shows that correct attention was paid to the location of the clips, lungs, and effusions. More attention was given to the bone structure, consistent with the skeleton distribution. These results suggest that the fusion of fine-grained knowledge enables the model to focus on important anatomical locations, image representations, and other information in radiology reports. This, in turn, helps improve the quality of reports automatically generated by the model.

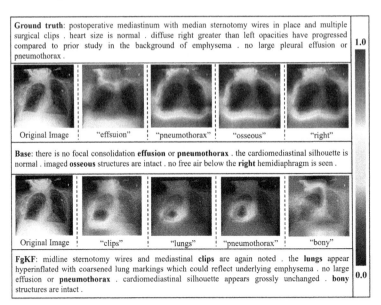

Fig. 4. Sample Attention Visualization by FgKF "Base" stands for the Transformer-base model, and "FgKF" stands for the model proposed by us. Colors ranging from blue to red indicate that the weights range from low to high.

5 Conclusion

In this paper, we propose a fine-grained knowledge fusion model for radiology report generation by fine-tuning the cross-modal pretrained model CLIP to perform a cross-modal retrieval process from images to reports using the MIMIC-CXR training set as a knowledge base. The radiological entities contained in the obtained similarity reports are used as fine-grained knowledge information. In the knowledge fusion process, a multi-attention mechanism for entity information enhancement and a knowledge fusion module are proposed to interact and align image features and report features to facilitate the fusion of different modality features and improve the quality of generated reports. Experiments on two datasets, IU X-Ray and MIMIC-CXR, demonstrate the effectiveness of the cross-modal retrieval procedure with the fine-grained knowledge fusion approach. In future work, we will attempt to edit and distill the fine-grained knowledge in the hidden layers of the neural network to guide the model in generating more accurate radiology reports.

Acknowledgements. This work was supported in part by the Science and Technology Innovation 2030- "New Generation of Artificial Intelligence" Major Project under Grant No. 2021ZD0111000, Zhengzhou City Collaborative Innovation Major Projects (20XTZX11020). We would like to thank the anonymous reviewers for their valuable comments and suggestions on the improvement of this paper.

References

1. Shen, D., Wu, G., Suk, H.I.: Deep learning in medical image analysis. Annu. Rev. Biomed. Eng. **19**, 221–248 (2017)
2. Topol, E.: Deep Medicine: How Artificial Intelligence Can Make Healthcare Human Again. Hachette, UK (2019)
3. Rosman, D.A., Bamporiki, J., Stein-Wexler, R., et al.: Developing diagnostic radiology training in low resource countries. Curr. Radiol. Rep. **7**, 1–7 (2019)
4. Otter, D.W., Medina, J.R., Kalita, J.K.: A survey of the usages of deep learning for natural language processing. IEEE Trans. Neural Netw. Learn. Syst. **32**(2), 604–624 (2021)
5. Demner-Fushman, D., Kohli, M.D., Rosenman, M.B., et al.: Preparing a collection of radiology examinations for distribution and retrieval. J. Am. Med. Inform. Assoc. **23**(2), 304–310 (2016)
6. Johnson, A.E.W., Pollard, T.J., Greenbaum. N.R., et al.: MIMIC-CXR-JPG, a large publicly available database of labeled chest radiographs (2019). arXiv preprint arXiv:1901.07042
7. Pan, J.Y., Yang, H.J., Duygulu, P., et al.: Automatic Image Captioning. In: 2004 IEEE International Conference on Multimedia and Expo (ICME) (IEEE Cat. No. 04TH8763), vol. 3, pp. 1987–1990. IEEE (2004)
8. Farhadi, A., et al.: Every picture tells a story: generating sentences from images. In: Daniilidis, K., Maragos, P., Paragios, N. (eds.) Computer Vision – ECCV 2010. ECCV 2010. LNCS, vol. 6314, pp. 15–29. Springer, Berlin, Heidelberg (2010). https://doi.org/10.1007/978-3-642-155 61-1_2
9. Li, S., Kulkarni, G., Berg, T., et al.: Composing simple image descriptions using web-scale N-grams. In: Proceedings of the Fifteenth Conference on Computational Natural Language Learning, pp. 220–228 (2011)
10. Cho, K., Van Merriënboer, B., Gulcehre, C., et al.: Learning phrase representations using RNN encoder-decoder for statistical machine translation (2014). arXiv preprint arXiv:1406. 1078
11. Sutskever, I., Vinyals, O., Le, Q.V.: Sequence to sequence learning with neural networks. Adv. Neural Inf. Process. Syst. **27** (2014)
12. Bahdanau, D., Cho, K., Bengio, Y.: Neural machine translation by jointly learning to align and translate (2014). arXiv preprint arXiv:1409.0473
13. Ji, J., Luo, Y., Sun, X., et al.: Improving image captioning by leveraging intra-and inter-layer global representation in transformer network. In: Proceedings of the AAAI Conference on Artificial Intelligence, vol. 35, no. 2, pp. 1655–1663 (2021)
14. Lu, J., Xiong, C., Parikh, D., et al.: Knowing when to look: Adaptive attention via a visual sentinel for image captioning. In: Proceedings of the IEEE Conference on Computer Vision and Pattern Recognition, pp. 375–383 (2017)
15. Vinyals, O., Toshev, A., Bengio, S., Erhan, D.: Show and tell: Lessons learned from the 2015 MSCOCO image captioning challenge. IEEE Trans. Pattern Anal. Mach. Intell. **39**(4), 652–663 (2016)
16. Vaswani, A., Shazeer, N., Parmar, N., et al.: Attention is all you need. Adv. Neural Inf. Process. Syst. **30** (2017)
17. Fang, Z., Wang, J., Hu, X., et al.: Injecting semantic concepts into end-to-end image captioning. In: Proceedings of the IEEE/CVF Conference on Computer Vision and Pattern Recognition, pp. 18009–18019 (2022)
18. Li, Y., Pan, Y., Yao, T., et al.: Comprehending and ordering semantics for image captioning. In: Proceedings of the IEEE/CVF Conference on Computer Vision and Pattern Recognition, pp. 17990–17999 (2022)

19. Radford, A., Kim, J.W., Hallacy, C., et al.: Learning transferable visual models from natural language supervision. In: International Conference on Machine Learning. PMLR, pp. 8748–8763 (2021)
20. Jing, B., Xie, P., Xing, E.: On the automatic generation of medical imaging reports. In: Proceedings of the 56th Annual Meeting of the Association for Computational Linguistics (Volume 1: Long Papers), pp. 2577–2586 (2018)
21. Li, Y., Liang, X., Hu, Z., et al.: Hybrid retrieval-generation reinforced agent for medical image report generation. Adv. Neural Inf. Process. Syst. **31** (2018)
22. Chen, Z., Song, Y., Chang, T.H., et al.: generating radiology reports via memory-driven transformer. In: Proceedings of the 2020 Conference on Empirical Methods in Natural Language Processing (EMNLP), pp. 1439–1449 (2020)
23. Zhang, Y., Wang, X., Xu, Z., et al.: When radiology report generation meets knowledge graph. In: Proceedings of the AAAI Conference on Artificial Intelligence, vol. 34, no. 07, pp. 12910–12917 (2020)
24. You, D., Liu, F., Ge, S., Xie, X., Zhang, J., Wu, X.: Aligntransformer: hierarchical alignment of visual regions and disease tags for medical report generation. In: de Bruijne, M., et al. (eds.) Medical Image Computing and Computer Assisted Intervention – MICCAI 2021. MICCAI 2021. LNCS, vol. 12903, pp. 72–82. Springer, Cham (2021). https://doi.org/10.1007/978-3-030-87199-4_7
25. Wang, J., Bhalerao, A., He, Y.: Cross-modal prototype driven network for radiology report generation. In: Avidan, S., Brostow, G., Cissé, M., Farinella, G.M., Hassner, T. (eds.) Computer Vision – ECCV 2022. ECCV 2022. LNCS, vol. 13695, pp. 563–579. Springer, Cham (2022). https://doi.org/10.1007/978-3-031-19833-5_33
26. He, K., Zhang, X., Ren, S., et al.: Deep residual learning for image recognition. In: Proceedings of the IEEE Conference on Computer Vision and Pattern Recognition, pp. 770–778 (2016)
27. Jain, S., Agrawal, A., Saporta, A., et al.: Radgraph: extracting clinical entities and relations from radiology reports. In: Proceedings of the 35th Neural Information Processing Systems (NeurIPS 2021) Track on Datasets and Benchmarks (2021)
28. Alsentzer, E., Murphy, J.R., Boag, W., et al.: Publicly available clinical BERT embeddings (2019). arXiv preprint arXiv:1904.03323
29. Lee, J., Yoon, W., Kim, S., et al.: BioBERT: a pre-trained biomedical language representation model for biomedical text mining. Bioinformatics **36**(4), 1234–1240 (2020)
30. Papineni, K., Roukos, S., Ward, T., et al.: Bleu: a method for automatic evaluation of machine translation. In: Proceedings of the 40th Annual Meeting of the Association for Computational Linguistics, pp. 311–318 (2002)
31. Denkowski, M., Lavie, A.: Meteor 1.3: automatic metric for reliable optimization and evaluation of machine translation systems. In: Proceedings of the Sixth Workshop on Statistical Machine Translation, pp. 85–91 (2011)
32. Lin, C.Y.: Rouge: a package for automatic evaluation of summaries. Text Summarization Branches Out, pp. 74–81 (2004)
33. Dosovitskiy, A., Beyer, L., Kolesnikov, A., et al.: An image is worth 16×16 words: Transformers for image recognition at scale (2020). arXiv preprint arXiv:2010.11929
34. Vinyals, O., Toshev, A., Bengio, S., et al.: Show and tell: a neural image caption generator. In: Proceedings of the IEEE Conference on Computer Vision and Pattern Recognition, pp. 3156–3164 (2015)
35. Rennie, S.J., Marcheret, E., Mroueh, Y., et al.: Self-critical sequence training for image captioning. In: Proceedings of the IEEE Conference on Computer Vision and Pattern Recognition, pp. 7008–7024 (2017)

36. Chen, Z., Shen, Y., Song, Y., et al.: Cross-modal memory networks for radiology report generation (2022). arXiv preprint arXiv:2204.13258
37. Liu, F., Wu, X., Ge, S., et al.: Exploring and distilling posterior and prior knowledge for radiology report generation. In: Proceedings of the IEEE/CVF Conference on Computer Vision and Pattern Recognition, pp. 13753–13762 (2021)

Automatic Generation of Discharge Summary of EMRs Based on Multi-granularity Information Fusion

Bingfei Zhao[1], Hongying Zan[1(✉)], Chengzhi Niu[2], Hongyang Chang[3],
and Kunli Zhang[1]

[1] Zhengzhou University, Zhengzhou, China
{iehyzan,ieklzhang}@zzu.edu.cn
[2] The First Affiliated Hospital of Zhengzhou University, Zhengzhou, China
[3] Unit 63893 of the People's Liberation Army, Luoyang, China

Abstract. Discharge summaries are a significant component of electronic medical records, playing a crucial role in follow-up treatment and scientific research. However, there are few researches on automated discharge summary generation based on deep learning, and there is also a lack of available datasets. To address this, in this paper, we construct a small-scale dataset containing various types of entity information for the task of automated discharge summary generation from electronic medical records. In order to make full use of the rich entity information implied in medical records, we design a generation model based on a T5 architecture that encodes various types of entity information and incorporates the information contained in the entities into the encoder using multi-granularity fusion methods. Meanwhile, we use pointer-generator networks to enhance the model's generalization capability. The experimental results show that the proposed dataset is challenging, and compared to the baseline models, the proposed model achieves significant improvements on the evaluation metrics. Additionally, ablation studies further demonstrate that incorporating entity information and pointer-generator networks positively contributes to the summarization quality of the model.

Keywords: Discharge Summary Generation · Entity Information · Multi-granularity Fusion · Pointer-generator Networks

1 Introduction

Automatic text summarization technology, also known as automatic summarization, uses short sentences to compress a large amount of text, retaining the key information in the text, solving the problem of redundant and complex content of the original text, which can effectively reduce the burden brought by a large amount of information and improve the speed of Internet users to obtain information, so as to replace manual work and save a lot of manpower and material resources. The application scope of automatic text summarization is very wide, such as in the news [10, 30, 31], public opinion analysis, opinion/emotional summary, scientific paper summary [4, 21] and other fields have important research value. Although there are a large number of studies on automatic summarization generation, they are mainly concentrated in the fields of economics and journalism, and there is little work in the clinical field. With the widespread adoption of electronic medical records in the medical field, each patient accumulates a large amount of medical history. While these records contain rich information about the patient, there is also a lot of redundancy. Doctors need to spend significant time going through all the records when writing discharge summaries for patients. Therefore, utilizing automatic summarization techniques to generate discharge summaries can effectively simplify the doctor's work and improve efficiency.

Currently, research in the medical field primarily focuses on tasks such as medical entity relationship extraction [18,36,52], disease risk prediction [19,27], medical imaging report generation [42,45], and auxiliary diagnosis [14]. Although some work has also viewed medical text generation as a summarization task, for example, summarizing radiology reports to generate clinical impressions [50]; summarizing patient health records to generate medical history [38] and extracting important clinical entities from radiology reports and inpatient records [9,40]. However, research has been predominantly focused on the English medical domain, with very few studies on discharge summary generation in the Chinese domain. To address this gap and provide researchers with sufficient data for training and evaluating models based on electronic medical record data in real-world healthcare settings, we have constructed a small-scale electronic medical record dataset (EMRDS) containing diverse entity information.

Considering that incorporating additional knowledge can improve summarization model performance [8,39,41], and electronic medical records contain abundant structured entity information such as diseases, symptoms, examinations, drug treatments, surgical procedures, etc., how to effectively utilize such key entity information to improve text generation quality is a promising direction to explore. Therefore, based on the constructed dataset for discharge summary generating from electronic medical records, this paper proposes an entity-enhanced model called DSGE for discharge summary generation from electronic medical records.

The main contributions of this paper can be summarized as follows:

- We construct an annotated dataset EMRDS for discharge summary generation from electronic medical records across three diseases. The dataset contains various types of entity information and is manually labeled.
- By introducing the method of multi-granularity fusion, DSGE enriches the semantic information of original text with various entity information from electronic medical records.
- To enhance the generation ability of sequence-to-sequence models, DSGE uses pointer-generation networks to enhance the generalization ability of models by using the information of the original text.
- Comparative experiments with various baseline models on the EMRDS dataset verify the effectiveness of the two proposed methods. Ablation studies are also conducted to analyze the impact of different numbers of entity types and two fusion approaches, as well as the effect of pointer-generator networks.

2   Related Work

2.1   Abstractive Summarization

Unlike extractive automatic summarization which produces summaries by simply concatenating content from the source text, abstractive automatic summarization generates summaries through understanding the semantics of the original text and utilizing natural language generation techniques. There are two issues with attention-based seq2seq model for abstractive summarization. First, During encoding, it only considers several preceding words when computing vector representations or hidden states for each word, leading to suboptimal results. Second, The UNK problem where words outside the vocabulary cannot be handled properly. To address the first issue, Zeng [48] proposed a read-again mechanism which reads the input sequence again before computing representations to identify key words. For the second issue, pointer-generator networks [39] are adopted to balance generation and copying, improving generalization capability. In addition to the implicit learning, existing work also focuses on explicit structure. In particular, explicit structure plays an important role in recent deep learning-based extraction and abstract summarization methods [20,26]. Different structures contribute to summarization from different aspects [5,43]. Dependency parse trees facilitate semantic understanding for summarizers, helping generate sentences with better semantic relevance [12]. In addition to sentence-level structure, document-level structure has also attracted widespread attention. Fernandes [6] constructed a simple graph consisting of sentences, tokens, and parts of speech for summary generation. By combining RST tree, Xu [44] proposed a discourse perception model to extract sentences. Besides, structure from semantic analysis is helpful, Abstract Meaning Representation (AMR) guide summary to better understand the input context [22].

2.2   Text Generation in Medical Field

The field of medical language generation has garnered growing research attention. For example, generating radiology reports from chest X-ray images [13,24,25], generating clinical records from emergency department medical records from discharge diagnosis coding [16], and mental health record generation [11]. For the medical generation field, most of the research has focused on the production of radiology reports [28,51]. In biomedical natural language processing, some domain-specific pre-trained language models (PLMs), such as BioBERT [15], SciBERT [2], and PubMedBERT [7], have been proposed by training domain-specific texts in PubMed/MEDLINE. These domain-specific models show remarkable performance on downstream tasks within the domain. Similarly, following the success of PLMs based generation encoder-decoders such as BART [17], T5 [35], and BERT2BERT [37], pre-trained biomedical generation models such as SciFive [33] and BioBART [47] have been proposed. These models can handle generative tasks in the biomedical field, such as clinical conversations, biomedical questions and answers, and biomedical text summaries.

However, as research has been more focused on the English language, in order to fill the gap in the Chinese medical domain, this paper conducts research on the Chinese medical domain using the proposed dataset.

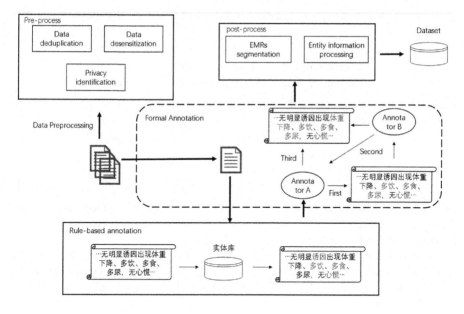

Fig. 1. EMRDS dataset construction details.

3   Dataset Construction

Due to high construction costs, Chinese EMR data is relatively scarce. This study collected EMRs from endocrinology, cardiology, and neurology departments at a top tier 3 hospital, and constructed an EMR discharge summary generation dataset (EMRDS). The EMRDS construction process had three main steps: preparation, annotation, and post-processing, as shown in Fig. 1. As the EMRs were from the same source and had an overall consistent structure, the data preprocessing, annotation system, and annotation specifications were generally consistent.

3.1   Preparatory Work

This paper refers to the existing electronic medical record annotation system and annotation specification [3,46] to guide the training of annotators and the physical annotation of electronic medical records.

EMRs for different diseases have slightly different structures, but generally contained admission records, first course of disease, ward round records, and discharge summaries. Analysis showed discharge summaries could be divided into five sections: admission situation, admission diagnosis, diagnosis basis, diagnosis and treatment process and discharge situation. Furthermore, analysis found each section of the discharge summary originated from other parts of the EMR, while the remaining parts were also interrelated. The relationships are shown in Table 1.

The left half of Table 1 can serve as the original text for the EMR discharge summary generation dataset, while the right half as the summary. Specifically, this study

Table 1. The correspondence of medical record data after segmentation.

Source	Target
Admission record	First course of disease
Admission record	Diagnostic basis
First course of disease	Admission diagnosis
First course of disease	Admission situation
Ward round record	Diagnosis and treatment process
Ward round record	Discharge situation

used the five discharge summary sections - admission situation, admission diagnosis, diagnosis basis, diagnosis and treatment course, and discharge situation from the EMRs. Finally, 1250 EMRs were selected for the dataset.

In order to improve the efficiency and quality of data annotation and facilitate the review of annotation progress, the entity and relationship annotation platform developed by Zhang [46] was adopted in this paper to manually annotate entities in electronic medical records.

3.2   Entity Information Annotation

Pre-annotation. EMRs annotation relied on medical expertise, the annotators were computer science graduate students. To ensure quality and consistency, annotators received pre-annotation training on platform operation, guidelines, and specifications. Trial annotation deployed same-source, same-type data to avoid trial errors impacting formal annotation yet ensure quality. Pre-annotation training and trial annotation ensured annotators thoroughly understood tasks and requirements, laying groundwork for subsequent formal annotation. This study emphasizes standardized annotation process management, adopting quality control measures to build high-quality dataset.

During analysis, we found admission records' general examination section contained dense, repetitive text with many entities. For such repetitive, entity-rich dense text, we used rule-based automatic pre-annotation before manual annotation. Rule-based pre-annotation can reduce human labor costs while facilitating overall annotation control for such content, improving efficiency and quality.

Formal Annotation. For dataset formal annotation, a multi-round cross-review strategy was used where each EMR was jointly annotated by two annotators. Annotator A did primary annotation, manually supplementing rules/dictionary omissions and recording issues for discussion, forming the first annotated file. Annotator B then reviewed the first file, modifying erroneous/missing annotations to produce the second file. Controversial issues were recorded and discussed jointly by A and B for resolution by A in a confirmation pass, finally producing the third annotated file.

After two rounds of multi-round annotation, entity annotation files were exported in entity-attribute pair format and checked for inconsistent annotations of the same entity and guideline violations. Finally, issues were fed back to A for rectification.

Table 2. Different lengths of medical record data.

Section	Length avg
First course of disease	652.56
Admission situation	349.55
Admission diagnosis	28.29
Diagnosis and treatment process	722.92
Diagnostic basis	550.08
Discharge situation	54.08

Table 3. Entity types and numbers of different diseases.

Entity types	Diabetes mellitus	Cardiovascular	Cerebral stroke
Symptoms	3682	5347	2118
Examinations	2049	1566	2035
Diseases	1039	1064	896
Drug therapy	1010	718	490
Decorate	456	544	466
Other treatment	392	428	321
Time	330	328	283
Body	242	504	868
surgical operation	155	96	204

3.3 Data Processing

Segmentation of Electronic Medical Records. As EMRs are typically long (avg 2358 words) and commonly used pre-trained models limit max input text to 512 tokens, the corresponding medical history and discharge summary sections can be split into multiple summary text pairs for model training and inference. This addresses overly long input while ensuring section correspondence, as shown in Table 1.

To facilitate limiting model input/output lengths, average section lengths were analyzed, with results shown in Table 2. The analysis shows the average lengths after splitting are close to the 512 maximum input text length limit of the model. This indicates splitting the EMRs into multiple summary pairs avoids losing original EMR data information, allowing the model to fully leverage the textual information.

Entity Information Processing. To enable entity information comparison across different disease EMRs, entity types and quantities were statistically analyzed for the three diseases. cerebral stroke EMRs contained 10,595 unique entities, diabetes mellitus 9,355, and cardiovascular 7,681 (Table 3). Symptoms, examinations, and diseases types accounted for 65% of all entities, likely due to the numerous examinations in the cases including general and disease/symptom-specific. Since diseases, symptoms, and examinations were the most relevant and numerous entities in the EMRs, only these three entity types were retained in the dataset.

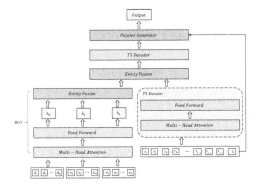

Fig. 2. DSGE Model Architecture.

Labeling Consistency Evaluation. To evaluate annotation quality, the initial and final annotated files were exported after dataset annotation completion for comparison of annotation consistency between the two rounds. Annotation consistency was calculated as:

$$P = \frac{A_1 \cap A_2}{A_1} \tag{1}$$

$$R = \frac{A_1 \cap A_2}{A_2} \tag{2}$$

$$F_1 = \frac{2 * P * R}{P + R} \tag{3}$$

where A_1 and A_2 refer to the annotation results for the same EMR in the initial and final annotated files, respectively, and $\cap$ denotes their intersection, i.e. the identical annotations between the two files. Artstein [1] stated annotation consistency values above 80% indicate trustworthy annotation results.

After calculation, the entity consistency rate for the dataset was 89.66%. The high consistency demonstrates the annotated content is reliable.

4   Model

Based on the constructed dataset, this study proposes an EMR discharge summary generation model enhanced by entity information. By improving multi-granularity information fusion, entity information is embedded into the encoder to obtain enriched encoded text representations. Since discharge summaries largely originate from the original text, the model utilizes a pointer-generator network to rewrite the decoded results after decoding to obtain the final outputs. The overall architecture of the DSGE model is shown in Fig. 2.

4.1   Multi-granularity Entity Information Fusion

To integrate different entity information and obtain more comprehensive, accurate results, one approach is direct concatenation of text contents as the fusion result. This is

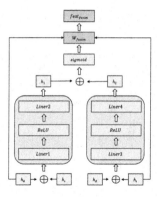

Fig. 3. Fusion Gate Structure Diagram.

simple to implement with little impact on original text, retaining existing semantics and syntax. However, concatenation cannot deeply fuse information, making it difficult to internalize new information, leading to inconsistent granularity and less fluent semantics. Therefore, this study adopts fusion gates to fuse different granularity information, with adjustments to commonly used fusion gates to suit the dataset.

We define the disease entity sequence $D = d_1, d_2, ..., d_n$, where n is the length of the disease entity sequence; the symptom entity sequence $S = s_1, s_2, ..., s_m$, where m is the length of the symptom entity sequence; the examination entity sequence $E = e_1, e_2, ..., e_k$, where k is the length of the examination entity sequence; and the original sentence sequence $T = t_1, t_2, ..., t_l$, where l is the length of the original sentence sequence. In this study, we chose the pretrained model Bert as the encoder for the entity information. During model training, the encoded three types of entity information are fed into Bert separately to obtain the latent vector representations for each,

$$h_x = Bert\,(x_1, x_2, \ldots, x_n)$$
$$where \quad x = d, s, e \tag{4}$$

where h_d, h_s, and h_e represent the encoded outputs for the disease, symptom, and examination entities respectively. To integrate information from different entities, we adopt an improved fusion gate strategy $Fusion_{gate}$ to fuse the three entity representations, with the structure shown in Fig. 3. Taking the latent vectors h_d and h_s as an example, we define $Fusion_{gate}(h_d, h_s)$ as:

$$h_1 = fusion\,(add\,(h_d, h_s)) \tag{5}$$

$$h_2 = fusion\,(add\,(h_d, h_s)) \tag{6}$$

$$W_{fusion} = sigmoid\,(add\,(h_1, h_2)) \tag{7}$$

$$feat_{fusion} = W_{fusion} * h_d + (1 - W_{fusion}) * h_s \tag{8}$$

where $fusion$ is a sequential module for non-linear feature extraction, implemented by combining two Linear layers with a $ReLU$ activation function. It is used to extract information from different representational subspaces to enhance the expressive capability

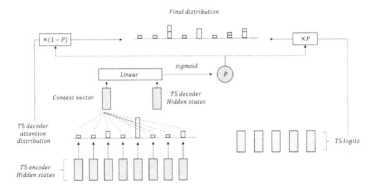

Fig. 4. Pointer-generator Network Decoder.

of features. $W_f usion$ represents the gating weights for fusing entity pair representations h_d and h_s. Let h_1 and h_2 denote the structural and content information respectively before fusion. The feature representation after fusing the three entity information sources is:

$$F_{fusion} = Fusion_{gate} \left(Fusion_{gate} \left(h_d, h_s \right), h_e \right) \tag{9}$$

The fused entity pair representation F_{fusion} is further fused with the text sequence representation h_t from the encoder in the same gated manner to obtain the final sequence feature h_m:

$$h_m = Fusion_{gate} \left(F_{fusion}, h_t \right) \tag{10}$$

4.2 Decoding Based on Pointer Network

Since abstractive summaries often contain content copied from the original text, a pointer-generator network decoder is constructed to enhance the sequence-to-sequence model's generation capability, as shown in Fig. 4. This decoder has a dual-channel architecture, consisting of a generation channel and a copying channel.

Specifically, let m_t be the decoder hidden state at time step t, and α_t be the attention distribution over the original sequence. The probability distribution of the copying channel is computed as:

$$P_{copy} = \sum_{i:w_i=w} \alpha_{t,i} \tag{11}$$

where w_i is the $i - th$ word in the original sequence, and $\alpha_(t, i)$ is the attention weight for the $i - th$ word at time step t. The final output $logits$ are a convex combination of the generation and copying distributions, fused by a gating unit g:

$$P\left(\text{w}\right) = g * P_{copy}\left(\text{w}\right) + \left(1 - g\right) * P_{gen}\left(\text{w}\right) \tag{12}$$

where g is obtained by mapping the decoder hidden state h_t and original context vector c_t from the attention mechanism through a single layer network with a *sigmoid* function:

$$g = sigmoid\left(W_g\left[h_t, c_t\right] + b_g\right) \tag{13}$$

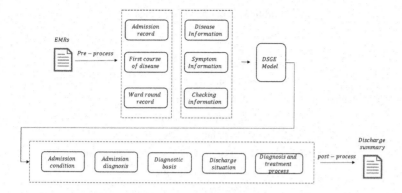

Fig. 5. Flow chart of electronic medical record discharge summary generation.

W_g and b_g are the weight and bias of the fully connected layer. This dual-channel decoder architecture allows the decoder to freely copy words from the input as well as generate novel words. This ensures both accuracy and generalizability, enhancing the generation capability of the model. During training, cross-entropy loss is computed between the decoder outputs and target sequences to end-to-end learn the parameters of the gating unit, achieving adaptive control over generation and copying. During inference, we search over both the target vocabulary and original sequence words, and output the most likely target sequence.

5 Experiment

5.1 Experimental Settings

To verify model effectiveness, we used the constructed EMR dataset. Specifically, when a new EMR is obtained, it is pre-processed to split into admission records, first course of disease and ward round records and extract contained entity information. The text and entities are then fed into the DSGE model to generate admission situation, admission diagnosis, diagnosis basis, diagnosis and treatment process and discharge situation. Finally, post-processing obtains the final discharge summary. The specific process is shown in Fig. 5.

The experiments were conducted on an NVidia GeForce RTX4090 GPU, using Pytorch 1.13.1 and CUDA 11.10.3. The hyperparameter settings for the experiments are shown in Table 4.

Since different diseases have varying data amounts, to prevent training and test distribution bias and better evaluate model generalization, equal disease data amounts were extracted for the test set (100 data total). The remaining data was split 9:1 into training and validation sets.

Table 4. Experimental Settings.

	Parameter	Value
	Epoch	15
	Batch size	4
Input Part	Admission records	512
	First course of disease	512
	Ward round records	512
Output Part	Admission situation	100
	Admission diagnosis	64
	Diagnosis and treatment process	512
	Diagnostic basis	512
	Discharge situation	448
	lr	1e-5
	Optimizer	AdamW
Entity information	Disease entity	512
	Symptom entity	512
	Examination entity	512

Table 5. Experimental results on the EMRDS dataset.

Model	R-1	R-2	R-3	Bleu	R-avg
TextRank	42.23	27.94	28.51	–	32.90
LEAD-3	45.89	33.40	31.27	–	36.85
T5	77.15	68.98	68.30	56.47	71.48
Prophet	77.86	69.57	69.77	59.56	72.40
Pegasus	79.86	72.16	72.16	61.17	74.72
T5-pegasus	80.31	71.33	74.11	61.81	75.24
DSGE	**82.82**	**75.84**	**75.39**	**63.77**	**78.02**

5.2 Baselines and Evaluation

To understand EMRDS dataset challenges and comprehensively evaluate the DSGE model, we trained and evaluated several common abstractive models including two unsupervised models, including LEAD-3 and TextRank [29]. In addition, we used the pretrained language models T5, Pegasus [49], ProphetNet [34], and T5-pegasus.

To verify summary quality, we adopted Rouge [23] and Bleu [32] metrics to compare model-generated discharge summaries against original EMR discharge summaries for matching degree.

5.3 Experimental Analysis

Analysis of Main Experiment Results. Table 5 shows the comparative experiment results on the DSGE dataset, where R-1, R-2, and R-L represent Rouge-1, Rouge-2,

Table 6. Ablation experiments with different methods.

Model	R-1	R-2	R-3	Bleu	R-avg
Baseline (T5)	77.15	68.98	68.30	56.47	71.48
+cp	79.39	71.72	71.43	60.54	74.18
+cp&en	82.82	75.84	75.39	63.77	78.02

and Rouge-L respectively, and R-avg represents the average of Rouge-1, Rouge-2, and Rouge-L.

The experimental results show that just fine-tuning pretrained models like T5 on the dataset can significantly outperform unsupervised models like TextRank and LEAD-3. This further validates the superior performance of pretrained language models on text summarization tasks. Compared to the T5 model, DSGE achieved improved results on the test set, with increases of 6.54% points on Rouge-avg and 7.30% points on BLEU. Moreover, DSGE outperformed unsupervised models, and compared to pretrained models Pegasus and Prophet, obtained 3.30 and 5.62% point gains on Rouge-avg, and 2.60 and 4.21% point gains on BLEU respectively. This sufficiently demonstrates the efficacy of the proposed method in improving text summarization quality.

The analysis is that the performance gains of DSGE can be attributed to the entity information providing multi-faceted understanding for the model, while the pointer-generator network utilizes statistical characteristics of the data itself, enabling the model to integrate local and global features. The organic combination of the two leads to remarkable improvement in model performance. Compared to Pegasus and Prophet models which rely more on the pretrained language model frameworks themselves, DSGE injects prior knowledge into the internal framework, tapping the potential of model capacity.

Ablation Experiments with Different Methods. To further analyze the necessity of incorporating multi-granularity entity information and pointer-generator networks in the model, ablation experiments were conducted on the dataset. The experimental results are shown in Table 6.

Where +cp represents adding pointer-generator network on top of the baseline model, and +cp&en denotes using both pointer-generator network and multi-information fusion on top of the baseline.

Compared to the baseline T5 model, adding pointer-generator network improved Rouge-avg by 2.70% points and Bleu by 4.07% points. This shows that employing pointer-generator networks can help the model copy key words and phrases from the original text more accurately, thus generating more fluent and logically clear text.

Furthermore, with pointer-generator network as the basis, adding multi-information fusion led to further significant improvements across metrics. This indicates that fusing different entity information can provide richer contextual support, enabling the model to learn better semantic matching relationships, and thus generate text more conforming to logic and semantics.

Table 7. Ablation experiments with different entity quantities and fusion modes.

Model	R-1	R-2	R-3	Bleu	R-avg
Baseline (T5+CP)	79.39	71.72	71.43	60.53	74.18
$+il$	80.90	73.71	73.22	60.93	75.94
$+sy$	80.09	72.46	71.68	59.20	74.74
$+ex$	80.36	72.98	72.50	59.71	75.28
$+il\&sy\&ex$	80.31	73.10	72.79	60.18	75.40
$+il \odot sy \odot ex$ (DSGE)	82.82	75.84	75.39	63.77	78.02

Ablation Experiments of Different Entity Quantities and Fusion Modes. This paper further analyzes the effect of different numbers of entity information and different fusion methods on the model, with experimental results shown in Table 7.

Where $+il$ represents incorporating disease information on top of the baseline model, $+sy$ represents incorporating symptom information, +ex represents incorporating examination information, $+il\&sy\&ex$ represents directly concatenating the three types of entity information on top of the baseline model, and $+il \odot sy \odot ex$ represents incorporating the three types via a fusion gate on top of the baseline model.

Comparing the results of $+il$, $+sy$, and +ex with the baseline T5+CP, incorporating different additional entity information on top of the baseline model can effectively enhance the summarization performance. The results show that using different entity information leads to varying degrees of improvement, indicating that incorporating different entity information into the baseline model can optimize the model to different extents.

Furthermore, directly concatenating ($+il\&sy\&ex$) and using a fusion gate ($+il \odot sy \odot ex$) were explored for integrating the three types of entity information. The former directly concatenates the information while the latter selectively aggregates information by learning weights. Experiments show that the fusion gate mechanism better utilizes the different types of entity information, leading to significant improvements on ROUGE and BLEU metrics. This demonstrates that the fusion gate can automatically learn the importance of different types of information, achieving better information fusion and providing an effective method for integrating multi-source heterogeneous information for text generation tasks.

6   Conclusion

This paper primarily introduces an application of text summarization in the medical domain - generating discharge summaries from electronic medical records. Due to the high cost of collecting medical data, a small-scale dataset EMRDS was constructed. To fully utilize the rich entity information in medical records, a multi-granularity information fusion summarization model is proposed. Specifically, the model incorporates various encoded entity information into the source text through an improved fusion gate, enriching the semantic information of the source. Furthermore, a pointer-generator network is added on top of the base model to enhance generalizability. Experiments show the proposed method is effective for discharge summary generation, and multi-granularity information fusion complements the pointer-generator network. Information fusion enriches the semantic representation, while the pointer-generator balances decoding to obtain better summaries. For future work, knowledge graphs could be considered to better incorporate information and further improve the generation performance of the model.

Acknowledgements. This research is supported by the key research and development and promotion project of Henan Provincial Department of Science and Technology in 2023 (232102211041, 232102211033) and the Science and Technology Innovation 2030-"New Generation of Artificial Intelligence" Major Project under Grant No.2021ZD0111000. We would like to thank the anonymous reviewers for their valuable comments and suggestions on the improvement of this paper.

References

1. Artstein, R., Poesio, M.: Inter-coder agreement for computational linguistics. Comput. Linguist. **34**(4), 555–596 (2008)
2. Beltagy, I., Lo, K., Cohan, A.: SciBERT: a pretrained language model for scientific text. arXiv preprint arXiv:1903.10676 (2019)
3. Chang, H., Zan, H., Ma, Y., Zhang, K.: Corpus construction for named-entity and entity relations for electronic medical records of cardiovascular disease. In: Tang, B., et al. (eds.) CHIP 2022. CCIS, vol. 1772, pp. 633–642. Springer, Singapore (2021). https://doi.org/10. 1007/978-981-19-9865-2_1 : (corpus construction for named-entity and entity relations for electronic medical records of stroke disease). In: Proceedings of the 20th Chinese National Conference on Computational Linguistics. pp. 633–642 (2021)
4. Cohan, A., Goharian, N.: Scientific document summarization via citation contextualization and scientific discourse. Int. J. Digit. Libr. **19**, 287–303 (2018)
5. Desai, S., Xu, J., Durrett, G.: Compressive summarization with plausibility and salience modeling. arXiv preprint arXiv:2010.07886 (2020)
6. Fernandes, P., Allamanis, M., Brockschmidt, M.: Structured neural summarization. arXiv preprint arXiv:1811.01824 (2018)
7. Gu, Y., Tinn, R., Cheng, H., Lucas, M., Usuyama, N., Liu, X., Naumann, T., Gao, J., Poon, H.: Domain-specific language model pretraining for biomedical natural language processing. ACM Trans. Comput. Healthc. (HEALTH) **3**(1), 1–23 (2021)
8. Gunel, B., Zhu, C., Zeng, M., Huang, X.: Mind the facts: knowledge-boosted coherent abstractive text summarization. arXiv preprint arXiv:2006.15435 (2020)
9. Hassanpour, S., Langlotz, C.P.: Information extraction from multi-institutional radiology reports. Artif. Intell. Med. **66**, 29–39 (2016)
10. Hermann, K.M., et al.: Teaching machines to read and comprehend. In: Advances in Neural Information Processing Systems, vol. 28 (2015)
11. Ive, J., et al.: Generation and evaluation of artificial mental health records for natural language processing. NPJ Digit. Med. **3**(1), 69 (2020)
12. Jin, H., Wang, T., Wan, X.: SemSUM: semantic dependency guided neural abstractive summarization. In: Proceedings of the AAAI Conference on Artificial Intelligence, vol. 34, pp. 8026–8033 (2020)
13. Jing, B., Xie, P., Xing, E.: On the automatic generation of medical imaging reports. arXiv preprint arXiv:1711.08195 (2017)

14. Kermany, D.S., et al.: Identifying medical diagnoses and treatable diseases by image-based deep learning. Cell **172**(5), 1122–1131 (2018)
15. Lee, J., et al.: BioBERT: a pre-trained biomedical language representation model for biomedical text mining. Bioinformatics **36**(4), 1234–1240 (2020)
16. Lee, S.H.: Natural language generation for electronic health records. NPJ Digit. Med. **1**(1), 63 (2018)
17. Lewis, M., et al.: BART: denoising sequence-to-sequence pre-training for natural language generation, translation, and comprehension. arXiv preprint arXiv:1910.13461 (2019)
18. Li, H., Chen, Q., Tang, B., Wang, X.: Chemical-induced disease extraction via convolutional neural networks with attention. In: 2017 IEEE International Conference on Bioinformatics and Biomedicine (BIBM), pp. 1276–1279. IEEE (2017)
19. Li, J., Wu, B., Sun, X., Wang, Y.: Causal hidden Markov model for time series disease forecasting. In: Proceedings of the IEEE/CVF Conference on Computer Vision and Pattern Recognition, pp. 12105–12114 (2021)
20. Li, W., Xiao, X., Lyu, Y., Wang, Y.: Improving neural abstractive document summarization with explicit information selection modeling. In: Proceedings of the 2018 Conference on Empirical Methods in Natural Language Processing, pp. 1787–1796 (2018)
21. Li, Y., et al.: CSL: a large-scale Chinese scientific literature dataset. arXiv preprint arXiv:2209.05034 (2022)
22. Liao, K., Lebanoff, L., Liu, F.: Abstract meaning representation for multi-document summarization. arXiv preprint arXiv:1806.05655 (2018)
23. Lin, C.Y.: ROUGE: a package for automatic evaluation of summaries. In: Text Summarization Branches Out, pp. 74–81 (2004)
24. Liu, F., Wu, X., Ge, S., Fan, W., Zou, Y.: Exploring and distilling posterior and prior knowledge for radiology report generation. In: Proceedings of the IEEE/CVF Conference on Computer Vision and Pattern Recognition, pp. 13753–13762 (2021)
25. Liu, F., You, C., Wu, X., Ge, S., Sun, X., et al.: Auto-encoding knowledge graph for unsupervised medical report generation. In: Advances in Neural Information Processing Systems, vol. 34, pp. 16266–16279 (2021)
26. Liu, Y., Titov, I., Lapata, M.: Single document summarization as tree induction. In: Proceedings of the 2019 Conference of the North American Chapter of the Association for Computational Linguistics: Human Language Technologies, Volume 1 (Long and Short Papers), pp. 1745–1755 (2019)
27. Lutz, C.S., et al.: Applying infectious disease forecasting to public health: a path forward using influenza forecasting examples. BMC Public Health **19**(1), 1–12 (2019)
28. MacAvaney, S., Sotudeh, S., Cohan, A., Goharian, N., Talati, I., Filice, R.W.: Ontology-aware clinical abstractive summarization. In: Proceedings of the 42nd International ACM SIGIR Conference on Research and Development in Information Retrieval, pp. 1013–1016 (2019)
29. Mihalcea, R., Tarau, P.: TextRank: bringing order into text. In: Proceedings of the 2004 Conference on Empirical Methods in Natural Language Processing, pp. 404–411 (2004)
30. Narayan, S., Cohen, S.B., Lapata, M.: Don't give me the details, just the summary! Topic-aware convolutional neural networks for extreme summarization. arXiv preprint arXiv:1808.08745 (2018)
31. Over, P., Dang, H., Harman, D.: Duc in context. Inf. Process. Manage. **43**(6), 1506–1520 (2007)
32. Papineni, K., Roukos, S., Ward, T., Zhu, W.J.: BLEU: a method for automatic evaluation of machine translation. In: Proceedings of the 40th Annual Meeting of the Association for Computational Linguistics, pp. 311–318 (2002)
33. Phan, L.N., et al.: SciFive: a text-to-text transformer model for biomedical literature. arXiv preprint arXiv:2106.03598 (2021)

34. Qi, W., et al.: ProphetNet: predicting future n-gram for sequence-to-sequence pre-training. arXiv preprint arXiv:2001.04063 (2020)
35. Raffel, C., et al.: Exploring the limits of transfer learning with a unified text-to-text transformer. J. Mach. Learn. Res. **21**(1), 5485–5551 (2020)
36. Ramamoorthy, S., Murugan, S.: An attentive sequence model for adverse drug event extraction from biomedical text. arXiv preprint arXiv:1801.00625 (2018)
37. Rothe, S., Narayan, S., Severyn, A.: Leveraging pre-trained checkpoints for sequence generation tasks. Trans. Assoc. Comput. Linguist. **8**, 264–280 (2020)
38. Scott, D., Hallett, C., Fettiplace, R.: Data-to-text summarisation of patient records: using computer-generated summaries to access patient histories. Patient Educ. Couns. **92**(2), 153–159 (2013)
39. See, A., Liu, P.J., Manning, C.D.: Get to the point: summarization with pointer-generator networks. arXiv preprint arXiv:1704.04368 (2017)
40. Shing, H.C., et al.: Towards clinical encounter summarization: learning to compose discharge summaries from prior notes. arXiv preprint arXiv:2104.13498 (2021)
41. Vinyals, O., Fortunato, M., Jaitly, N.: Pointer networks. In: Advances in Neural Information Processing Systems, vol. 28 (2015)
42. Wang, X., Peng, Y., Lu, L., Lu, Z., Summers, R.M.: TieNet: text-image embedding network for common thorax disease classification and reporting in chest x-rays. In: Proceedings of the IEEE Conference on Computer Vision and Pattern Recognition, pp. 9049–9058 (2018)
43. Xu, J., Durrett, G.: Neural extractive text summarization with syntactic compression. arXiv preprint arXiv:1902.00863 (2019)
44. Xu, J., Gan, Z., Cheng, Y., Liu, J.: Discourse-aware neural extractive text summarization. arXiv preprint arXiv:1910.14142 (2019)
45. Xu, L., Zhou, Q., Gong, K., Liang, X., Tang, J., Lin, L.: End-to-end knowledge-routed relational dialogue system for automatic diagnosis. In: Proceedings of the AAAI Conference on Artificial Intelligence, vol. 33, pp. 7346–7353 (2019)
46. Ye, Y., Hu, B., Zhang, K., Zan, H.: Construction of corpus for entity and relation annotation of diabetes electronic medical records. In: Proceedings of the 20th Chinese National Conference on Computational Linguistics, pp. 622–632 (2021)
47. Yuan, H., Yuan, Z., Gan, R., Zhang, J., Xie, Y., Yu, S.: BioBART: pretraining and evaluation of a biomedical generative language model. arXiv preprint arXiv:2204.03905 (2022)
48. Zeng, W., Luo, W., Fidler, S., Urtasun, R.: Efficient summarization with read-again and copy mechanism. arXiv preprint arXiv:1611.03382 (2016)
49. Zhang, J., Zhao, Y., Saleh, M., Liu, P.: PEGASUS: pre-training with extracted gap-sentences for abstractive summarization. In: International Conference on Machine Learning, pp. 11328–11339. PMLR (2020)
50. Zhang, Y., Ding, D.Y., Qian, T., Manning, C.D., Langlotz, C.P.: Learning to summarize radiology findings. arXiv preprint arXiv:1809.04698 (2018)
51. Zhang, Y., Merck, D., Tsai, E.B., Manning, C.D., Langlotz, C.P.: Optimizing the factual correctness of a summary: a study of summarizing radiology reports. arXiv preprint arXiv:1911.02541 (2019)
52. Zhou, H., Lang, C., Liu, Z., Ning, S., Lin, Y., Du, L.: Knowledge-guided convolutional networks for chemical-disease relation extraction. BMC Bioinform. **20**(1), 1–13 (2019)

An Unsupervised Clinical Acronym Disambiguation Method Based on Pretrained Language Model

Siwen Wei[1], Chi Yuan[1(✉)], Zixuan Li[1], and Huaiyu Wang[2]

[1] School of Computer and Information, Hohai University, Nanjing 211100, China
{siwenwei,chiyuan,zixuanli}@hhu.edu.cn
[2] School of Traditional Chinese Medicine, Beijing University of Chinese Medicine, Beijing 100029, China
wanghuaiyuelva@126.com

Abstract. Clinical concept normalization plays a vital role in extracting information from clinical documents, specifically clinical notes. The presence of abbreviations within these texts has a substantial impact on concept normalization performance. To address this issue, our objective is to propose an unsupervised learning approach for automatic disambiguation of clinical abbreviations. Our proposed pipeline consists of three main modules: a) Prompt-based contextualized token prediction, b) embedding-based semantic similarity calculation , and c) candidate ranking and selection. Our method achieves accuracies of 73.6% and 74.3% on two distinct clinical datasets, respectively. An ablation study demonstrates the beneficial contributions of all modules within our pipeline for acronym disambiguation. Our study highlights the effectiveness of the prompt-based unsupervised method in the clinical acronym disambiguation task, showcasing its potential application within existing clinical NLP pipelines for entity concept normalization.

Keywords: Acronym disambiguation · Clinical concept normalization · Clinical natural language processing

1 Introduction

Doctors usually write clinical notes with abbreviations and shorthand that are difficult to decipher [1]. Although the usage of abbreviations can make writing clinical notes more efficient [2], it adversely affects the comprehension and normalization of the clinical text [3]. These clinical abbreviations can be clinical jargon, ambiguous terms that require expertise to disambiguate, or domain-specific vernacular. With the wide application of electronic health record (EHR) systems, the reuse of historical clinical data can facilitate clinical practice and research. As abbreviations are broadly used in clinical records and most of them have over one meaning, it is significant to determine the right sense of an abbreviation [4]. For example, an abbreviation like 'mg' could be expanded to 'myasthenia gravis (a disease) or 'milligrams' (a unit of measure) [5]. Moreover, a sentence often has more than one abbreviation, such as 'ba at a dosage of only about percent ld mg kg', containing four abbreviations, 'ba', 'ld', 'mg,' and 'kg'.

Furthermore, abbreviations commonly appear in clinical notes and no corresponding expansions are followed, which results in confusion and misinterpretations of the information extraction process. It requires medical knowledge and contextual information to predict the full name of those acronyms precisely [6–8]. Besides, medical terminology may only include the standard concept name of some medical terms instead of their abbreviation format. For instance, in LOINC [9] there is only 'Hemoglobin A1c [Mass/volume] in Blood' (41995-2) for the Lab Test class. It may influence the compatibility of string-matching-based concept normalization methods. Consequently, identifying the exact full name of abbreviations in the clinical text would benefit the current clinical NLP pipeline, especially for information extraction and information retrieval tasks.

Currently, a variety of models have been trained for disambiguating abbreviations in clinical notes, including naïve Bayes [10], support vector machines [11], convolutional neural networks [5], profile-based approaches [12], long short-term memory networks [13,14], encoder-based transformers [15], latent meaning cells [16], and decoder-based transformers [17]. Supervised learning methods to solve clinical concept normalization always require a large quantity of human-labeled training data which is time-consuming to create. In this paper, we proposed a purely unsupervised pipeline that did not require manual annotation data and represents abbreviations with contextualized information, to solve clinical abbreviation disambiguation. It can be helpful in semantic analysis with abstract meaning representation parsing, and so on. And it can be employed in many aspects such as machine translation, information retrieval, text analysis, automatic summarization, and knowledge mining.

2   Related Work

Abbreviation sense disambiguation usually contains two key parts: abbreviation inventory creation, and abbreviation recognition and disambiguation. Many researchers have made attempts to solve the problem from the perspective of natural language processing.

2.1   Abbreviation Inventory Creation Depending on Clinical Textual Material

Selecting or building a word sense inventory is critical in linking acronyms to their expansions based on clinical texts. Sungrim Moon et al. [18] created a sense inventory for clinical abbreviations using clinical notes and medical dictionary resources. It used the most frequently occurring abbreviations and acronyms from 352 267 dictated clinical notes. This work could be used as a foundational resource with semi-automated techniques that aim to scale the disambiguation of abbreviations for real-world use in the clinical field. Liu et al. [8] presented a deep database of medical abbreviations, the Medical Abbreviation and Acronym Meta-Inventory. A systematic harmonization of eight source inventories across multiple healthcare specialties and settings identified 104,057 abbreviations with 170,426 corresponding senses. The Meta-Inventory demonstrated high completeness or coverage of abbreviations and senses in new clinical text, a substantial improvement over the next largest repository (6–14% increase in abbreviation coverage; 28–52% increase in sense coverage). Grossman et al. [19] presented an automated method for harmonization of clinical abbreviation sense inventories. The method involves integrating multiple source sense inventories into one centralized inventory and cross-mapping redundant entries to establish synonymy. It may help generalize sense inventories to medical institutions that lack the resources to develop them.

2.2 Abbreviation Recognition and Disambiguation for Clinical Texts

Abbreviations often contain important clinical information that must be recognizable and accurate in health records [20]. Proper ways are needed to recognize and disambiguate abbreviations. Yu et al. [7] developed two methods of mapping defined and undefined abbreviations. For defined abbreviations, they developed a set of pattern-matching rules to map an abbreviation to its full form and implemented the rules into a software program, AbbRE (for 'abbreviation recognition and extraction'). Besides, the application of machine learning also appears in the solution strategy. Kim et al. [21] developed an abbreviation disambiguation tool for clinical text in the context. Their semi-supervised abbreviation disambiguation method with 12 abbreviations reached over 90% accuracy with five-fold cross-validation. Wu et al. [22] developed an open-source framework for clinical abbreviation recognition and disambiguation (CARD). It can be used to generate corpus-specific sense inventories and can improve the performance of an existing NLP system (MetaMap) on recognition and disambiguation of clinical abbreviations, thereby improving its performance on the disorder NER task. Improving the method of selecting datasets can also effectively enhance the quality of the method. Skreta et al. [23] proposed a novel data augmentation technique that utilizes information from related medical concepts, which improves the model's ability to generalize.

3 Methods

3.1 Pipeline

The pipeline of the proposed method mainly consists of three modules: contextualized token predicting, semantic similarity calculation, and candidate ranking (Fig. 1). The sentence, the location of abbreviation were the inputs of our pipeline. The most possible long form was the output.

Contextualized Token Predicting. Inspired by the training method used in the contextual language model, BERT, the pre-trained language model could predict the masked word in the sentence. As shown in Fig. 2, the abbreviation, 'VAD', was replaced with a contextualized token '[MASK]', and then the sentence was put into the module contextualized token predicting.

To capture the contextual information of original abbreviations, we took advantage of the pre-trained language model, BERT which could predict the tokens where the '[MASK]' was located. Considering the unsupervised training process of the BERT-based model had already optimized the parameters of the model for masked token prediction, the token was highly determined by contextual semantics. We called the predicted results 'contextualized tokens'. After the processing of the BERT pipeline, a list of contextualized tokens was generated with their confidence scores.

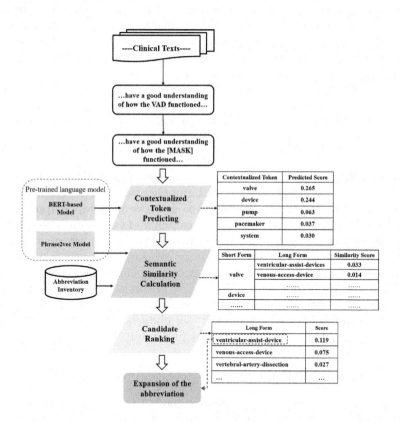

Fig. 1. The whole pipeline of the study containing three modules.

Semantic Similarity Calculation. After the generation of contextualized tokens, we designed a semantic similarity calculation module to filter out the most semantically similar word or phrase with the tokens (Fig. 3). To compare the semantic similarities between tokens and long forms of abbreviations, we employed the word2vec-based method to represent word/phrase semantic meaning with a fixed dimension vector. The semantic similarity would be quantified by the cosine distance between vectors. The pre-trained word2vec model could generate distributed representations in many NLP tasks. However, each word only has one representation vector after the pre-trained processing of word2vec. It would be a barrier for comparing the semantics of abbreviations with their different long forms directly. To tackle this problem, we employed various contextualized tokens for abbreviations to represent different meanings in different scenarios. The semantic comparison between the abbreviation and its long forms was turned into the comparison between contextualized tokens and long-form candidates. Additionally, while word2vec has achieved a breakthrough in word representations, it only contains words and cannot handle the operation of phrases. To overcome the weakness and enlarge the scope it acts on, a concept embedding model called PubMedPhrase2vec model [24] was trained on all PubMed abstracts with the same algorithm as word2vec. An open set of coherent medical phrases, PubMed Phrase, was employed to contain a vast phrase vocabulary. In the training corpus of the embedding model, multi-word expressions are formatted as hyphenated connectives. Phrases can be treated as word concepts by adding hyphens to connect words. Semantic similarity scores could be calculated for the next module.

Candidate Ranking. In the last module of our pipeline, the long form of the abbreviation in the clinical text was the output according to the candidate ranking (Fig. 4). Considering the results of the first two modules comprehensively, we defined a parameter to represent the possibility of expansion. The parameter is the product of the confidence score in contextualized token predicting and the similarity score from semantic similarity calculation. The score of each contextual token was multiplied by its corresponding similarity scores one by one. As we got five words in contextualized token predicting for each prediction, we would get five groups of products in this module. Then, these five groups were merged and sorted from high to low by the products. At last, the long form in the pair with the highest product was the final result.

3.2   Evaluation Method

We conducted two kinds of evaluation methods to study the accuracy of the whole pipeline for the abbreviation disambiguation and the necessity of every module. In the first experiment, we tested four pre-trained language models in contextualized token predicting and five abbreviation sense inventories in semantic similarity calculation to test the whole pipeline. In the second experiment, we kept the first module and the second module respectively to do the ablation experiment. We used accuracy as the main performance measure. Here, accuracy was defined as the fraction of abbreviation instances for which the word sense

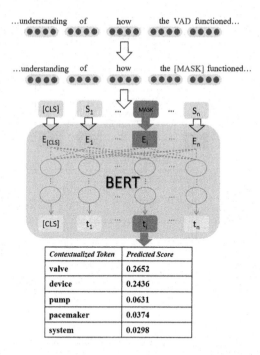

Fig. 2. An example of contextualized token predicting utilizing pre-trained language models.

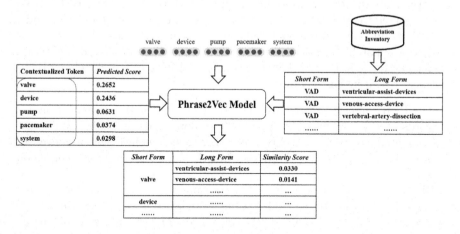

Fig. 3. An example of semantic similarity calculation.

was correctly predicted out of the total abbreviation instances in the test set with more than one sense.

$$accuracy = \frac{number\ of\ correctly\ predicted\ abbrevations}{total\ number\ of\ instances\ in\ the\ datasets} \tag{1}$$

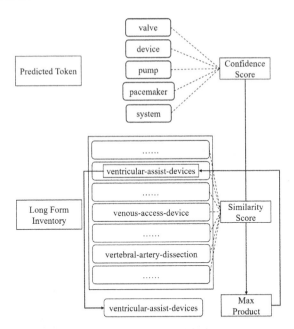

Fig. 4. An example of candidate ranking.

Comparison of Pre-trained Language Models. Pretrained BERT-based models served to predict the masked word in the clinical notes. Language models trained on different corpora may result in various performances. To evaluate the predicting capability of models trained with corpus from different domains, four models, BERT [25], BioBERT [26], Bio_ClinicalBERT [27], and PubMedBERT [28] were tested in this section.

- The BERT model, presented by Devlin et al., was pretrained on 800 million words of BooksCorpus [29] and 2,500 million words of English Wikipedia. They used a document-level corpus rather than a shuffled sentence-level corpus such as the Billion Word Benchmark [30] to extract long contiguous sequences.
- BioBERT model was pretrained with the same algorithm but on the corpus of 2.5 billion words in the general domain of English Wikipedia, 0.8 billion words in the general domain of Book Corpus, 4.5 billion words in the biomedical domain of PubMed Abstracts, 3.5 billion words in the biomedical domain of PMC Full-text articles.
- Bio_ClinicalBERT model was initialized from BioBERT and trained on all notes from MIMIC III, a database containing electronic health records from ICU patients at the Beth Israel Hospital in Boston, MA.
- PubMedBERT model was pretrained from scratch using abstracts from PubMed and full-text articles from PubMedCentral, including 14 million abstracts with 3 billion words (21 GB), which achieves state-of-the-art perfor-

mance and holds the top score on many biomedical NLP tasks (e.g., Named Entity Recognition).

Comparison of Abbreviation Sense Inventories. The abbreviation sense inventory is another external source for our pipeline. The completeness and redundancy of the inventory would significantly influence the candidate generation in the last two modules. Five abbreviation sense inventories are compared as follows:

- The metathesaurus proposed by Grossman et al. as a trimmed version of the source sense inventories described below includes 52519 abbreviations, and 89298 full names [20].
- The source sense inventories are from UMLS LRABR [31], ADAM [32], Berman, Vanderbilt Discharge Summaries, Vanderbilt Clinical Notes, Stetson, Columbia OBGYN, Wikipedia. There are 376270 SF/LF pairs in the inventories, including 97789 abbreviations and 157819 corresponding full forms.
- Clinical sense inventory version 1 (hereinafter referred to as VERSION 1) is proposed by Sungrim Moon et al., containing 440 common abbreviations and 24156 corresponding full forms. It includes exact mappings of lexical forms for each of the long forms from a given resource.
- Clinical sense inventory version 2 (hereinafter referred to as VERSION 2) is proposed by Sungrim Moon et al., containing 440 common abbreviations and 13027 corresponding full forms. It includes mappings of forms for each resource after merging forms using Lexical Variant Generation (LVG)(2) normalization and then performing semantic mappings [18].
- Anonymized Clinical Abbreviations And Acronyms Data Set(hereinafter referred to as CASI) is proposed by Sungrim Moon et al. The inventory includes 75 abbreviations and their corresponding 352 full forms. And each abbreviation has 500 examples.

4   Evaluation

4.1   Datasets

To evaluate the performance of the proposed pipeline and modules in this work, we used two datasets for testing. The first was randomly selected 500 sentences from Clinical Abbreviation Sense Inventory (CASI) dataset [18], including 30 abbreviations and their corresponding 73 full forms. We also use the sample which contains 268 sentences with 126 abbreviations and 143 expansions in total from Medical Dataset for Abbreviation Disambiguation for Natural Language Understanding (MeDAL) presented by Wen et al. [33] for testing. A majority of sentences in the dataset have more than three abbreviations, so these sentences were tested many times for different abbreviations. The whole dataset (MeDAL) can be used for pre-training natural language understanding models. It contained 5,886 abbreviations and 24,005 pairs of mappings.

4.2   Results of the Whole Pipeline

As shown in Table 1, for the sample of CASI, PubMedBERT performed best at 73.6% accuracy, while BERT performed worst at 63.2% accuracy. The accuracy rates of the other two models were 64.2% and 67.6% from low to high. Since the BERT model was a pre-trained model on the raw texts only and not trained specifically in one aspect, it cannot predict tokens accurately compared to other models trained on the medical corpus. BioBERT was a domain-specific language representation model pretrained on large-scale biomedical corpora. So, despite the same architecture across tasks, it largely outperformed BERT. Bio_ClinicalBERT model was initialized from BioBERT, but there is robust evidence that the clinical embeddings are superior to the general domain or BioBERT-specific embeddings for non-de-ID tasks, and that using note-type specific corpora could induce further selective performance benefits. Thus, its ability to predict tokens was slightly higher than BioBERT. Compared with the first three models, the PubMedBERT model was the most domain-specific model in the medical field and it performed best to predict the highly relevant tokens.

The accuracy achieved the highest at 73.6%, with the application of CASI compared with the other four inventories. The pairs of abbreviations and long forms in the inventory achieved a higher homology rate with the content in the dataset. Therefore, it was more conducive to finding the correct long form in the inventory. VERSION 2 got the lowest rate 21.4%. Compared with VERSION 1, 37.8%, it has fewer long terms, meaning a lower possibility to match irregular forms, which resulted in poorer results. Source sense inventory had a modest performance, 50%, due to quite a large quantity of entries. However, a large quantity probably means that some irregular or obscure long forms will interfere with the calculation of similarity due to the training method of the Phrase2Vec model. Same with VERSION 2, Metathesaurus performed worse than the source sense inventory, and its accuracy was 37.4%.

Table 1. Results of CASI for different language models and abbreviation inventories.

	BERT	BioBERT	Bio_ClinicalBERT	PubMedBERT
Grossman's metathesaurus	25.40%	27.00%	25.40%	37.40%
Source sense inventories	30.40%	30.20%	31.40%	50.00%
Moon's inventory v1 (VERISON1)	24.40%	26.60%	23.60%	37.80%
Moon's inventory v2 (VERISON2)	13.80%	13.20%	15.40%	21.40%
CASI	63.20%	64.20%	67.60%	73.60%

Skreta et al. used reverse substitution (RS) with replacement and augmentation with related medical concepts as well as global context to train models to do abbreviation disambiguation. For the classification task, they built one model for each abbreviation. They used 65 abbreviations from CASI. On average, each abbreviation had 4 expansions with 459 test sentences. And they labeled the abbreviation with the expansion having the largest probability. They considered two forms of accuracy: Micro accuracy was the total number of abbreviations correctly disambiguated divided by the total number of samples in the test set across all abbreviation disambiguation abbreviations with two or more possible expansions. Macro accuracy was the average of individual abbreviation accuracies. The two accuracies of their concept model trained as described above on test sets from CASI were both 0.760.

As shown in Table 2, for the sample of MeDAL, PubMedBERT still performed best among the four models at 74.3% accuracy, but the worst performance for this dataset was Bio_ClinicalBERT instead of BERT, at 45.1% accuracy. Considering the analysis in the previous paragraph, the possible reason was the lack of sufficient training data for Bio_ClinicalBERT, and its generalization ability for this sample was weaker than BERT's. It seemed that source sense inventories covered the most acronyms and corresponding expansions among the five inventories (The acronyms in this sample had a very low crossover rate in CASI, so the results were not for reference.). In this table, there were 14 cells with two results. The former result in each cell included acronyms that could not be found in the sense inventories, but the latter did not. And the lowest accuracy was 9.3% with the application of VERSION 2. However, if abbreviations which missed in the inventories were not classified as an error but eliminated, the accuracy was much higher at 47.2%. This might be due to inventories' coverage of acronyms and whether acronyms in the test set were common in medical scenes.

Table 2. Results of MeDAL for different language models and abbreviation inventories.

	ERT	BioBERT	Bio_ClinicalBERT	PubMedBERT
Grossman's metathesaurus	30.60%/35.30%	37.70%/44.90%	27.60%/32.90%	42.90%/85.80%
Source sense inventories	54.10%/–	63.10%/64.80%	45.10%/46.40%	74.30%/–
Moon's inventory v1 (VERISON1)	10.40%/50.00%	12.70%/64.10%	9.70%/49.00%	16.00%/76.80%
Moon's inventory v2 (VERISON2)	10.80%/51.80%	12.70%/64.10%	9.30%/47.20%	16.40%/78.60%

4.3   Ablation Experiments

To ensure the effectiveness of each module in our pipeline, we conducted ablation experiments. And to ensure the high probability validity of each dictionary, we chose the CASI dataset for the ablation experiments and analysis. We only kept contextualized token predicting module, the accuracy was only 6.6%. When using the same model, the result was 67% lower than the 73.6% obtained with the entire process. And when we only kept the semantic similarity calculation module, the accuracy was 51.8%. Using the same inventory, the result was 21.8% lower than the 73.6% obtained with the entire process. As shown in Table 3, without either of the two modules, it gave rise to poor results. Without contextualized token predicting, acronyms lost their meanings in context, and we could not find a contextual expansion from a large number of long forms. Without semantic similarity calculation, we did not have a measurable way to find the long form with the closest meaning. All in all, both modules were necessary.

Table 3. Results of ablation experiments.

Module Name	Model	Accuracy
Contextualized	BERT	2.20%
Token	BioBERT	2.60%
Predicting	Bio_ClinicalBERT	2.60%
(only)	PubMedBERT	6.60%
Semantic	Grossman's metathesaurus	1.40%
Similarity	Source sense inventories	7.00%
Calculation	Moon's inventory v1	2.20%
(only)	Moon's inventory v2	1.00%
	CASI	51.80%
Full pipeline	PubMedBERT+CASI	73.60%

5   Discussion

By incorporating clinical acronym disambiguation within the NLP pipeline, several benefits can be realized. First, it improves the accuracy of clinical concept normalization, ensuring that the intended meanings of acronyms are correctly identified and associated with their respective full forms. This enhances the interoperability and semantic understanding of clinical data, facilitating data integration and exchange between healthcare systems and applications.

Furthermore, clinical acronym disambiguation aids in reducing ambiguity and potential errors in downstream clinical NLP tasks, such as named entity recognition, information extraction, and clinical coding. It enhances the precision of these tasks by providing unambiguous references to clinical entities, thereby improving the overall quality and reliability of automated clinical text analysis.

Additionally, accurate disambiguation of clinical acronyms contributes to the development of comprehensive clinical knowledge bases and ontologies. It supports the creation of standardized terminologies and controlled vocabularies, enabling consistent representation and interpretation of clinical information across different healthcare settings and systems.

Clinical acronym disambiguation serves as a valuable component in the clinical NLP pipeline, facilitating more accurate and meaningful analysis of clinical texts, improving healthcare decision support, and fostering advancements in clinical research and knowledge discovery. In this section, we analyzed errors in detail. Besides, limitations and future work were outlined.

5.1 Error Analysis

The results indicated that our method still has space in progress. As shown in Table 4, for the contextualized token predicting module, among all the incorrectly predicted long forms, 4.01% of errors were caused by the format of predicted tokens. When the predicted tokens were digit, it was difficult to calculate similarity scores precisely. Besides, 10.3% of errors were due to predicted tokens that were not even words, such as '##dine', and symbols like '.', '(', '-'. They were generally meaningless, resulting in subsequent calculation deviations. These errors were related to the vocabulary and training strategy of the BERT-based model. Since the dataset used for pre-training could not cover a certain aspect, the predicted tokens were more likely to be meaningless, which would affect the similarity calculation in the next module.

For the semantic similarity calculation module, there were some errors due to inconsistent parts of speech. For instance, the true long form was 'intramuscular', an adjective, while the final output was 'intramuscularly', an adverb. Moreover, the correct long form was composed of several words side by side, and there were separators between them, such as 'cyclophosphamide, vincristine, prednisone'. Also, the initials of words that made up the long form were not related to acronyms in the abbreviation inventory. For example, 'Biochemical' became an extended form of the abbreviation 'PSA'. Moreover, a qualified inventory needed sufficient abbreviations and corresponding expansions to test. if not, it would adversely affect semantic similarity calculation, and the final result might not come up.

Table 4. Illustration of error analysis. The second column of the first module means what was predicted in the part. For the second module, the column 'Error analysis' demonstrates some reasons of errors.

Module Name	Error analysis	Example
Contextualized	Digit	predicted token: 1, 2, 3...
Token	Incomplete words	predicted token: '##dine'
Predicting	Symbols	predicted token: '-', '.', '('...
Semantic	Inconsistent parts of speech	ground truth 'intramuscular'; final result: 'intramuscularly'
Similarity	Non-standard form of expansion	'cyclophosphamide, vincristine, prednisone'
Calculation	Initials of expansions differing from acronyms	expansion: 'Biochemical'; abbreviation:'PSA'

5.2   Limitations and Future Work

This work still has several limitations. First, most current pre-trained language models were not able to predict phrases for the masked token, but a number of abbreviations have extended forms that are phrases. If the predicted token is a phrase instead of one word, it will match more closely with possible candidates. Consequently, the accuracy of similarity score calculation will be improved a lot.

Besides, the irregularity of acronyms and their standard forms can harm the performance of the method. Domain-oriented inventory might be helpful and more efficient for candidate generation. Pre-trained language models for our pipeline were task-specific and domain-specific. For example, the frequently used acronyms in clinical notes might be different from those used in clinical trials. The separation of clinical notes-oriented inventory and clinical trial-oriented inventory would benefit both domains and improve the performance of our method.

In the whole pipeline, predicting contextual tokens by the pre-trained language model is a downstream task. Sometimes the downstream tasks do not fully utilize the knowledge in the model, perhaps because of bias caused by word frequency, case, subword, etc. in BERT's native model, and the layers of BERT itself do not correct this problem. Based on the training process of BERT models, the addition of prompt learning can help to adjust the downstream task to accommodate the model, thus utilizing the knowledge in each layer of BERT more effectively.

6   Conclusion

In this work, we proposed a pipeline to disambiguate abbreviations in clinical texts, which was an early attempt to adopt a pure unsupervised pre-trained language model for abbreviation expansion. It replaced the abbreviation in the sentences with the contextualized token, which enabled the representation of different semantics in different scenarios and solved the problem of multiple meanings of the same abbreviation. With the evaluation on the two datasets, it proved that the method could be potentially applied in the existing clinical NLP pipeline for the acronym disambiguation.

Acknowledgements. This project was sponsored by Fundamental Research Funds for the Central Universities (B220201032, B220202076).

References

1. Rajkomar, A., et al.: Deciphering clinical abbreviations with a privacy protecting machine learning system. Nat. Commun. **13**(1), Art. no. 1 (2022). https://doi.org/10.1038/s41467-022-35007-9
2. Janssen, S.L., Venema-Taat, N., Medlock, S.: Anticipated benefits and concerns of sharing hospital outpatient visit notes with patients (open notes) in dutch hospitals: mixed methods study. J. Med. Internet Res. **23**(8), e27764 (2021). https://doi.org/10.2196/27764

3. Pakhomov, S.: Semi-supervised Maximum Entropy based approach to acronym and abbreviation normalization in medical texts. In: Proceedings of the 40th Annual Meeting on Association for Computational Linguistics - ACL 2002, Philadelphia, Pennsylvania, p. 160 (2001). https://doi.org/10.3115/1073083.1073111
4. Jaber, A., Martínez, P.: Disambiguating clinical abbreviations using pre-trained word embeddings. In: Proceedings of the 14th International Joint Conference on Biomedical Engineering Systems and Technologies, Online Streaming, – Select a Country –, pp. 501–508 (2021). https://doi.org/10.5220/0010256105010508
5. Joopudi, V., Dandala, B., Devarakonda, M.: A convolutional route to abbreviation disambiguation in clinical text. J. Biomed. Inform. **86**, 71–78 (2018). https://doi.org/10.1016/j.jbi.2018.07.025
6. Okazaki, N., Ananiadou, S., Tsujii, J.: Building a high-quality sense inventory for improved abbreviation disambiguation. Bioinform. Oxf. Engl. **26**(9), 1246–1253 (2010). https://doi.org/10.1093/bioinformatics/btq129
7. Yu, H., Hripcsak, G., Friedman, C.: Mapping abbreviations to full forms in biomedical articles. J. Am. Med. Inform. Assoc. JAMIA **9**(3), 262–272 (2002). https://doi.org/10.1197/jamia.m0913
8. Grossman Liu, L., et al.: A deep database of medical abbreviations and acronyms for natural language processing. Sci. Data **8**(1), 149 (2021). https://doi.org/10.1038/s41597-021-00929-4
9. Briscoe, T.: LOINC version 2.73 is now available-LOINC%. LOINC (2022). https://loinc.org/news/loinc-version-2-73-is-now-available/. Accessed 18 Dec 2022
10. Moon, S., Pakhomov, S., Melton, G.B.: Automated disambiguation of acronyms and abbreviations in clinical texts: window and training size considerations. In: AMIA Annual Symposium Proceedings, AMIA Symposium, vol. 2012, pp. 1310–1319 (2012)
11. Wu, Y., Xu, J., Zhang, Y., Xu, H.: Clinical abbreviation disambiguation using neural word embeddings. In: Proceedings of BioNLP 2015, Beijing, China, pp. 171–176 (2015). https://doi.org/10.18653/v1/W15-3822
12. Xu, H., Stetson, P., Friedman, C.: Combining corpus-derived sense profiles with estimated frequency information to disambiguate clinical abbreviations. In: AMIA Annual Symposium Proceedings, AMIA Symposium (2012). https://www.semanticscholar.org/paper/Combining-Corpus-derived-Sense-Profiles-with-to-Xu-Stetson/58bcd4bdc30bc6ca2f4222509d1fe0246aacc28f. Accessed 18 Dec 2022
13. Li, I., et al.: A neural topic-attention model for medical term abbreviation disambiguation. arXiv (2019). https://doi.org/10.48550/arXiv.1910.14076
14. Pesaranghader, A., Matwin, S., Sokolova, M., Pesaranghader, A.: deepBioWSD: effective deep neural word sense disambiguation of biomedical text data. J. Am. Med. Inform. Assoc. **26**(5), 438–446 (2019). https://doi.org/10.1093/jamia/ocy189
15. Jaber, A., Martínez, P.: Disambiguating clinical abbreviations using a one-fits-all classifier based on deep learning techniques. Methods Inf. Med. **61**(S 01), e28–e34 (2022). https://doi.org/10.1055/s-0042-1742388
16. Adams, G., Ketenci, M., Bhave, S., Perotte, A., Elhadad, N.: Zero-shot clinical acronym expansion via latent meaning cells. arXiv (2020). https://doi.org/10.48550/arXiv.2010.02010
17. Agrawal, M., Hegselmann, S., Lang, H., Kim, Y., Sontag, D.: Large language models are zero-shot clinical information extractors. arXiv (2022). http://arxiv.org/abs/2205.12689. Accessed 20 Mar 2023
18. Moon, S., Pakhomov, S., Liu, N., Ryan, J.O., Melton, G.B.: A sense inventory for clinical abbreviations and acronyms created using clinical notes and medical

dictionary resources. J. Am. Med. Inform. Assoc. **21**(2), 299–307 (2014). https://doi.org/10.1136/amiajnl-2012-001506

19. Grossman, L.V., Mitchell, E.G., Hripcsak, G., Weng, C., Vawdrey, D.K.: A method for harmonization of clinical abbreviation and acronym sense inventories. J. Biomed. Inform. **40**(2), 150–159 (2007). https://doi.org/10.1016/j.jbi.2006.06.001

20. Yu, H., Kim, W., Hatzivassiloglou, V., Wilbur, W.J.: Using MEDLINE as a knowledge source for disambiguating abbreviations and acronyms in full-text biomedical journal articles. J. Biomed. Inform. **40**(2), 150–159 (2007). https://doi.org/10.1016/j.jbi.2006.06.001

21. Kim, Y., Hurdle, J., Meystre, S.M.: Using UMLS lexical resources to disambiguate abbreviations in clinical text. In: AMIA Annual Symposium Proceedings, AMIA Symposium, vol. 2011, pp. 715–722 (2011)

22. Wu, Y., et al.: A long journey to short abbreviations: developing an open-source framework for clinical abbreviation recognition and disambiguation (CARD). J. Am. Med. Inform. Assoc. **24**(e1), e79–e86 (2017). https://doi.org/10.1093/jamia/ocw109

23. Skreta, M., et al.: Automatically disambiguating medical acronyms with ontology-aware deep learning. Nat. Commun. **12**(1), Art. no. 1 (2021). https://doi.org/10.1038/s41467-021-25578-4

24. Yuan, C., Wang, Y., Shang, N., Li, Z., Zhao, R., Weng, C.: A graph-based method for reconstructing entities from coordination ellipsis in medical text. J. Am. Med. Inform. Assoc. JAMIA **27**(9), 1364–1373 (2020). https://doi.org/10.1093/jamia/ocaa109

25. Devlin, J., Chang, M.-W., Lee, K., Toutanova, K.: BERT: pre-training of deep bidirectional transformers for language understanding. arXiv (2019). https://doi.org/10.48550/arXiv.1810.04805

26. Lee, J., et al.: BioBERT: a pre-trained biomedical language representation model for biomedical text mining. Bioinformatics btz682 (2019). https://doi.org/10.1093/bioinformatics/btz682

27. Alsentzer, E., et al.: Publicly available clinical BERT embeddings. arXiv (2019). https://doi.org/10.48550/arXiv.1904.03323

28. Gu, Y., et al.: Domain-specific language model pretraining for biomedical natural language processing. ACM Trans. Comput. Healthc. **3**(1), 1–23 (2022). https://doi.org/10.1145/3458754

29. Zhu, Y., et al.: Aligning books and movies: towards story-like visual explanations by watching movies and reading books. arXiv (2015). https://doi.org/10.48550/arXiv.1506.06724

30. Chelba, C., et al.: One billion word benchmark for measuring progress in statistical language modeling. arXiv (2014). https://doi.org/10.48550/arXiv.1312.3005

31. UMLS® Reference Manual. National Library of Medicine (US) (2009)

32. Zhou, W., Torvik, V.I., Smalheiser, N.R.: ADAM: another database of abbreviations in MEDLINE. Bioinforma. Oxf. Engl. **22**(22), 2813–2818 (2006). https://doi.org/10.1093/bioinformatics/btl480

33. Wen, Z., Lu, X.H., Reddy, S.: MeDAL: medical abbreviation disambiguation dataset for natural language understanding pretraining. In: Proceedings of the 3rd Clinical Natural Language Processing Workshop, pp. 130–135 (2020). https://doi.org/10.18653/v1/2020.clinicalnlp-1.15

Healthcare Data Mining
and Applications

TIG-KIGNN: Time Interval Guided Knowledge Inductive Graph Neural Network for Misinformation Detection from Social Media

Shaowei Zhang, Tongxuan Zhang$^{(\boxtimes)}$, and Guiyun Zhang

Tianjin Normal University, No. 393, Binshui West Road, Xiqing District, Tianjin, China
2111090044@stu.tjnu.edu.cn, {zhangguiyun,txzhang}@tjnu.edu.cn

Abstract. Since the emergence of social media, misinformation has become prevalent and is propagated through various social media platforms. Time plays a crucial role in verifying the source and authenticity of information, especially when it comes to detecting misinformation. Although current research on misinformation detection often focuses on timestamps for temporal analysis, it tends to overlook the time interval between an event's occurrence and its reporting, which can provide valuable insights. To address this gap, we propose the Time Interval Guided Knowledge Inductive Graph Neural Network (TIG-KIGNN) for detecting health-related misinformation. Our approach leverages time interval features in social media texts and integrates domain expertise from the knowledge graph into the semantic features of the texts, thereby enhancing the detection process. Moreover, to improve efficiency and minimize resource consumption, we employ inductive graph neural networks to optimize feature representation and update by neighboring nodes during training and when adding new nodes. We validate the effectiveness of our model using a real-world dataset and demonstrate significant improvements over existing methods based on experimental results.

Keywords: Graph Neural Network · Knowledge Graph · Misinformation · Social Media · Time Interval

1 Introduction

With the increasing popularity of social media, people are increasingly relying on it as a source of information. However, there is a significant amount of false news that can potentially mislead people. According to Darwish, O. et al. [8], information from social media is highly susceptible to manipulation due to contextual conventions, and the credibility of its source is constantly questioned. This makes users on social media more prone to being misled by false information. Since the outbreak of COVID-19, there has been significant attention given to the detection of misinformation from social media [3,4,14,15]. People often share false information about COVID-19 without thoroughly considering its accuracy [24].

H. Xu et al. (Eds.): CHIP 2023, CCIS 1993, pp. 287–300, 2024.
https://doi.org/10.1007/978-981-99-9864-7_19

Misinformation not only deprives people of the right to know the truth [24] but also has a negative impact on the stability of society and undermines official credibility. Therefore, there is a clear need for effective misinformation detection to combat its widespread dissemination.

According to Muhammed T S et al. [21], verifying false news takes time. Most current research on the temporal dimension focuses on specific points in time, such as the publication time of news articles. However, using a single point in time as temporal information does not fully capture the temporal dynamics. In the medical field, medical knowledge is crucial for assessing the validity of news, and there are various graph neural network models [7,31] for knowledge fusion. Several studies [7,11,30] combine transductive graph neural network (GNN) models with knowledge graphs for misinformation detection tasks. However, in many cases, the graph evolves with changing network structures and the emergence of new nodes. These methods often require loading the entire graph for information updates, which may introduce noise that negatively affects the accuracy of predictions.

Addressing the aforementioned issues, we propose a novel method called TIG-KIGNN (Time Interval Guided Knowledge Inductive Graph Neural Network) for misinformation detection. This method effectively captures the temporal dimension by using time intervals as a feature representation. To improve the efficiency of graph loading during training, the method combines domain expertise with an inductive Graph Neural Network. Specifically, the method enhances the semantic information of articles by incorporating entities extracted from the knowledge graph and employs the inductive graph neural network to optimize the feature representation of each article by utilizing a subset of neighboring articles in the article-article bipartite graph. This approach enables more efficient learning of article features while reducing noise introduced by unnecessary data.

In a nutshell, our contributions are listed as follows:

· We extract the interval between the time mentioned in the article and the time the article was published as the time feature information of the article.
· We apply an inductive graph neural network to optimize the article feature representation for information-containing knowledge graphs.
· We use a real-world dataset called ReCOvery. Our experiments have demonstrated the effectiveness of TIG-KIGNN. The report results show that TIG-KIGNN has achieved the best results in terms of precision, recall and F1 score.

2   Related Work

2.1   Misinformation Detection

Kumar S et al. [18] conducted a survey on misinformation, discussing various categories of misinformation, existing methods for detecting it, and potential future directions. Shin J et al. [27] focused on investigating misinformation in interdisciplinary fields. Their research can be divided into four main aspects: examining false knowledge that can deceive people, analyzing writing styles, studying propagation patterns, and evaluating the credibility of individuals who spread misinformation. Dou Y et al. [10] developed models that combine content-based and graph-structure-based approaches for detecting fake news. They considered users' spreading performance as an endogenous factor in their analysis. Shu K et al. [28] constructed hierarchical propagation networks to distinguish between genuine news and false news. They analyzed network features, including structural, temporal, and linguistic aspects, to detect misinformation.

2.2 Time Interval

When it comes to misinformation detection task, the time dimension is a crucial piece of information which can help the task to be carried out more effectively. Most of the studies in the time dimension are now studies based on timestamp. Ji J et al. [16] has studied the feature effectiveness at different time points. However, according to Galli A et al. [12], they argue that the spurious news meaning has evolved over the time. Rastogi S et al. [25] provides an overview of misinformation detection tasks that include a temporal dimension, but they consider points in time and do not take into account time intervals as a temporal dimension. We adopt the interval between the time mentioned in the article and the time of the news release as the article's temporal characteristic.

2.3 Graph Neural Network

Since the proposal of the graph neural network model [26], it has been widely utilized. Cui L et al. [7] applied the graph neural network to the misinformation detection task, achieving better performance and providing more possible solutions for misinformation detection. Some solutions have explored the utilization of Graph Neural Networks [20, 29]. Li J et al. [20] proposed models based on GCN for misinformation detection, while Song C et al. [29] utilized GAT to detect misinformation on social media. However, transductive graphs require loading the entire graph with vertex and edge information, which consumes significant resources and time. If the task requires updating information for specific vertices, the entire graph needs to be updated. Hamilton W et al. [13] proposed a model that eliminates the need to re-process the entire graph. Inspired by Brennen J S et al. [2] and S.B. Parikh et al. [22], our method focuses on the paragraph level of article features.

3 Method

Our proposed method consists of three components, shown in Fig. 1.

3.1 Time Encoder Layer

The time information is an essential part of our model. To guide our model in extracting more efficient time information, we provide 2 possible time information for model. Firstly, there is the case of article with publication date, in which

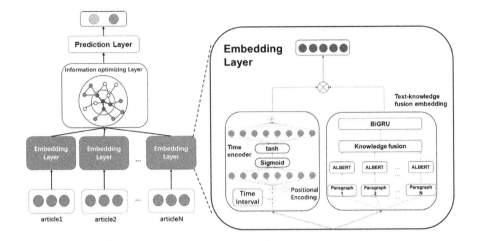

Fig. 1. Schematic overview of the proposed methodology.

case we can extract the time interval information directly from the article. The can be expressed as $t\_interval_i$

$$t\_interval_i = Interval(t\_post_i, min\{t_1, ..., t_n\}) \quad (1)$$

where $t\_interval_i$ means the extracted article interval information, represents the article posting time information and $\{t_1, ...t_n\}$ represents the set of events time mentioned in the article. For each article S_i, we obtain its post time t_post_i along with a time set $\{t_1, ..., t_n\}$. We then regularize the time information. Finally, we subtract the minimum value of the time set $\{t_1, ..., t_n\}$ from the post time t_post_i to obtain $t\_interval_i$.

To obtain the positional embedding, the obtained time interval information is encoded with the original text. Then normalize it to acquire the time interval representation. The t_rep_i can be expressed as:

$$t\_rep_i = tanh(Sigmoid(t\_interval_i)) \quad (2)$$

where t_rep_i serves as the time interval representation.

3.2   Information Embedding Layer

In our method, we focus on paragraph-level feature representation. The contextual representations are concatenated from paragraph-level feature representation.

Contextual Embedding. Each paragraph-level feature representation is obtained via ALBERT [19]. Based on BERT [9], ALBERT solves the problem of a large number of model parameters in BERT. We use the pre-training model of ALBERT on huggingface to obtain article features at the paragraph-level. To fully capture the feature representation of each article, we use Bidirectional Gating Recurrent Unit (BiGRU) [1] to encode paragraph-level feature representation a_i.

Knowledge Embedding. The knowledge embedding in TIG-KIGNN is based on a knowledge graph. The knowledge graph can effectively organize and represent knowledge so that it can be efficiently utilized in advanced applications [6]. For example, 2019-nCoV (entity) is one of (relation) coronavirus (entity), and its representation is (2019-nCoV, one of, coronavirus).

Knowledge embedding aims to obtain the entities in knowledge graph. To obtain the knowledge representation in the article, we can consider methods to match entities of the knowledge graph and article. For each article S_i, the knowledge representation k_rep_i can be expressed as:

$$k\_rep_i = getKnowledge(S_i, KnowledgeGraph) \tag{3}$$

In Eq. (3), for each article S_i, extract its entities and attempt to find a match with in the knowledge graph. Once a match is found, we leverage the relationships of these entities in the knowledge graph to further extract relevant knowledge information from the article.

In our work, we mainly focus on the final article representation, the knowledge graph will provide additional information for the article. We model this knowledge information into the article. The structures of the knowledge graph are shown in Fig. 2 and Fig. 3:

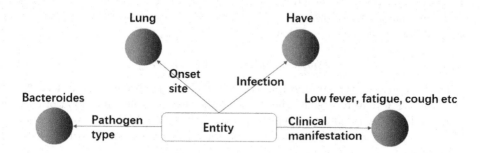

Fig. 2. Properties of one entity in knowledge graph.

The final article representation f_i can be expressed as:

$$f_i = concat(a_i, k\_rep_i, t\_rep_i) \tag{4}$$

where a_i represents the article feature, k_rep_i represents the knowledge embedding and t_rep_i represents time interval feature representation.

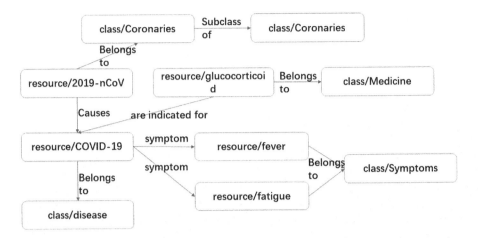

Fig. 3. Relations of entities in knowledge graph partly.

3.3 Information Optimizing Layer

In our work, we use an inductive graph neural network graphSAGE [13] to reach the goal. It generates embeddings by sampling and aggregating features from a vertex's neighborhood. It means that instead of learning the embedding of all vertexes on a graph, graphSAGE learns a mapping that generates the embedding for each vertex.

GraphSAGE. We use an inductive graph neural network graphSAGE (sample and aggregate) to optimize each article feature. The output of the graphSAGE embedding generation is as follows:

$$Output = graphSAGE(G, f, K, W^k) \tag{5}$$

where G represents the input graph structure $G(V, \varepsilon)$, f represents input features set $\{f_i, \forall i \in V\}$, K represents the depth of the searching neighborhood of each node and W^k represents the weight matrices $\forall k \in \{1, ..., K\}$. The pseudocode of the graphSAGE embedding generation forward propagation algorithm is as follows:

For each aggregated neighbor operation, we have:

$$h_{N(i)}^k = AGGREGATE_k(\{h_{u'}^{h-1}, \forall u \in N_k(V)\}) \tag{6}$$

$$h_i^k = \sigma(W^k \cdot CONCAT(h_i^{k-1}, h_{N(i)}^k)) \tag{7}$$

where the $h_{N(i)}^k$ represents the results of each layer of aggregation via aggregator functions $AGGREGATE_k, \forall k \in \{1, ..., K\}$ and h_i^k represents the final result of aggregation of a node by the neighborhood function N:$i \rightarrow 2^V$.

Sampling and Aggregation. We choose a two-layer network centered on a specific node. From this node, we select up to 20 neighbors, aggregate their features, and then update the feature of the center node. The aggregation function we use mean aggregator, the algorithm is as follows:

$$h_i^k = \sigma(W \cdot MEAN(\{h_i^{h-1}\} \cup \{h_u^{k-1}, \forall u \in N(i)\}))$$ (8)

The aggregator function is the mean operator, which takes the elementwise mean of the vectors in $\{h^{(k-1)}, \forall u \in N(i)\}$. The aggregator function is used to convert a collection of unordered vectors into a vector, where $N(i)$ represents the set of neighboring nodes of node i. And the mean aggregator function algorithm is as follows:

$$AGGREGATE = \sum_{u \in N(i)} \frac{h^l}{N(i)}$$ (9)

Update. After obtaining an aggregated representation based on the neighbors of node i, update the current node i using a combination of its previous representation and the aggregated representation. The update algorithm is as follows:

$$h_i^k = UPDATE(h_N^k(i), h_i^{k-1})$$ (10)

the $UPDATE$ function only needs to be differentiable, in our task, we use the mean function $MEAN$ as the $UPDATE$ method.

3.4   Prediction Layer

We next feed the embedding to a softmax layer for classification as follows, where $\hat{y}$ is the predicted result, compared to Softmax, LogSoftmax solves the problem of possible Softmax overflow.

$$\hat{y} = LogSoftmax(h_i^k)$$ (11)

4   Experiment

4.1   Dataset

We use the dataset ReCOvery [33]. The dataset investigated about 2000 news publishers, from which 60 are identified with extreme (high or low) levels of credibility.

The dataset provides multimodal information on news articles on COVID-19, including textual, visual, temporal, and network information, in our work, we will use textual information only. The credibility of the website that published each article contains 9 parts and each score of the part was from an authoritative website NewsGuard.

The general statistics on ReCOvery are presented in Table 1:

Table 1. statistics on ReCOvery

	Reliable	Unreliable	Total
News articles	1364	665	2029
Tweets	114402	26418	140820
Users	78659	17323	93761

4.2   Knowledge Graph

As a knowledge graph in the COVID-19 domain, we use the open-sourced knowledge graph openKG which contains 108298 examples and 298663 tripes collected from 5 encyclopedias. We use Medical Encyclopedia and English Encyclopedia of it, while the Medical Encyclopedia contains 26852 examples, and 31031 triples and English Encyclopedia contains 11051 examples, and 56864 triples.

4.3   Settings

To evaluate the performance of our model, we use the following metrics, which are commonly used to evaluate classifiers: Precision (P), Recall (R), and F1-score (F1).

We implement our model with PyTorch. The dataset is divided into training and testing datasets with a proportion of 4:1. After merging the paragraph embeddings into article embedding. We tested the depth of optimizing layer $K = 1, 2, 3$.

For TIG-KIGNN, we use SGD for the optimizer and the training epoch is set as 2000 to find the best-performing models and observe the convergence situation.

5   Results

5.1   Baseline Methods

During the experiment, we use the same training and testing data as the work on the proposed dataset. The following methods are involved as our baselines.

DT [5]: DT (Decision Transformer) is an autoregressive model and its advantage is that it performs well for sparse problems in reinforcement learning.

LIWC [23]: LIWC (Linguistic Inquiry and Word Count) is a widely-accepted psycholinguistic lexicon, which can classify words into many classes about psychology.

RST [17]: RST (Rhetorical Structure Theory) generates article content as a tree structure that captures the rhetorical relation among its phrases and sentences.

Text-CNN [32]: Text-CNN is a classic text classifier using a convolutional neural network, which can capture different granularity of text features with multiple convolution filters.

SAFE [34]: SAFE is a method that utilizes multimodal information for mis-information detection, where article feature is learned by article and image information.

BERT [9]: BERT provides a powerful foundational model for various natural language processing tasks by learning contextually rich language representations through pre-training and fine-tuning, which enhances the accuracy and effectiveness of the model in understanding and processing natural language.

5.2 Performance Evaluation

We show the precision, recall, and F1-score to compare with the baselines in Table 2.

Table 2. Performance on ReCOvery dataset.

Method	Reliable news			Unreliable News		
	P	R	F1	P	R	F1
LIWC [23]+DT [5]	0.779	0.771	0.775	0.540	0.552	0.545
RST [5]+DT	0.721	0.705	0.712	0.421	0.441	0.430
Text-CNN [32]	0.746	0.782	0.764	0.522	0.472	0.496
SAFE [34]	0.836	0.829	0.833	0.667	0.677	0.672
BERT [9]	0.746	**0.966**	0.841	0.868	0.407	0.554
TIG-KIGNN	**0.900**	0.945	**0.920**	**0.874**	**0.776**	**0.822**

· In Table 2, LIWC combined with Decision Trees (LIWC+DT) outperforms due to LIWC's enhancement of informational content. However, as a psychological lexicon, LIWC is less effective for sentiment analysis, a divergence from misinformation detection. Rhetorical Structure Theory (RST), while structuring article content, becomes complex and noisy with longer texts, impacting classification. Text-CNN excels in capturing semantic details locally but overlooks the valuable insights from inter-article relationships crucial for comprehensive understanding.

· In Table 2, BERT demonstrates enhanced recall for reliable news, owing to its adept learning of their semantics, reinforced by their prevalence in the dataset. Its ability to grasp contextually rich linguistic representations enables precise, fact-focused comprehension, leading to accurate predictions.

· Among the methods based on time interval, article contents, and knowledge graph, our method TIG-KIGNN consistently outperforms other methods in terms of Precision, Recall, and F1-score on the ReCOvery dataset. TIG-KIGNN shows an improvement of 6.4%, 11.6%, and 8.7% on reliable news, and 20.7%, 9.9%, and 15% on unreliable news, respectively.

5.3   Ablation Studies

In this section, to prove the efficiency of our model and the influence of each module, we show the ablation studies in Table 3 and Table 4.

Table 3. Ablation experiment results on reliable news.

Method	P	R	F1	△F1
TIG-KIGNN	**0.900**	**0.945**	**0.920**	–
(w/o) time interval	0.859	0.938	0.896	−0.024
(w/o) knowledge graph	0.866	0.926	0.895	−0.025
(w/o) graphSAGE	0.865	0.881	0.873	−0.047
(w/o) graphSAGE + time interval	0.800	0.930	0.860	−0.060
(w/o) Knowledge Graph + time interval	0.875	0.890	0.883	−0.037

Table 4. Ablation experiment results on unreliable news.

Method	P	R	F1	△F1
TIG-KIGNN	**0.874**	**0.776**	**0.822**	–
(w/o) time interval	0.844	0.687	0.757	−0.065
(w/o) knowledge graph	0.828	0.711	0.765	−0.057
(w/o) graphSAGE	0.734	0.705	0.719	−0.103
(w/o) graphSAGE + time interval	0.840	0.600	0.700	−0.122
(w/o) Knowledge Graph + time interval	0.706	0.675	0.691	−0.131

Tables 3 and 4 reveal a marked 8.9% decline in recall for unreliable news when excluding time intervals, attributed to the brief gap between event occurrence and news release, compromising authenticity. Furthermore, removing the GraphSAGE module degrades the performance for both news types due to the absence of neighbor-informed node optimization.

5.4   Comparison of K

In our work, we use a graph to optimize the information in each article. Therefore, we should consider the effect of the depth of graph aggregation on the classification results.

Table 5 shows the performance and training time with each node's neighborhood in depth $K = 1, 2, 3$ on reliable news and unreliable news. When $K = 2$, the model obtains the best result. The results are as Table 5.

Table 5. Result of different depth of aggregation.

Depth of aggregation	Reliable news			Unreliable news		
	P	R	F1	P	R	F1
K = 1	0.868	0.914	0.890	0.818	0.736	0.774
K = 2	**0.900**	**0.945**	**0.920**	**0.874**	**0.776**	**0.822**
K = 3	0.880	0.862	0.871	0.777	0.803	0.790

Table 5 shows that aggregating with depth K = 1, encompassing only the current node and its immediate neighbors, may lead to inadequate information for robust node analysis. Conversely, a depth of K = 3, which aggregates information from a broader network, risks introducing noise that can hinder misinformation detection, while also prolonging training time. This highlights the necessity of balancing aggregation depth with information quality and computational efficiency.

5.5 Case Study

TIG-KIGNN's proficiency in managing time intervals, expertise, and contextual semantics is highlighted in Fig. 4, which compares its attention to post content against baseline models. Notably, TIG-KIGNN assigns darker shades, indicative of greater attention, to time and expertise-related elements, signaling its potential for higher accuracy in results.

5.6 Error Analysis

In our study, TIG-KIGNN shows limitations in accurately predicting data-driven content, such as in the sentence reporting COVID-19 cases, where it fails to dis-

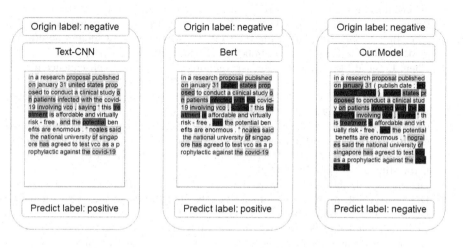

Fig. 4. Schematic overview of the proposed methodology.

cern fabricated data. Instead of relying on data truthfulness, the model assesses news authenticity through contextual semantics and external knowledge, analyzing the article's overall structure.

6   Conclusions

We introduce TIG-KIGNN, a Time Interval Guided Knowledge Inductive Graph Neural Network, tailored for COVID-19 misinformation detection. It utilizes time interval data and a specialized COVID-19 knowledge graph to enrich article embeddings, further optimized by neighboring node analysis. Validated with a real-world dataset, TIG-KIGNN surpasses existing methods. However, it faces limitations like dependence on the knowledge graph, interpretability challenges, and an imbalanced dataset. Future enhancements will consider author credibility to refine its efficacy.

Fundings. This work was supported by Tianjin Research Innovation Project for Postgraduate Students (2022SKYZ275) and the Natural Science Foundation of China (No. 62306213).

Data Availability. The datasets analysed during the current study are available in the ReCOvery repository, http://coronavirus-fakenews.com.

References

1. Bahdanau, D., Cho, K., Bengio, Y.: Neural machine translation by jointly learning to align and translate. arXiv preprint arXiv:1409.0473 (2014)
2. Brennen, J.S., Simon, F.M., Howard, P.N., Nielsen, R.K.: Types, sources, and claims of COVID-19 misinformation. Ph.D. thesis, University of Oxford (2020)
3. Brindha, D., Jayaseelan, R., Kadeswaran, S.: Social media reigned by information or misinformation about COVID-19: a phenomenological study (2020)
4. Chen, K., Luo, Y., Hu, A., Zhao, J., Zhang, L.: Characteristics of misinformation spreading on social media during the COVID-19 outbreak in China: a descriptive analysis. Risk Manag. Healthc. Policy 1869–1879 (2021)
5. Chen, L., et al.: Decision transformer: reinforcement learning via sequence modeling. Adv. Neural Inf. Process. Syst. **34**, 15084–15097 (2021)
6. Chen, X., Jia, S., Xiang, Y.: A review: knowledge reasoning over knowledge graph. Expert Syst. Appl. **141**, 112948 (2020)
7. Cui, L., Seo, H., Tabar, M., Ma, F., Wang, S., Lee, D.: Deterrent: knowledge guided graph attention network for detecting healthcare misinformation. In: Proceedings of the 26th ACM SIGKDD International Conference on Knowledge Discovery & Data Mining, pp. 492–502 (2020)
8. Darwish, O., Tashtoush, Y., Bashayreh, A., Alomar, A., Alkhaza'leh, S., Darweesh, D.: A survey of uncover misleading and cyberbullying on social media for public health. Clust. Comput. **26**(3), 1709–1735 (2023)
9. Devlin, J., Chang, M.W., Lee, K., Toutanova, K.: Bert: pre-training of deep bidirectional transformers for language understanding. arXiv preprint arXiv:1810.04805 (2018)

10. Dou, Y., Shu, K., Xia, C., Yu, P.S., Sun, L.: User preference-aware fake news detection. In: Proceedings of the 44th International ACM SIGIR Conference on Research and Development in Information Retrieval, pp. 2051–2055 (2021)
11. Dun, Y., Tu, K., Chen, C., Hou, C., Yuan, X.: KAN: knowledge-aware attention network for fake news detection. In: Proceedings of the AAAI Conference on Artificial Intelligence, vol. 35, pp. 81–89 (2021)
12. Galli, A., Masciari, E., Moscato, V., Sperlí, G.: A comprehensive benchmark for fake news detection. J. Intell. Inf. Syst. **59**(1), 237–261 (2022)
13. Hamilton, W., Ying, Z., Leskovec, J.: Inductive representation learning on large graphs. Adv. Neural Inf. Process. Syst. **30** (2017)
14. Himelein-Wachowiak, M., et al.: Bots and misinformation spread on social media: implications for COVID-19. J. Med. Internet Res. **23**(5), e26933 (2021)
15. Hussain, W.: Role of social media in COVID-19 pandemic. Int. J. Front. Sci. **4**(2), 59–60 (2020)
16. Ji, J., Zhu, Y., Chao, N.: A comparison of misinformation feature effectiveness across issues and time on Chinese social media. Inf. Process. Manag. **60**(2), 103210 (2023)
17. Ji, Y., Eisenstein, J.: Representation learning for text-level discourse parsing. In: Proceedings of the 52nd Annual Meeting of the Association for Computational Linguistics (volume 1: Long papers), pp. 13–24 (2014)
18. Kumar, S., Shah, N.: False information on web and social media: a survey. arXiv preprint arXiv:1804.08559 (2018)
19. Lan, Z., Chen, M., Goodman, S., Gimpel, K., Sharma, P., Soricut, R.: Albert: a lite Bert for self-supervised learning of language representations. arXiv preprint arXiv:1909.11942 (2019)
20. Li, J., Ni, S., Kao, H.Y.: Meet the truth: leverage objective facts and subjective views for interpretable rumor detection. arXiv preprint arXiv:2107.10747 (2021)
21. Muhammed, T.S., Mathew, S.K.: The disaster of misinformation: a review of research in social media. Int. J. Data Sci. Anal. **13**(4), 271–285 (2022)
22. Parikh, S.B., Atrey, P.K.: Media-rich fake news detection: a survey. In: 2018 IEEE Conference on Multimedia Information Processing and Retrieval (MIPR), pp. 436–441. IEEE (2018)
23. Pennebaker, J.W., Boyd, R.L., Jordan, K., Blackburn, K.: The development and psychometric properties of liwc2015. Technical report (2015)
24. Pennycook, G., McPhetres, J., Zhang, Y., Lu, J.G., Rand, D.G.: Fighting COVID-19 misinformation on social media: experimental evidence for a scalable accuracy-nudge intervention. Psychol. Sci. **31**(7), 770–780 (2020)
25. Rastogi, S., Bansal, D.: A review on fake news detection 3t's: typology, time of detection, taxonomies. Int. J. Inf. Secur. **22**(1), 177–212 (2023)
26. Scarselli, F., Gori, M., Tsoi, A.C., Hagenbuchner, M., Monfardini, G.: The graph neural network model. IEEE Trans. Neural Netw. **20**(1), 61–80 (2008)
27. Shin, J., Jian, L., Driscoll, K., Bar, F.: The diffusion of misinformation on social media: temporal pattern, message, and source. Comput. Hum. Behav. **83**, 278–287 (2018)
28. Shu, K., Mahudeswaran, D., Wang, S., Liu, H.: Hierarchical propagation networks for fake news detection: investigation and exploitation. In: Proceedings of the International AAAI Conference on Web and Social Media, vol. 14, pp. 626–637 (2020)
29. Song, C., Shu, K., Wu, B.: Temporally evolving graph neural network for fake news detection. Inf. Process. Manag. **58**(6), 102712 (2021)

30. Vedula, N., Parthasarathy, S.: FACE-KEG: fact checking explained using knowledge graphs. In: Proceedings of the 14th ACM International Conference on Web Search and Data Mining, pp. 526–534 (2021)

31. Wang, Y., Liu, Z., Fan, Z., Sun, L., Yu, P.S.: DSKReG: differentiable sampling on knowledge graph for recommendation with relational GNN. In: Proceedings of the 30th ACM International Conference on Information & Knowledge Management, pp. 3513–3517 (2021)

32. Zhang, Y., Wallace, B.: A sensitivity analysis of (and practitioners' guide to) convolutional neural networks for sentence classification. arXiv preprint arXiv:1510.03820 (2015)

33. Zhou, X., Mulay, A., Ferrara, E., Zafarani, R.: Recovery: a multimodal repository for COVID-19 news credibility research. In: Proceedings of the 29th ACM International Conference on Information & Knowledge Management, pp. 3205–3212 (2020)

34. Zhou, X., Wu, J., Zafarani, R.: SAFE: similarity-aware multi-modal fake news detection. In: Lauw, H.W., Wong, R.C.-W., Ntoulas, A., Lim, E.-P., Ng, S.-K., Pan, S.J. (eds.) PAKDD 2020. LNCS (LNAI), vol. 12085, pp. 354–367. Springer, Cham (2020). https://doi.org/10.1007/978-3-030-47436-2_27

Double Graph Convolution Network with Knowledge Distillation for International Media Portrait Analysis of COVID-19

Xingyu Yu[1], Jingjian Gao[1], Hongfei Lin[2], and Yijia Zhang[1]([✉])

[1] School of Information Science and Technology, Dalian Maritime University, Dalian 116026, Liaoning, China
{yuxy,1120221482,zhangyijia}@dlmu.edu.cn
[2] School of Computer Science and Technology, Dalian University of Technology, Dalian 116024, Liaoning, China
hflin@dlut.edu.cn

Abstract. Global media with international influence play a crucial role in shaping international public opinion related to China. These media report on objective events and shape people's perceptions and viewpoints. So, we are studying how international public opinion forms are crucial for constructing a positive national image, improving the international public opinion environment, and resisting various forms of ideological infiltration. This paper focuses on conducting an international media portrait analysis of China during the COVID-19 pandemic as a typical case study. The task involves fine-grained sentiment classification through aspect-based sentiment analysis. Due to the complexity of online comments and inaccurate parsing results, improving the accuracy of this task presents significant challenges. We propose a KD-Dual-GCN model based on knowledge distillation and dual graph convolutional networks to address these challenges, considering both syntactic structure and semantic correlation. Our SynGCN module leverages rich syntactic knowledge to mitigate dependency parsing errors, and our SemGCN module incorporates a self-attention mechanism to capture semantic correlation. Additionally, we employ knowledge distillation to reduce model latency and network parameters. The results from experiments conducted on three standard datasets show that our KD-Dual-GCN model outperforms existing methods, validating the effectiveness of our proposed approach.

Keywords: COVID-19 · media portrait · knowledge distillation

1 Introduction

Against unprecedented global changes in a century, the world is undergoing structural reforms, and public opinion has emerged as a significant power source. The development and integration of online social platforms have created a new communication ecosystem, emphasizing the increasing importance of international media in shaping the evolving international environment [1]. In this context, studying China's latest developments

H. Xu et al. (Eds.): CHIP 2023, CCIS 1993, pp. 301–316, 2024.
https://doi.org/10.1007/978-981-99-9864-7_20

and trends in overseas media coverage can help us understand the dominant forces in international public opinion, enhance our communication capabilities, and foster a favorable external environment for China's reform, development, and stability.

International public opinion analysis primarily focuses on the emotional tendencies and language styles of news texts published by the media, aiming to reveal their opinions and attitudes toward specific events. Traditional international public opinion research methods heavily rely on manual reading and data statistics, which consume significant time and resources and are prone to subjective bias. However, with the explosive growth of new information online, relying solely on traditional qualitative analysis has become impractical, making accurate and efficient data processing challenging. As machine learning and deep learning methods such as extensive data analysis continue to advance, constructing portraits of network media has become a commonly used approach for studying the evolution of public opinion. Analyzing online public opinion using big data and exploring hot topics and trends in international mainstream media can provide relevant government departments with timely, comprehensive, and accurate insights into the direction of international public opinion. Analyzing online public opinion is crucial in establishing an international discourse power that aligns with China's comprehensive national strength and international status [2].

In sentiment analysis, employing deep learning architectures to analyze the emotional stance of international media typically requires a large amount of labeled data [3]. Considering the substantial volume of news data, annotating all the collected data would demand significant human and material resources. Furthermore, the model's performance may decrease due to distributional shifts during training, testing, and practical operations. Domain adaptation methods effectively address this issue by learning the differences between data from the source and target domains, allowing the model trained on the source domain to transfer well to the target domain and maintain optimal performance [4]. However, adversarial learning in the domain adaptation process may lead to knowledge forgetting because of the disparities in data between the source and target domains and the unavailability of target domain labels. To overcome this challenge, knowledge distillation techniques widely used in natural language processing allow the injection of external knowledge into the model [5]. By leveraging a teacher model, knowledge can be better transferred to the student model, mitigating knowledge forgetting during adversarial training. Initially, this technology involved applying temperature scaling to teacher predictions for specific instances. Subsequently, Li and Caraga [6] introduced a novel method of dynamic temperature scaling for knowledge extraction, aiming to fine-tune the teacher's predictions at each step of the generation process. These advancements contribute to emotional stance detection tasks and knowledge extraction methods.

We propose a public opinion analysis model that incorporates knowledge distillation and dual graph convolutional networks to detect the emotional tendencies of mainstream international media. Since the outbreak of the COVID-19 pandemic, Western media outlets and politicians, led by the United States, have distorted facts, disregarded the significant sacrifices and efforts made by the Chinese government and people in handling the crisis, and exploited the pandemic to launch an offensive against our country, attacking our socialist system. The behavior of Western media poses a grave threat to our ideological security. Therefore, this paper utilizes the GDELT database as the data source, crawling articles published by international mainstream media during the COVID-19 epidemic to construct a comprehensive profile of international media sentiment.

Our contributions are highlighted as follows:

1) We made a media portrait of the international media during the COVID-19 epidemic and obtained many profound results.
2) We propose orthogonal and differential regularizers to address the challenges of reducing model latency and compressing network parameters through knowledge distillation. The orthogonal regularizer promotes the learning of an orthogonal semantic attention matrix within the SemGCN network. In contrast, the differential regularizer encourages the SemGCN network to develop semantic features distinct from the syntactic features built by the SynGCN network.
3) The experimental results demonstrate the effectiveness of our KD-Dual-GCN model. Additionally, we constructed a GDELT and Twitter-based dataset suitable for ABSA tasks.

2 Related Work

2.1 Research on Media Portraits

The construction of media portraits aims to describe the characteristics and evolving trends of public opinion of a media outlet or a group of media outlets by analyzing the themes, emotions, and language styles of their news articles [9]. Within the field of communication, theories on media effects and emotional analysis have provided a theoretical foundation for the development of media portraits. Research has shown that media impacts public attitudes, beliefs, and behaviors [10], while emotions are crucial in driving human thinking and behavior [11]. In summary, media profiling is a practical approach to understanding the characteristics and emotional tendencies of the media, providing a basis for in-depth analysis and comprehension of media public opinion.

Sentiment analysis involves determining the emotional polarity of a text and is an essential task in media portraits. Taboada et al. [12] employed a semantic-based approach to analyze the emotional orientation of words in a text. They utilized these orientations to assess the overall emotional orientation of the text. Socher et al. [13] adopted a machine learning-based sentiment analysis method, training a model using a large dataset and then applying it to classify new samples based on sentiment. While semantic-based methods offer fine-grained analysis, they are often constrained by resources such as sentiment dictionaries. On the other hand, machine learning-based approaches are relatively objective but heavily rely on training data.

Theme modeling uses deep learning techniques to extract and represent underlying themes from textual data [14]. This represents another important aspect of constructing media portraits. For instance, Wu Peng et al. [15] employed the latent dirichlet allocation (LDA) topic model to analyze the evolution of policy-related themes during the COVID-19 pandemic, providing insights into government emergency management strategies. Yang Jiayun et al. [16] integrated thematic and emotional information to construct a thematic-emotional model, exploring the emotional evolution of online public opinion and identifying hot topics of negative public sentiment during sudden public health events. Researchers have recently explored using LDA and other deep learning technologies for public opinion analysis. For example, Zeng Ziming et al. [17] used an LDA and Bi-LSTM attention model to analyze online public opinion's thematic and emotional evolution during the COVID-19 pandemic.

2.2   Research on Public Opinion of Google News Database GDELT

The Global Database of Events, Language, and Tone (GDELT) is currently the world's largest open-source political event database. Since 1979, GDELT has been recording a wide range of significant events from global news media. It monitors news events from television, radio, and online news sources in over 100 languages across various countries and regions worldwide. The database is updated in real-time, with new data available every 15 min. GDELT provides daily media coverage data in three formats: the event database (event), the global knowledge graph (GKG), and the event mention table (element). Within international relations research, many scholars and research institutions are utilizing the GDELT database as a primary data source for studying the evolution of public opinion worldwide. For instance, Chi Zhipei [23] conducted a quantitative study on the China-US bilateral relationship using GDELT, while Qin Kun [24] employed complex network theory and methods to analyze international relations based on the network data available in GDELT.

3   Methods

This paper proposes a public opinion analysis model KD-Dual-GCN to study international public opinion during the COVID-19 epidemic. The model focuses on detecting international emotional positions through a ternary classification task. The model's overall structure is illustrated in Fig. 1 and consists of three main components. First, the model conducts pretraining on the source encoder and classifier using target data. This step aims to establish baseline performance by training the encoder and classifier with data from the target domain. Next, adversarial training is performed on the target encoder using a domain adaptive model with knowledge distillation. This process aligns the feature representation of the target data with the representation of the source data. The model enhances its ability to handle diverse data sources by reducing the domain discrepancy. Finally, the hidden representations of sentences are fed into the SynGCN and SemGCN modules. These modules capture syntactic and semantic information, enabling the model to understand the nuances of public opinion. To facilitate adequate information flow, we propose a BiAffine module. The representations from the SynGCN and SemGCN modules are aggregated through pooling and concatenation to form the final aspect representation.

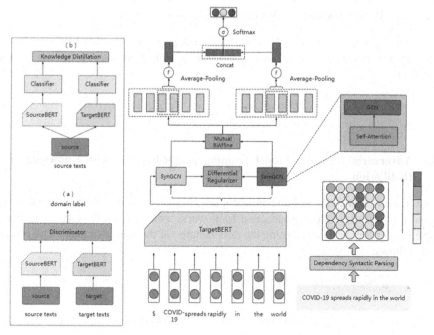

Fig. 1. The overall structure of the KD-Dual-GCN model

3.1 Word Encoding Layer

The word encoding layer uses a large pretrained language model, BERT, to encode and extract corresponding features from news segments. Assuming formulas represent the labeled source domain data (1), (2), and (3):

$$X_S = \{(x_s^i)\}_{i=0}^{N_S} \tag{1}$$

$$Y_S = \{(y_s^i)\}_{i=0}^{N_S} \tag{2}$$

$$(x_s, y_s) \sim (X_s, Y_s) \tag{3}$$

Formulas represent the unlabeled target domain data (4) and (5):

$$X_T = \left\{\left(x_t^i\right)\right\}_{i=0}^{N_t} \tag{4}$$

$$x_t \sim X_T \tag{5}$$

where N_S represents the number of samples in the source domain and N_t represents the number of samples in the target domain. Input the given source data X_S and target data X_S into the BERT encoder in the form of "$[CLS]x_{i1}, x_{i2}, \ldots x_{im}$" $i \in [S, T]$. Assuming that the target data share the same label space as the source data, the source encoder is represented by function $E_{s(x)}$, where x represents the input of the network and $E_{t(x)}$ represents the target encoder. In addition, C represents the source classifier function, and D represents the target classifier function.

3.2 Fine-Tuning the Source Domain Encoder and Classifier

By accessing source data (X_s, Y_s), fine-tune source encoder E_s and classifier C using the standard cross entropy loss function, and fine-tune them using the cross entropy loss function:

$$\min_{E_s, C} \mathcal{L}_s(X_s, y_s) = E_{(x_s, y_s)} - \sum_{k=1}^{K} 1_{[k=y_s]} \, logC(E_s(x_s)) \tag{6}$$

3.3 Adversarial Adaptive Model Training Target Encoder with Knowledge Distillation

First, the target encoder and discriminator are alternately trained in the original adversarial network of the domain adaptive framework, which allows the target encoder to have greater flexibility in learning the data features of the source domain. The process is as follows:

$$\min_{D} \mathcal{L}_{dis}(X_S, X_T) = E_{x_s} - logD(E_s(x_s)) + E_{x_t} - log(1 - D(E_t(x_t))) \tag{7}$$

$$\min_{E_t} \mathcal{L}_{gen}(X_T) = E_{x_t} - logD(E_t(x_t)) \tag{8}$$

In the context of limited access to labeled target data and the inherent dissimilarity between the target domain task and the source domain, feature forgetting may occur, resulting in random classification. This paper introduces the concept of knowledge distillation loss. The goal of incorporating knowledge distillation is to provide the model with enhanced flexibility in adversarial adaptation while retaining important class information. It is achieved using a knowledge distillation technique that leverages a maximum temperature value of t. The process can be summarized as follows:

$$\mathcal{L}_{KD}(X_s) = t^2 \times E_{x_s} \sum_{k=1}^{K} -softmax(z_k^s/t) \times log\,(softmax(z_k^T/t)) \tag{9}$$

where $z^s = C(E_s(x_s))$ and $z^T = C(E_t(x_s))$. Therefore, the final objective function used for training the target encoder becomes:

$$\min_{E_t} \mathcal{L}_T(X_s, X_T) = \mathcal{L}_{gen}(X_T) + \mathcal{L}_{KD}(X_s) \tag{10}$$

We developed a self-attention mechanism with orthogonal regularization to enhance the capture of semantic relationships in reports and short text comments. This module generates an attention score matrix by calculating the weights using Eq. (11). Equation (11) represents the weight calculation formula, which determines the importance of each token in the context based on its relevance to other tokens. By incorporating orthogonal regularization, the self-attention mechanism promotes the independence and diversity of the attention weights, leading to a better representation of the semantic relationships within the text. This approach improves the ability to capture and model the intricate semantic connections in reports and short text comments through the self-attention mechanism with orthogonal regularization. Equation (11) underpins the weight calculation process that determines the significance of each token in the context:

$$A = softmax\left(\frac{QW^Q \times (KW^K)^T}{\sqrt{d}}\right) \tag{11}$$

where Q and K are graph representation matrices, and W^Q and W^K are learnable weight matrices.

An orthogonal regularizer is applied to the initial attention score matrix to enhance the semantic representation. By incorporating the orthogonal regularizer, we aim to ensure that the attention scores assigned to different words are mutually independent and diversified. It helps capture a more comprehensive range of semantic information and improves the overall quality of the representation. Equation (12) reflects the equation used for the orthogonal regularization:

$$R = \left\|A^s A^{sT} - I\right\|_F \tag{12}$$

where I is the identity matrix. The subscript F represents the Frobenius norm. Minimize each nondiagonal element of A to maintain the orthogonality of the matrix Asem.

The attention score matrix is fed into the GCN module for feature fusion. This step leverages the strengths of the self-attention module and the semantic-based graph convolution. The self-attention module captures the semantic relationships among words in a sentence, providing flexibility in understanding their interconnections beyond syntactic structures. Meanwhile, semantic-based graph convolution can adapt to online comments that may not heavily rely on syntactic information. By combining these two modules, the GCN module generates a sentiment probability distribution. This distribution represents the likelihood of different sentiment categories for the given input. A normalization function is applied to the output to ensure a valid probability distribution. A loss function is defined to train the model, as shown in Eq. (13). This loss function guides learning by measuring the discrepancy between the predicted sentiment probability distribution and the ground truth labels. Minimizing this loss improves the model's ability to predict sentiment accurately. In summary, the attention score matrix is utilized in the GCN module for feature fusion. The combined strength of the self-attention module and the semantic-based graph convolution allows for a more comprehensive understanding of the input.

$$L_T = L_C + \lambda_1 R + \lambda_2 \|\theta\|_2 \tag{13}$$

$$L_C = -\sum_{(s,a)\in D} \sum_{c\in C} \log p(a) \tag{14}$$

where λ_1, λ_2 is the regularization coefficient, θ for all trainable model parameters. C is the standard cross entropy loss (14). Among them, D contains all sentence pairs, and C is a set of different emotional polarities.

4 Experiment

4.1 Dataset

We used Web Crawler to obtain 735,566 pieces of original data from GDELT from December 5, 2021, to January 5, 2022, then deleted 381,040 pieces of invalid data with empty titles and content, and finally obtained 354,526 pieces of valid data, with a crawl success rate of 48.20%. We selected 3,000 pieces of data to label as the GDELT dataset manually. We conduct experiments on three public standard datasets. The Restaurant and Laptop datasets are made public from the SemEval ABSA challenge. All three datasets have three sentiment polarities: positive, negative, and neutral. Each sentence in these datasets is annotated with marked aspects and their corresponding polarities. Statistics for the three datasets are shown in Table 1.

Table 1. Statistics for the three experimental datasets.

Dataset	Division	# Positive	# Negative	# Neutral
GDELT	Training	566	751	441
	Testing	356	542	344
Restaurant	Training	2164	807	637
	Testing	727	196	196
Laptop	Training	976	851	455
	Testing	337	128	167

4.2 Baseline Methods

We conducted a comparison between KD-Dual-GCN and several state-of-the-art baseline models. Here is a brief description of each model:

1) kumaGCN [19]: This model incorporates a latent graph structure to complement syntactic features for better performance.
2) InterGCN [20]: InterGCN utilizes a graph convolutional network (GCN) over a dependency tree to learn aspect representations, leveraging syntactic information.
3) R-GAT [21]: R-GAT proposes an aspect-oriented dependency tree structure and then encodes new dependency trees using a relational graph attention network (GAT).
4) DGEDT [22]: DGEDT introduces a dependency graph-enhanced dual-transformer network that considers flat and graph-based representations jointly.
5) RGAT-BERT [23]: RGAT-BERT reshapes and prunes the original dependency tree to generate a unified aspect-oriented dependency tree. It then applies a relational graph attention network for tree encoding.
6) T-GCN [24]: T-GCN designs a type-aware GCN, explicitly utilizing dependency type information for aspect-based sentiment analysis (ABSA).

7) BERT4GCN [25]: BERT4GCN enhances the dependency graph using attention weights from intermediate layers in BERT. It then applies GCNs over the augmented dependency graph.

8) DR-BERT [26]: DR-BERT learns dynamic aspect-oriented semantics by employing a dynamic reweighting adapter. This adapter selects the most important words at each step and updates the semantics accordingly.

These models represent the current state-of-the-art approaches in sentiment analysis and aspect-based sentiment analysis. By comparing KD-Dual-GCN with these baselines, we aim to assess its performance and demonstrate its advancements in tackling sentiment analysis tasks.

4.3 Comparison Results

We adopted accuracy and macroscopic average F1 score as the primary evaluation metrics to evaluate the ABSA model. The experimental results are presented in Table 2, and our KD-Dual-GCN model consistently outperforms all other attention and syntax-based methods on the Restaurant, Laptop, and GDELT datasets. These outcomes demonstrate that our KD-Dual-GCN effectively integrates syntactic knowledge and semantic information, improving performance on formal, informal, and complex comments. Compared with attention-based methods, our KD-Dual-GCN model utilizes syntactic knowledge to establish dependency relationships between words, thereby avoiding any noise or limitations resulting from attention mechanisms. This feature enables our model to capture the sentiment of the input text more accurately.

Table 2. Experimental results comparison on three publicly available datasets.

Models	GDELT		Restaurant		Laptop	
	Accuracy	F1	Accuracy	F1	Accuracy	F1
kumaGCN (Chen et al., 2020)	71.22	69.64	81.43	73.64	76.12	72.42
InterGCN (Liang et al., 2020)	72.23	69.12	82.23	74.01	77.86	74.32
R-GAT (Wang et al., 2020)	80.3	73.05	83.3	76.08	77.42	73.76
DGEDT (Tang et al., 2020)	78.9	70.06	83.9	75.1	76.8	72.3
RGAT-BERT (Wang et al., 2020)	81.6	75.05	86.6	81.35	78.21	74.07
T-GCN (Tian et al., 2021)	79.16	71.85	86.16	79.95	80.88	77.03
BERT4GCN (Xiao et al., 2021)	70.01	69.95	73.01	77.11	77.49	73.01
DR-BERT (Zhang et al., 2022)	81.72	79.3	87.72	82.31	**81.45**	78.16
KD-Dual-GCN (Ours)	**82.59**	**80.5**	**88.25**	**83.02**	80.45	**79.23**

4.4 Ablation Study

We conducted extensive ablation studies to further delve into the role of modules in the KD-Dual-GCN model. These studies revealed that removing one or both regularizers responsible for orthogonal and differential correlations caused a substantial decrease in model performance, particularly on the Restaurant and Laptop datasets. Specifically, KD-Dual-GCN w/o RO&RD indicates that we removed both the orthogonal and differential regularizers, while KD-Dual-GCN w/o RO or RD denotes that we removed only one. The experimental results showed that both regularizers play a crucial role in encouraging the KD-Dual-GCN to capture semantic correlations accurately. Overall, our KD-Dual-GCN model with all modules achieved the best performance. These findings demonstrate the effectiveness of the orthogonal and differential regularizers in improving the model's ability to capture complex semantic relationships (Table 3).

Table 3. Experimental results of the ablation study.

Models	GDELT		Restaurant		Laptop	
	Accuracy	F1	Accuracy	F1	Accuracy	F1
KD-Dual-GCN w/o RO&RD	79.16	71.85	82.93	75.79	76.58	72.03
KD-Dual-GCN w/o Ro	70.01	69.95	83.56	77.43	76.58	72.78
KD-Dual-GCN w/o RD	81.72	79.3	83.65	76.34	77.53	73.72
KD-Dual-GCN (Ours)	**82.59**	**80.5**	**88.25**	**83.02**	**80.45**	**79.23**

4.5 International Public Opinion Analysis in the COVID-19 Pandemic

We proposed a calculation method for social media influence. We filtered the attribute data of seven social media accounts through specific fields, including the New York Times, BBC News, CNN International, CBC News, MFA Russia, DW News, and RFI. We evaluate media influence (IF) in three aspects: transmission power (TP), guidance (GD), and degree of trust (DT).

Transmission power reflects the ability of a social media account to spread information. It is evaluated by the number of tweets (TS) the account posts. Protected (PR) indicates whether the account has privacy protection. In Formula (15), the value of PR is only 0 and 1. If the account has privacy protection, we consider the media to have no transmission power. At this time, the value of PR is 0. Otherwise, it is 1. The value of parameter α is $1*10^4$.

$$TP = \frac{TS}{\alpha} \cdot PR \tag{15}$$

Public participation in tweeting calculation: Select random tweets, calculate the public participation of each tweet, and then take the average value as the final result. Public participation in tweets is the product of the number of replies (RE), followers (FL), and forward (FW) of this tweet. In formula (16), the parameter t is the number of tweet samples, and our value is 5. In addition, the value of parameter β is $1*10^7$.

$$GD = \frac{FS}{\beta} \cdot \sum_{i=1}^{t} RE \cdot FL \cdot FW \tag{16}$$

The degree of trust reflects the credibility of a social media account. It is evaluated by the number of lists (LS) associated with the account. Verified (VD) is used to indicate whether the media account has passed official verification. If the account does not pass the verification, we consider this media has no credibility. In Formula (17), the value of VD is only 0 and 1. If the account fails to pass official verification, we consider the media to have no guiding force. At this time, the value of VD is 0. Otherwise, it is 1. The value of parameter γ is $1*10^4$.

$$DT = \frac{LS}{\gamma} \cdot VD \tag{17}$$

As shown in Fig. 2, the New York Times's indicators are superior to other media's. All BBC indicators are relatively balanced. Through this study, media portraits can be carried out to provide data support for public opinion analysis. This study provides a reference for countermeasures to enhance the influence of the media.

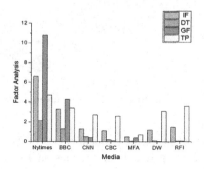

Fig. 2. Media influence and its parameters

Based on the previous work, we selected two special periods to conduct sentiment analysis of seven media on the timeline. They are the declining period of tweets (3.21–3.24) and the stable period (3.28–4.08). Then, based on the tweets of these seven media accounts, we screened out tweets related to the Chinese epidemic and analyzed their sentiment (as shown in Fig. 3).

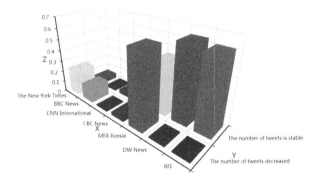

Fig. 3. Sentiment analysis in two special periods

During the period of an increasing number of cases in China, most media accounts were pessimistic about the epidemic. When the epidemic situation in China improved, media accounts were more optimistic about the epidemic in China. We classify Twitter users' replies to seven social media accounts. They were divided into three categories: economic, political, and military.

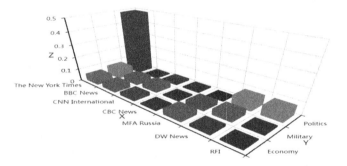

Fig. 4. Sentiment analysis in three aspects

As shown in Fig. 4, except for the political tweets of the New York Times, users' replies to all accounts were negative. Users' replies on Twitter are not subject to any restrictions, while those on mainstream media are different. Therefore, the results of this part of the emotional analysis are more realistic. It can more genuinely reflect the genuine attitude of Western public opinion toward the epidemic in China.

We selected the top 20 media according to the number of articles published. We took the media as the research object to analyze the sentiment tendency of different media outlets toward the epidemic in China.

According to the sentiment analysis results of all the news items in Fig. 5, different colors represent different sentiments. The length of a certain color determines the proportion of the sentiment. We choose the longest as the final result of sentiment tendency, which is the last column of Table 4.

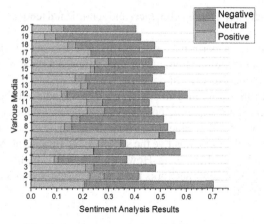

Fig. 5. Sentiment tendency of different media

Table 4. Media portrait data results

Media	Sentimental indicator	Media influence	Sentimental tendency
msn	0.2863	0.3629	negative
bignewsnetwork	0.0917	0.1015	positive
menafn	0.0275	0.0884	negative
bnnbloomberg	0.1779	0.0574	negative
sina	0.0947	0.0367	negative
forbes	0.2391	0.0406	positive
prnewswire	0.4321	0.0325	positive
chinanationalnews	0.2427	0.0255	negative
cnn	0.1679	0.0326	negative
indiatimes	0.0319	0.0239	positive
iol.co.za	0.0309	0.0219	positive
thehill	0.3481	0.0246	negative
shanghaisun	0.1064	0.0223	negative
thestar	0.0888	0.0251	negative
beijingbulletin	0.0446	0.0208	negative

We calculate the absolute value of the positive and negative scores of the article as an indicator of the article's sentiment indicator. The calculation method of media influence here is different from that of Twitter. The influence of mainstream media is calculated by media scope and media activity. Media scope refers to the number of topics covered by the article. Media activity refers to the number of articles published by the media. We took sentimental indicators, media influence, and sentimental tendency as the parameters of media portraits.

Table 4 shows media portraits for 15 media. We focused on the top five media regarding the number of publications. After that, we used a radar map to make a more critical comparative analysis of their data.

Figure 6 shows the difference in five mainstream media attribute values on five evaluation indicators. The farther the point representing each value is from the center of the radar chart, the greater the value. Regarding the attribute of sentiment analysis, the farther the distance is, the more positive the sentiment is. In general, MSNs have a more substantial media influence than others. However, its article is highly subjective. Among the five media, only large news networks have positive sentiments toward China, while the other four are negative.

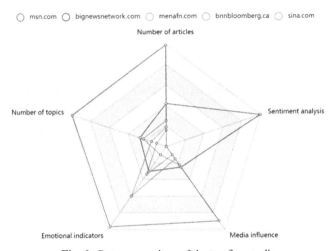

Fig. 6. Data comparison of the top five media

5 Conclusion

In this paper, we propose a novel architecture called KD-Dual-GCN, which effectively tackles the limitations of attention-based and dependency-based methods in ABSA tasks. Our proposed KD-Dual-GCN model integrates syntactic knowledge and semantic information by incorporating SynGCN and SemGCN modules. Additionally, to address concerns regarding model size and latency and compress network parameters, we employ knowledge distillation techniques. Through extensive experiments conducted on benchmark datasets, we demonstrate that our KD-Dual-GCN model surpasses baseline approaches and achieves superior performance.

Research and analysis have revealed that China garners significant attention from international mainstream media. However, emotional analysis indicates that biases toward China persist in Western countries, leading to a negative attitude in most foreign mainstream media outlets. In light of these findings, we must adopt suitable communication strategies, reporting angles, and timing, all guided by the principles governing the dissemination of international public opinion. By promptly responding to distorted reports from Western media and actively working to eliminate misunderstandings, we can mitigate the impact of biased narratives. Engaging in effective communication that addresses misconceptions and presents a balanced and accurate portrayal of China's perspectives and actions is imperative. Doing so can foster a more nuanced and comprehensive understanding among international audiences.

Acknowledgment. This work is supported by a grant from the Social and Science Foundation of Liaoning Province (No. L20BTQ008).

References

1. Fan, H., Zheng, X., Re, Z.A., et al.: Research on multidimensional knowledge discovery in standard literature based on knowledge graph. Intell. Theory Pract. **46**(9), 175–184 (2023)
2. Qingwen, J.: Research on interpretability techniques and evaluation methods in intelligence analysis. Intell. Data Work **44**(4), 24–34 (2023)
3. Zuying, M., Daqing, P., Huan, L., et al.: Analysis of the false information problem and root causes of AIGC from the perspective of information quality. J. Libr. Inf. Sci. **40**(4), 32–40 (2023)
4. Gheisari, M., Baghshah, M.S.: Unsupervised domain adaptation via representation learning and adaptive classifier learning. Neurocomputing **165**, 300–311 (2015)
5. Hosseini, M., Caragea, C.: Distilling knowledge for empathy detection. In: Findings of the Association for Computational Linguistics, EMNLP 2021, pp. 3713–3724 (2021)
6. Li, Y., Caragea, C.: Distilling calibrated knowledge for stance detection. In: Findings of the Association for Computational Linguistics: ACL 2023, pp. 6316–6329 (2023)
7. Hong, Y., Ziqing, Q.: Research on the generation mechanism and simulation of public participation behavior based on the value realization of government open data: exploration under the moa framework. Intell. Inf. Work **44**(4), 54–65 (2023)
8. Lin, W., Liyu, M.: The key to enhancing the value of open data - data service institutions. Intell. Inf. Work **44**(4), 105–112 (2023)
9. Shijie, S., Yuxiang, Z., Qinghua, Z.: From ELIZA to ChatGPT: AI generated content (AIGC) credibility evaluation in human intelligence interactive experience. Intell. Data Work **44**(4), 35–42 (2023)
10. Taboada, M., Brooke, J., Tofiloski, M., et al.: Lexicon-based methods for sentiment analysis. Comput. Linguist. **37**(2), 267–307 (2011)
11. Socher, R., Perelygin, A., Wu, J.Y., et al.: Recursive deep models for semantic compositionality over a sentiment treebank. In: Proceedings of the Conference on Empirical Methods in Natural Language Processing (EMNLP), pp. 1631–1642 (2013)
12. Zhenqing, Z., Wei, S.: Research on interdisciplinary topic recognition based on feature measurement and PhraseLDA model - Taking the application of nanotechnology in agricultural environment as an example *. Data Anal. Knowl. Discov. **7**(7), 32–45 (2023)
13. Wu, P., Zhang, M., Suo, J.: Policy theme mining and hierarchical diffusion characteristics analysis of COVID-19 based on spatiotemporal big data evolution. Inf. Theory Pract. **46**(5), 185–192, 153 (2023)

14. Jiayun, Y., Huiming, Z.: Research on the evolution of network public opinion in sudden public health events based on theme emotion fusion analysis. Intell. Explor. **08**, 18–28 (2021)

15. Ziming, Z., Siyu, C.: Analysis of the evolution of network public opinion in sudden public health events based on LDA and BERT BiLSTM attention models. Intell. Theory Pract. **46**(09), 158–166 (2023)

16. Shangyuan, S., Junping, Q.: Research on the evaluation mechanism of philosophy and social sciences research projects based on socialization recommendation. Libr. Inf. Knowl. **40**(4), 92–98 (2023)

17. Kun, Q., Ping, L., Borui, Y.: GDELT data network mining and international relationship analysis. J. Earth Inf. Sci. **21**(1), 14–24 (2019)

18. Zhipei, C., Na, H.: Quantitative research on big data and bilateral relations: taking GDELT and Sino US relations as an example. Int. Polit. Sci. **4**(02), 67–88 (2019)

19. Chenhua, C., Zhiyang, T., Yue, Z.: Inducing target-specific latent structures for aspect sentiment classification. In: Proceedings of the 2020 Conference on Empirical Methods in Natural Language Processing (EMNLP), pp. 5596–5607, Online. Association for Computational Linguistics (2020)

20. Liang, B., Yin, R., Gui, L., Du, J., Xu, R.: Jointly learning aspect-focused and interaspect relations with graph convolutional networks for aspect sentiment analysis. In: Proceedings of the 28th International Conference on Computational Linguistics, pp. 150–161, Barcelona, Spain (Online). International Committee on Computational Linguistics (2020)

21. Wang, K., Shen, W., Yang, Y., Quan, X., Wang, R.: Relational graph attention network for aspect-based sentiment analysis. In: Proceedings of the 58th Annual Meeting of the Association for Computational Linguistics, pp. 3229–3238, Online. Association for Computational Linguistics (2020)

22. Tang, H., Ji, D., Li, C., Zhou, Q.: Dependency graph enhanced dual-transformer structure for aspect-based sentiment classification. In: Proceedings of the 58th Annual Meeting of the Association for Computational Linguistics, pp. 6578–6588, Online. Association for Computational Linguistics (2020)

23. Wang, K., Shen, W., Yang, Y., Quan, X., Wang, R.: Relational graph attention network for aspect-based sentiment analysis. In: Proceedings of the 58th Annual Meeting of the Association for Computational Linguistics, pp. 3229– 3238, Online. Association for Computational Linguistics (2020)

24. Tian, Y., Chen, G., Song, Y.: Aspect-based sentiment analysis with type-aware graph convolutional networks and layer ensemble. In: Proceedings of the 2021 Conference of the North American Chapter of the Association for Computational Linguistics: Human Language Technologies, pp. 2910–2922, Online. Association for Computational Linguistics (2021)

25. Xiao, Z., Wu, J., Chen, Q., Deng, C.: BERT4GCN: using BERT intermediate layers to augment GCN for aspect-based sentiment classification. In: Proceedings of the 2021 Conference on Empirical Methods in Natural Language Processing, pp. 9193–9200, Online and Punta Cana, Dominican Republic. Association for Computational Linguistics (2021)

26. Zhang, K., et al.: Incorporating dynamic semantics into pretrained language model for aspect-based sentiment analysis. In: Findings of the Association for Computational Linguistics: ACL 2022, pp. 3599–3610, Dublin, Ireland. Association for Computational Linguistics (2022)

Research on Double-Graphs Knowledge-Enhanced Intelligent Diagnosis

Yu Song, Dongming Dai, Kunli Zhang[✉], Hongying Zan, Bin Hu, Pengcheng Wu,
and Chenkang Zhu

College of Computer and Artificial Intelligence, Zhengzhou University, Zhengzhou, China
{ieysong,ieklzhang,iehyzan}@zzu.edu.cn

Abstract. Intelligent diagnosis is an effective method to assist doctors in disease diagnosis. Integrating domain knowledge graphs into the intelligent diagnosis process can enhance diagnostic effect. The enhancement effects of different knowledge in the knowledge graph are different. The knowledge introduced based on electronic medical record text can explain medical terms, extract hidden relations, and enrich text representation. However, this method is prone to generating noise and affecting the diagnostic results. Disease is our diagnostic goal, introducing external knowledge centered around diseases can not only obtain richer and more professional disease-related information, but also make the introduced knowledge more accurate and reduce the impact of external knowledge noise. Therefore, this paper proposes a Double-Graphs Knowledge-Enhanced Intelligent Diagnosis Model (DGKE). Firstly, we extract the knowledge related to electronic medical record text from the knowledge graph and construct a text subgraph. At the same time, we obtain the knowledge associated with the disease to be diagnosed and construct a disease subgraph. Then, the two graph representations are fused using a light-attention to obtain an external knowledge representation for the disease to be diagnosed. Finally, the disease-oriented knowledge representation is fused with the hierarchical information-enhanced text representation to obtain the knowledge-enhanced text representation, which is mapped to the disease list space to be diagnosed for prediction. Experiments are conducted on the COEMRs (Chinese Obstetric Electronic Medical Records) and the C-EMRs (Chinese Electronic Medical Records). Compared with models without disease knowledge enhancement, the F1_micro increase by 0.65% and 1.44% respectively and the F1_macro increase by 4.06%, 2.23% respectively.

Keywords: Electronic Medical Records · Knowledge Graph · Knowledge Enhancement

1 Introduction

Intelligent diagnosis refers to using of artificial intelligence technology to analyze the patterns of patient's symptoms, learn medical knowledge, simulate the reasoning process of doctors, and provide preliminary diagnostic results [1]. Combining artificial intelligence technology with medical diagnosis and treatment to create an auxiliary diagnosis

© The Author(s), under exclusive license to Springer Nature Singapore Pte Ltd. 2024
H. Xu et al. (Eds.): CHIP 2023, CCIS 1993, pp. 317–332, 2024.
https://doi.org/10.1007/978-981-99-9864-7_21

system is one of the effective ways to alleviate the current shortage, unreasonable allocation of medical resources and the difficulty of people seeing a doctor [2]. Since the release of the "Basic Specifications for Electronic Medical Records (Trial)" [3], the medical informatization has developed rapidly, a large amount of electronic medical record data has been made public and available, and data-driven research methods have gradually become the mainstream of disease diagnosis [4].

The early development process of intelligent diagnosis research can be divided into expert systems, intelligent diagnosis based on statistical machine learning, and intelligent diagnosis based on deep learning. However, these methods are limited by the training corpus and model capabilities, limited knowledge memory, and are extremely dependent on the quantity and quality of electronic medical records [5]. With the rise of knowledge graphs, researchers have begun to apply them to the organization and expression of medical information. Knowledge graphs incorporate medical knowledge mapping into knowledge service systems. Compared with traditional knowledge representation, KG has wider coverage, can represent different semantic information, and quickly replicates the domain knowledge and clinical experience of medical experts. Intelligent diagnosis based on medical knowledge graphs has also become an important research direction [6].

In the past few years, many tasks have used knowledge graph fusion methods to enhance the representation capabilities of the model. According to the stage of knowledge enhancement in the model, it can be divided into: (1) Knowledge learning in the pre-training stage. The given text and external knowledge are input into the model as pre-training corpus for retraining. This method broadens the knowledge coverage of the model, which well extends the language model training tasks and simultaneously learns language representation and knowledge representation with context, such as SMed-BERT [7], ERNIE [8], DialoKG [9], etc. However, these methods require retraining, require a large amount of data, and have higher requirements for experimental conditions. (2) Knowledge combination in the task-related stage. The knowledge introduced in this stage is usually closely related to the specific text and task. The knowledge is more accurate, and the original pre-training model parameters are directly called without re-doing. It can be roughly divided into: a) Adding knowledge to the input data for enhancement, such as K-BERT [10] and KEGCN [11]. b) Add new fusing module. This method decouples the knowledge enhancement process from the data flow of the original PLM, and interact with modules outside the model to obtain knowledge, such as KEDA [12] and GSKN [13]. These methods introduce a wealth of external knowledge to the model, provide expert interpretations of complex or critical terms, dig deeper into hidden relations in the data, but also introduce noise that can interfere with the final diagnosis. However, in the task of disease diagnosis as the core, constructing disease subgraphs centered around diseases can provide rich disease-related information as diagnostic basis, and can make the introduced knowledge more accurate and reduce the impact of external knowledge noise. Therefore, this paper proposes the Double-Graphs Knowledge-Enhanced Intelligent Diagnosis Model (DGKE). The main contributions of this article are as follows:

1) We extract electronic medical record text and knowledge related to the disease to be diagnosed from the knowledge graph, and construct text subgraphs and disease

subgraphs respectively, then use a light-attention to fuse the vector representations of the two subgraphs to obtain external knowledge representations for the disease to be diagnosed.

2) We propose a fusion mechanism based on interactive attention to fuse disease-oriented knowledge representation with hierarchical information enhanced text representation, and obtain the knowledge enhanced text representation, then map it to the list space of the diseases to be diagnosed for diseases prediction.

2 Methods

2.1 Overview

The overall structure of DGKE is shown in Fig. 1, which can be divided into text representation (TR) module, knowledge representation (KR) module, and Fusion Module. A hierarchical information enhanced text representation was obtained in the TR module.

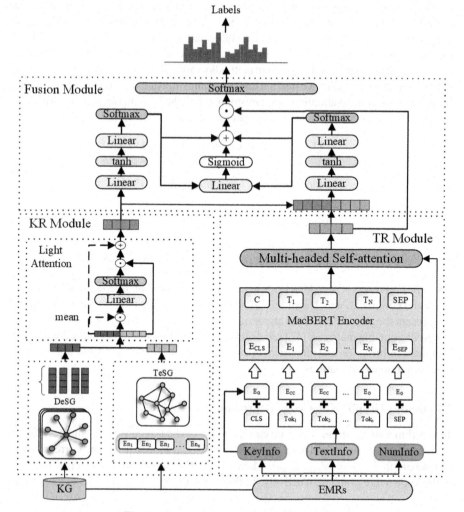

Fig. 1. The architecture of the DGKE model.

A knowledge representation for the disease to be diagnosed was obtained in the KR module. In the fusion module, the knowledge-enhanced text representation is obtained and mapped to the disease list space for diseases prediction.

2.2 Text Representation Module

Due to the fact that ours electronic medical records mainly contain Chinese textual information, we used MacBERT, which performs well on various Chinese datasets, as our pretraining model. We extract disease course records (text information), chief complaint and numerical information from electronic medical records for intelligent diagnosis based on the diversity of electronic medical record data types and the degree of impact on diagnostic results. The chief complaint is a description of the patient's main symptoms or signs (about 20 words). For the numerical information appearing in the text, such as the number "6" in "menopause for more than 6 months", the non-enumerability of numerical features during training makes it difficult to capture numerical features, resulting in numerical sparsity. Drawing on the success of hierarchical information enhancement in electronic medical records [14], the DGKE model adds a separate layer of KeyInfo Embedding containing the main complaint information to the embedding of MacBERT, and then adds it to the rest of the Embedding as input. For the numerical information in the text, we use the min-max and zero-mean methods to normalize and standardize it to obtain numerical features. Finally, we fuse the text-encoding information and numerical features through the multi-head attention mechanism to obtain the final hierarchical information-enhanced text representation $[C']$. The specific formula is shown in Eqs. (1)–(4).

$$Q = K = V = Concat([C]; Nums) \tag{1}$$

$$Attention(Q, K, V) = softmax(QK^T/\sqrt{d_k})V \tag{2}$$

$$head_i = Attention(QW_i^Q, KW_i^K, VW_i^V) \tag{3}$$

$$[C'] = Concat(head_0, \dots, head_i)W^O \tag{4}$$

where $[C]$ represents the hidden layer representation marked in the MacBERT enhanced with chief complaint, which contains information of the entire input sequence. Q, K, and V represent the parameters of the attention mechanism, respectively. W^Q, W^K, W^V, W^O represent trainable matrices, $[C']$ represents the text representation enhanced with chief complaint information and numerical information enhancement, and $Nums$ represent the processed numerical features.

2.3 Double Graphs Knowledge Representation Module

Text Subgraph Module. For a given electronic medical record text sequence $Seq_i = (s_0, s_1, \dots, s_{n-1})$ and knowledge graph $KG = (V, E)$, we construct the corresponding text subgraph $TeSG = (V_{sub}, E_{sub})$, where V and E represent all entities and relations in the knowledge graph, respectively. In the text subgraph, V_{sub} represents the entities and E_{sub} represents relations between entities in V_{sub}. The text subgraph construction process is as follows. First, we use the disease set in CSKB [15], ICD10 [16] and the symptom, disease, drug entity set in the knowledge graph to construct the vocabulary Voc. Then, we use the bidirectional maximum matching method based on Voc to obtain the n candidate entities $Entities_i = (e_0, e_1, ..., e_{n-1})$ with the highest scores from Seq_i. Next, due to the diversity of electronic medical record writing, a multi-strategy similarity weighting algorithm [17] is used to calculate the similarity between entities ei and the entities in V, and all entities with scores above the threshold are added to the entity set $Entitie\ s'_i$. Then, according to each entity in $Entitie\ s'_i$, m triples matched from KG $Triples_i = \{(h_0, r_0, t_0), (h_1, r_1, t_1), ..., (h_{m-1}, r_{m-1}, t_{m-1})\}$ which are used to construct text subgraphs. Finally, these triples are constructed as subgraphs $TeSG_i$ by connecting the same entities and maintaining relations as edges.

We construct an adjacency matrix A based on TeSG. Since the representation of the node itself can affect the representation of the next layer of nodes, the identity matrix I is added based on A. In order to avoid the distortion problem of the graph neural network when aggregating neighbor information, the adjacency matrix $\overline{A}$ is normalized with the help of the degree matrix D. Finally, we use GCN for calculation, and the mean_node algorithm is used in the last layer of the graph neural network to read out the entire graph. The output is a vector K, which is the knowledge representation result corresponding to TeSG. The formulas are shown in (5–9).

$$A_{ij} = A_{ji} = \begin{cases} 1, (v_i, v_j) \in E_{sub} \\ 0, (v_i, v_j) \notin E_{sub} \end{cases}, \forall v_i, v_j \in V_{sub} \tag{5}$$

$$\overline{A} = A + I \tag{6}$$

$$D_{ij} = \begin{cases} \sum_k \overline{A}_{ik}, i = j \\ 0, i \neq j \end{cases} \tag{7}$$

$$\hat{A} = D^{-\frac{1}{2}} A D^{-\frac{1}{2}} \tag{8}$$

$$H^{(l+1)} = f(H^{(l)}, \hat{A}) = \sigma(\hat{A} H^{(l)} W_0^{(l)} + b_0^{(l)}) \tag{9}$$

where $v_i \in V_{sub}$ represents the i-th entity in the graph, $(v_i, v_j) \in E_{sub}$ represents the relation between entity i and entity j, $H^{(l)}$ represents the representation of the text subgraph at the l-th layer, f represents the specific inference formula, $H^{(0)}$ obtained by the TransR model, and $W_0^{(l)}, b_0^{(l)}$ are the trainable parameters of the l-th layer of GCN, σ represents the activation function, and in this paper, the ReLU activation function is chosen.

Disease Subgraph Module. Linking knowledge graphs with the diseases to be diagnosed as the center can construct disease subgraphs which can provide rich disease-related information for the diagnosis process, and can make the introduced knowledge more accurate and reduce the impact of external knowledge noise. The example of the disease subgraph we introduced is shown in Fig. 2. The disease subgraph is constituted by the diseases and its characteristic entities.

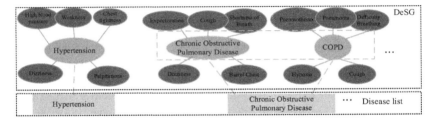

Fig. 2. The example of the disease subgraph

We identify the corresponding disease subgraph DeSG from the knowledge graph based on the set of diseases to be diagnosed in the EMRs. The construction process is as follows: First, we identify all the list of diseases to be diagnosed $Diseases = (dis_0 \ldots dis_i \ldots dis_{n-1})$. However, the description of the same disease may differ. For example, "chronic obstructive pulmonary disease" is also called "COPD". We need to obtain relevant symptoms through these two diseases as nodes for COPD. Therefore, the disease dictionary $Dict = \{dis_0{:}sy_0, \ldots Dis_i{:}sy_i, \ldots, dis_{n-1}{:}sy_{n-1}\}$ is constructed, and sy_i represents the synonym list of dis_i. Then, according to dis_i and sy_i, several triples are matched in the knowledge graph and extract several triples $D\_Triples_i$ used to construct the subgraph corresponding to dis_i. Next, for dis_i, the $D\_Triples_i$ obtained through the above steps is based on dis_i and sy_i. Therefore, using each entity in $D\_Triples_i$ as a node and the relations as edges can obtain the disease subgraph $DeSG_i$ corresponding to dis_i. Finally combine $DeSG_i$ into a graph structure to obtain the disease subgraph $DeSG$.

The disease subgraph DeSG has n connected subgraphs. In order to reduce the number of parameters of the model and training time, we set shared parameters for the n connected subgraphs. With the batch operation provided by Deep Graph Library [18], the n connected subgraphs can be established into a graph batch, and then the graph convolutional neural network is used to dynamically update the n connected subgraphs. The formula is as follows: (10–12) shown. The final disease subgraph can be obtained by splitting the entire batch of images to obtain the updated disease subgraph $DeSG' = (DeSG'_0, DeSG'_1, \ldots, DeSG'_{n-1})$. Read out the disease subgraphs one by one to obtain the final vector representation of the disease subgraph $De = (e_0, e_1, \ldots, e_{n-1})$, where e_i represents the vector representation corresponding to the i-th subgraph $DeSG_i$.

$$Disease_i^{(l+1)} = \sigma(b_1^{(l)} + \sum_{j \in N(i)} \frac{h_j^{(l)} W_1^{(l)}}{c_{ji}} + \frac{Disease_i^{(l)} W_2^{(l)}}{c_{ii}}) \tag{10}$$

$$h_j^{(l+1)} = \sigma(b_2^{(l)} + \frac{Disease_i^{(l)} W_3^{(l)}}{c_{ij}} + \frac{W_4^{(l)} h_j^{(l)}}{c_{jj}}) \tag{11}$$

$$c_{ij} = c_{ji} = \sqrt{|N(j)|}\sqrt{|N(i)|} \tag{12}$$

where $N(i)$ represents the set of neighbor nodes of node i, $Disease_i^{(l)}$ is the representation of the i-th disease in the l-th layer of GCN, and $h_j^{(l)}$ is the representation of the j-th non-disease node in the l-th layer of GCN. $Disease_i^{(0)}$ and h_j^0 are the initial vectors of TransR, and $W_1^{(l)}$, $W_2^{(l)}$, $W_3^{(l)}$, $W_4^{(l)}$, $b_1^{(l)}$, $b_2^{(l)}$ are the trainable parameters in the l-th layer of GCN. σ is the activation function, Relu is selected, and the product of the square root of the node degree, which is represented by c_{ij}.

Double-Graphs Fusion Module. DGKE fuses disease subgraph representation and text subgraph representation based on a light-attention [19]. Compared with the multi-head self-attention mechanism in Transformer, the light-attention has fewer parameters and better fusion effects. Advantages of better results. The light-attention divides information into original global features and global features to be updated. The original features are defined as shown in Eq. (13).

$$\tilde{K} = mean(K + De) \tag{13}$$

where K represents the text subgraph representation, De represents the disease subgraph representation, and $\tilde{K}$ represents the original global features. The global features to be updated $\overline{K}$ are obtained through a weight matrix W_e, K, De, and the calculation process is as shown in Eqs. (14)–(16).

$$Com = Concat(\tilde{K} \odot K; \tilde{K} \odot De) \tag{14}$$

$$W_e = softmax(W_5 Com + b_5) \tag{15}$$

$$\overline{K} = W_e * Concat(K; De) \tag{16}$$

where W_5 represents the trainable parameter matrix and b_5 represents the offset. W_e is a weight that measures the importance of K and De for subsequent updates, which is obtained by normalizing the dot product, K, De.

The final output of the knowledge representation module K_i' is obtained by weighted sum of the global features to be updated $\overline{K}$ and the original global features $\tilde{K}$. Where $w_1 \in 0, 1]$, $w_2 \in [0, 1][0, 1]$ is a hyperparameter that measures the relative importance between $\overline{K}$ and $\tilde{K}$ in each update.

$$K_i' = w_1 * \overline{K} + w_2 * \tilde{K} \tag{17}$$

Similar to Transformer's multi-head self-attention mechanism, the light-attention also supports multi-head operations. The multi-head light-attention calculation process is shown in Eqs. (18)–(19). The K_i' of each disease can be used as head $head_i'$ for multi-head attention calculation, and we finally obtain the knowledge representation for diseases K'.

$$head_i' = w_1^* \tilde{K} + w_2^* \tilde{K} \tag{18}$$

$$K' = Concat(head_0', \ldots, head_{n-1}')W_6 + b_6 \tag{19}$$

where W_6 represents the trainable parameter matrix and b_6 represents the offset.

2.4 Fusion Module

Through the above modules, we can obtain text representation $[C']$ that integrates chief complaint information, numerical information, and disease-oriented knowledge representation K'. We propose a fusion mechanism based on interactive attention to fuse $[C']$ and K', which can be divided into knowledge self-attention mechanism, knowledge-text attention mechanism and gated fusion mechanism.

Knowledge Self-attention Mechanism. In order to measure the impact of knowledge representation on the final diagnosis result, The light-attention is used to perform self-attention calculation. The process is shown in Eq. (20). Where W_7, W_8 represent the trainable parameter matrixs, and b_7, b_8 represent the offsets. α_i can be viewed as a weight matrix obtained from the global features to be updated. The process can be regarded as a feature selection, in which relatively important knowledge has a larger weight and unimportant knowledge tends to 0.

$$\alpha_i = softmax(W_8 tanh(W_7 K' + b_7) + b_8) \tag{20}$$

Knowledge-Text Attention Mechanism. In the process of integrating knowledge into text, although the knowledge representation has integrated information related to the disease to be diagnosed, knowledge noise may still be generated. DGKE uses a knowledge-text attention mechanism to measure the correlation between text and knowledge. The calculation process is shown in Eq. (21). Among them, W_9, W_{10} represents the trainable parameter matrixs, and b_9, b_{10} represents the offsets.

$$\beta_i = softmax(W_{10} tanh(W_9 Concat(K'; [C']) + b_9) + b_{10}) \tag{21}$$

Gated Fusion Mechanism. In order to further alleviate the problem of knowledge noise, the gated mechanism is used to identify and filter it. The specific calculation process is as shown in Eqs. (22)–(24). Which W_{11} represents the trainable parameter matrix, b_{11} represents the offset, and out represents the output result of the final model. $Weight_2$ can further measure the impact of knowledge representation and text representation on the final output result.

$$weight_2 = sigmoid(W_{11} Concat(\alpha_i; \beta_i) + b_{11}) \tag{22}$$

$$weight_2' = (1 - weight_2) \odot \alpha_i + weight_2 \odot \beta_i \tag{23}$$

$$G = weight_2' \odot [C'] \tag{24}$$

The final prediction result can be obtained by mapping the final hidden representation to the disease space. The process is shown in Eq. (25).

$$output = \sigma(W^G G) \tag{25}$$

where W^G represents the trainable parameter matrix and σ represents the sigmoid activation function.

3 Experiments

3.1 Datasets

The experiments use the multi-label Chinese Obstetric Electronic Medical Records (COEMRs) and the single-label Chinese Electronic Medical Records(C-EMRs) [20]. The basic information of the two experimental datasets is shown in Table 1. In this paper, the Chinese Obstetric Knowledge Graph (COKG) [21] is chosen as the knowledge source for COEMRs, and the Chinese Medical Knowledge Graph (CMeKG) [22] is chosen as the knowledge source for C-EMRs. The basic information of the two knowledge graphs is shown in Table 2. In order to better verify the performance of the model, the entire dataset is divided into training and testing sets in a 9:1 ratio, ensuring that the label sets of the training and testing sets are consistent.

Table 1. The statistical results of COEMRs and C-EMRs.

Dataset	Total	Training Set	Test Set	Total Diseases	Multilabel
COEMRs	24,339	21,905	2,434	73	yes
C-EMRs	18,331	16,498	1,833	10	no

Table 2. The statistical results of COKG and CMeKG.

Dataset	Total Number of Entities	Number of Relations
COKG	10,674	15,249
CMeKG	16,498	1,833

COEMRs is a dataset of real electronic medical records from multiple hospitals in China. After going through preprocessing such as de-privacy, standardization, and structuring, there are a total of 24,339 data samples. After dividing into training and testing sets with a ratio of 9:1, there are 21,905 train samples and 2,434 test samples. The number of diseases to be diagnosed is 73. The frequency of diseases in COEMRs is shown in Fig. 3 (only the top 35 diseases are displayed here). Due to the large number of diseases, it is not feasible to embed the entire disease subgraph in the knowledge reasoning process, so only 16 diseases with lower occurrence frequencies are selected.

After data cleaning and filtering, the EMRs dataset retains 18,331 data samples. After dividing into train and test sets with a ratio of 9:1, there are 16,498 train samples and 1,833 test samples. The diagnostic results are in a single-label format, and there are 10 diseases to be diagnosed. The disease distribution is shown in Fig. 4.

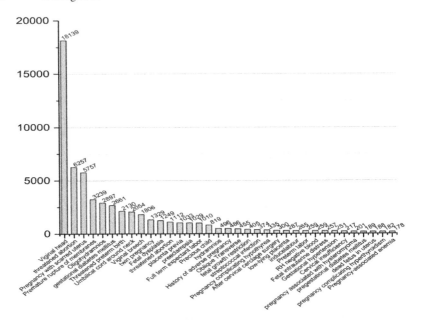

Fig. 3. Distribution of diseases in the COEMRs

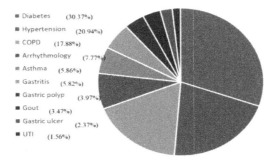

Fig. 4. Distribution of diseases in C-EMRs

3.2   Experimental Results and Analysis

Experimental Results on COEMRs. The experimental results of using COKG as external medical knowledge on COEMRs are shown in Table 3.

The experimental results show that compared to traditional CNN, RNN, and their derivative deep learning models, the pre-trained model has learned more knowledge during the training process and outperforms traditional deep learning models in various performance indicators. Similar to the doctor's diagnostic process, KAIE [23] fusing medical knowledge in triples and GKSN fusing graph structure knowledge both obtain further performance improvement based on BERT. DGKE integrates hierarchical information enhanced text representation and double-graph knowledge representation, and the experimental results show the F1_micro increase of 0.65% compared to GSKN. Due

Table 3. The results on COEMRs.

Model	F1_micro (%)	P (%)	R (%)	F1_macro (%)	AP (%)	HL
TextRNN	42.87	73.81	30.04	1.17	40.57	0.02732
TextCNN	59.64	82.81	46.29	11.34	68.63	0.02138
TextRCNN	65.81	78.70	56.55	13.76	71.25	0.02005
TextRNN + Att	58.21	78.36	46.31	7.78	65.08	0.02268
DPCNN	68.76	80.10	60.23	19.50	73.13	0.01867
MacBERT	80.50	86.98	73.93	31.82	72.53	0.02230
KAIE	80.83	81.44	80.22	47.59	81.99	0.01298
GSKN	81.16	83.20	78.33	41.86	82.18	0.01241
DGKE	**81.81**	85.95	78.06	45.92	**82.65**	**0.01184**

to the complexity of the labels in COEMRs, it is difficult to make accurate judgments on all diseases to be diagnosed based on related symptoms in the knowledge graph. However, GSKN with graph neural network-based knowledge reasoning has a certain degree of decline in F1_macro compared to KAIE, its performance is still higher than the baseline MacBERT. In comparison with GSKN, DGKE adds corresponding label enhancement to the knowledge reasoning part based on GCN, which slightly alleviates the above situation, so the F1_macro of DGKE is closer to KAIE. Meanwhile, our DGKE shows the best performance in Hamming Loss, which evaluated the error classification score, Average Precision, which summarized the accuracy under different thresholds and F1_micro.

To further analyze the experimental results, GSKN and DGKE were further compared. By analyzing the F1 value of each disease diagnosis, it is found that among the 73 diseases to be diagnosed, the F1 value of 34 diseases has been further improved, and the F1 value of 25 diseases remains unchanged, we conducted statistics on 16 diseases that were enhanced with disease subgraphs, and the specific results are shown in Table 4. Among the 16 diseases added with disease subgraph enhancement, the F1 value of 11 diseases has been improved, and the F1 value of 3 diseases remains unchanged.

From the model perspective, on the one hand, the knowledge reasoning based on GCN confers more accurate and comprehensive external medical knowledge to MacBERT. On the other hand, adding disease subgraph enhancement to the knowledge reasoning process can help the model learn related knowledge of the diseases to be diagnosed, thereby increasing the accuracy of the model.

Experimental Results on C-EMRs. In order to further verify the effectiveness of DGKE, a comparative experiment was conducted on C-EMRs, as shown in Table 5. Since the diseases covered in C-EMRs are relatively broad, the more general CMeKG was selected as the external knowledge graph for the experiment.

Due to the single-label dataset nature of C-EMRs, and the much smaller number and imbalance of labels compared to COEMRs, traditional deep learning models also show strong performance. The experimental results of the DGKE model on C-EMRs are

Table 4. Impact of disease subgraph enhancement on various diseases in COEMRs.

Disease	DGKE (%)	GSKN (%)	Changing (%)
Arrhythmia	80.00	0.00	+80.00
Anemia in pregnancy	45.45	27.27	+18.18
Preeclampsia	30.77	16.22	+13.55
Group B streptococcal infection	23.00	18.18	+5.82
Preterm prelabor rupture of membranes	88.60	85.00	+2.60
Placenta previa	82.81	80.75	+2.06
Gestational diabetes mellitus	86.04	83.79	+1.25
Oligohydramnios	81.14	80	+1.14
Twin pregnancy	92.85	92.20	+0.65
Uterine fibroids in pregnancy	63.11	63.00	+0.11
Polyhydramnios	72.65	72.60	+0.05
Hyperemesis gravidarum	92.33	92.33	+0.00
Macrosomia	0.00	0.00	+0.00
Gastrointestinal dysfunction	0.00	0.00	+0.00
Twin-to-twin transfusion	72.73	72.00	−0.27
syndrome	96.77	97.10	−0.33
Premature rupture of membranes	80.00	0.00	+80.00

Table 5. The results on C-EMRs.

Model	F1_micro (%)	P (%)	R (%)	F1_macro (%)
TextRNN	63.63	79.97	53.23	30.38
TextCNN	75.53	87.50	66.45	55.24
TextRCNN	76.32	87.01	67.98	57.70
TextRNN + Att	73.70	85.56	66.28	52.76
DPCNN	77.79	82.90	72.50	61.26
MacBERT	89.37	89.85	87.36	88.33
KAIE	89.70	83.50	92.56	87.49
GSKN	89.95	87.85	85.92	86.77
DGKE	91.39	90.86	87.40	89.00

better than those of the comparison models. Since the public dataset C-EMRs has only 10 label categories, it is easier to obtain disease features, and the fused text subgraphs and disease subgraphs are more accurate, resulting in more improvement in F1_micro.

At the same time, since the single-label dataset does not have couplings, the diagnosis of a certain disease will not affect the diagnosis of other diseases, so the DGKE model also achieved the highest results in F1_macro.

To further verify the effectiveness of the DGKE model, we visualize the F1 values of the DGKE, GSKN, and MacBERT models on C-EMRs dataset for each disease, as shown in Fig. 5. It can be seen from the figure that DGKE achieves the highest F1 values in six diseases, including "Hypertension" and "Diabetes". For the three diseases of "Gastritis", "Gastric polyp", and "Gastric ulcer", since the corresponding symptoms have a high similarity, it is unable to effectively distinguish them based on symptoms during the knowledge enhancement process, so the F1 values of the MacBERT model are slightly higher than those of the GSKN model with knowledge added. For "urinary tract infection (UTI)", since the knowledge related to it in the knowledge graph is quite different from the content included in the electronic medical records, the F1 values of both GSKN and DGKE are lower than MacBERT. Among these four diseases, the DGKE model with double graph knowledge enhancement has a much better performance improvement compared to the GSKN model. The experimental results on C-EMRs dataset further prove the effectiveness of the DGKE model.

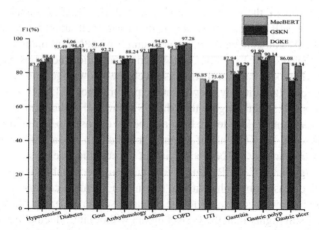

Fig. 5. F1 values of DGKE model for each disease on C-EMRs

Ablation Experiments. To evaluate the effectiveness of knowledge enhancement and the light-attention in graph neural networks, we conduct ablation experiments as shown in Table 6. In these experiments, NoGCN represents the knowledge enhancement module for removing text subgraphs. MSHA represents using the multi-head self-attention mechanism in Transformer to replace the light-attention. NoAtt represents the removal of the light-attention. Since DGKE that removes the entire disease subgraph enhancement module is similar to GSKN, which can be used to represent DGKE that removes the disease subgraph enhancement content.

From the experimental results, it can be seen that when the text subgraph module is removed, the evaluation indicators of the DGKE on COEMRs and C-EMRs datasets all have a significant decline, which indirectly proves the necessity of introducing double

Table 6. The ablation experiments results of DGKE.

Dataset	Model	F1_micro (%)	P (%)	R (%)	F1_macro (%)	AP (%)	HL
COEMRs	DGKE	81.81	85.95	78.06	45.92	82.65	0.01184
	NoGCN	81.38	85.22	77.88	43.76	82.24	0.01216
	MSHA	81.40	85.64	77.55	43.92	82.96	0.01209
	NoAtt	81.29	87.44	75.95	38.95	81.31	0.01193
C-EMRs	DGKE	91.39	90.86	87.40	89.00	–	–
	NoGCN	90.93	90.58	87.10	88.60	–	–
	MSHA	90.96	89.40	87.68	88.37	–	–
	NoAtt	90.54	88.00	87.93	87.85	–	–

graph knowledge enhancement in intelligent diagnosis tasks. When the light-attention is replaced with the multi-head self-attention mechanism in Transformer, the evaluation indicators of DGKE on COEMRs and C-EMRs all have a certain degree of decline. During the experiment, the light-attention has a total of 4,202,512 trainable parameters and requires 16.81MB of memory, while the multi-head self-attention mechanism has a total of 16,789,504 trainable parameters and requires 67.58MB of memory, demonstrating the effectiveness of the light-attention. When the attention mechanism is completely removed, DGKE model can not distinguish well the knowledge in disease subgraphs and text subgraphs. It intuitively shows that the performance of DGKE has a significant decline, but it is still slightly higher than the GSKN model without introducing disease knowledge enhancement. Due to the high number of diseases to be diagnosed in multi-label COEMRs, the DGKE without attention mechanism has a 6.97% decline in the F1_macro, lower than the GSKN model without introducing disease subgraph enhancement. In the single-label C-EMRs, due to the small number of labels and independence, Integrating the disease subgraphs without relying on attention can also effectively pay attention to the knowledge related to the disease, so the F1_macro has declined by 1.15%, but it is still higher than the GSKN model without introducing disease subgraph enhancement.

4 Conclusion

We propose a DGKE model for intelligent diagnosis. Firstly, we obtain text subgraphs and disease subgraphs from the knowledge graph. Then we fuse the GCN embedding representations of the two subgraphs through a light-attention mechanism to obtain a knowledge representation for the diseases to be diagnosed. Afterwards, we propose a fusion mechanism based on interactive attention that integrates knowledge representation and hierarchical information enhancement for text representation, and obtained a knowledge enhanced text representation. Finally, we map this representation to the disease space for prediction. We conducted experiments on the COEMRs and the C-EMRs to verify the effectiveness of the DGKE model. In the future, we will study the impact of different types of knowledge on model performance, introduce knowledge more precisely, and pay less cost while improving model performance. We will also combine cutting-edge path inference methods to improve the interpretability of the model.

Acknowledgements. We thank the anonymous reviewers for their constructive comments, and this work was supported in part by the Science and Technology Innovation 2030- "New Generation of Artificial Intelligence" Major Project under Grant No. 2021ZD0111000, Henan Science and Technology Research Project (222102210231) and Zhengzhou City Collaborative Innovation Major Projects (20XTZX11020).

References

1. National Health and Family Planning Commission of the P. R. C., Guiding opinions of The General Office of the State Council on promoting the construction and development of medical consortium, Bulletin of The State Council of the People's Republic of China, 2017
2. Li, Y., Du, L., Xu, F., Li, Y., Qiao, E.: Big data and artificial intelligence in medicine. Med. J. Peking Union Med. Coll. Hosp. **14**(1), 184–189 (2023)
3. The Ministry of Health issued the Basic Standard of Electronic Medical Records (Trial). China Med. Rec. **11**(03), 64–65 (2010)
4. Dong, H., Jun, C.: Artificial intelligence: commercialization and practical applications. Tsinghua University Press (2018)
5. Yin, Z., et al.: Do Large Language Models Know What They Don't Know? Findings of ACL 2023
6. Fensel, D., Şimşek, U., Angele, K., et al.: Introduction: what is a knowledge graph? Knowl. Graphs Methodol. Tools Sel. Use Cases 1–10 (2020)
7. Zhang, T., Cai, Z., Wang, C., et al.: SMedBERT: a knowledge-enhanced pre-trained language model with structured semantics for medical text mining (2021). arXiv preprint arXiv:2108. 08983
8. Zhang, Z., Han, X., Liu, Z., et al.: ERNIE: Enhanced Language Representation with Informative Entities (2019). CoRR, abs/1905.07129
9. Rony, M.R.A.H., et al.: DialoKG: Knowledge-Structure Aware Task-Oriented Dialogue Generation. NAACL 2022
10. Liu, W., Zhou, P., Zhao, Z., et al.: K-BERT: enabling language representation with knowledge graph. In: AAAI, pp. 2901–2908 (2020)
11. Ting, W., Xiaofei, Z., Tang, G.: Text classification based on knowledge-enhanced graph convolutional neural network. J. Zhejiang Univ. (Eng. Edit.) **56**(02), 322–328 (2022)
12. Zh, K., Zh, X., Zh, L., et al.: Knowledge-enabled diagnosis assistant based on obstetric EMRs and knowledge graph. In: Sun, M., Li, S., Zhang, Y., Liu, Y., He, S., Rao, G. (eds.) Chinese Computational Linguistics. CCL 2020. LNCS, vol. 12522, pp. 444–457. Springer, Cham (2020). https://doi.org/10.1007/978-3-030-63031-7_32
13. Zhang, K., Hu, B., Zhou, F., et al.: Graph-based structural knowledge-aware network for diagnosis assistant. Math. Biosci. Eng. **19**, 10533–10549 (2022)
14. Zhang, K., Hu, B., Zhao, X., et al.: A HIE-BERT model for diagnosis assistant based on Chinese obstetric EMRs. In: 2021 IEEE 9th International Conference on Healthcare Informatics (ICHI), pp. 489–490. IEEE (2021)
15. Zan, H., Han, Y., Fan, Y., et al.: Construction and analysis of symptom knowledge base in Chinese. J. Chin. Inf. Process **34**, 30–37 (2020)

16. WHO Collaborating Centre for Classification of Diseases, Beijing, International Statistical Classification of Diseases and Related Health Problems, 10 rd ed. (ICD-10), vol. 2. Beijing: People's Medical Publishing House, 2008
17. Song, Y., Dai, D., Hu, C., et al.: Research on partition block-based multi-source knowledge fusion for knowledge graph construction. In: 2022 IALP, pp. 458–463. IEEE (2022)
18. Wang, M., Zheng, D., Ye, Z., et al.: Deep graph library: a graph-centric, highly-performant package for graph neural networks (2019). arXiv preprints arXiv: 1909.01315
19. Hu, F., Chen, A., Wang, Z., et al.: Lightweight attentional feature fusion: a new baseline for text-to-video retrieval. In: European Conference on Computer Vision, pp. 444–461 (2022)
20. Yang, Z., Huang, Y., Jiang, Y., et al.: Clinical assistant diagnosis for electronic medical recordbased on convolutional neural network. Sci. Rep. **8**(1), 1–9 (2018)
21. Zhang, K., Hu, C., Song, Y., et al.: Construction of Chinese obstetrics knowledge graph based on the multiple sources data. In: Dong, M., Gu, Y., Hong, J.F. (eds.) Chinese Lexical Semantics. CLSW 2021. LNCS, vol. 13250, pp. 399–410. Springer, Cham (2022). https://doi.org/10.1007/978-3-031-06547-7_31
22. Byambasuren, O., Yang, Y., Sui, Z., et al.: An exploratory study on the construction of Chinese medical knowledge graph CMeKG. J. Chin. Inf. Process. **33**(10), 1–9 (2019)
23. Kunli, Z., Xu, Z., Lei, Z., et al.: Knowledge-enabled diagnosis assistant based on obstetric EMRs and knowledge graph. In: Sun, M., Li, S., Zhang, Y., Liu, Y., He, S., Rao, G. (eds.) Chinese Computational Linguistics. CCL 2020. LNCS, vol. 12522, pp. 444–457. Springer, Cham (2020). https://doi.org/10.1007/978-3-030-63031-7_32

Multilevel Asynchronous Time Network for Medication Recommendation

Jinyu Shi, Lei Wang, and Yijia Zhang[✉]

School of Information Science and Technology, Dalian Maritime University, Dalian 116026,
China
zhangyijia@dlmu.edu.cn

Abstract. Medication recommendation is a pivotal task for AI in the realm of healthcare. Previous works have primarily focused on recommending medication for intricate medical conditions solely based on patients' electronic health records (EHR).Although extensive progress has been made, current research still faces the following limitations: ignoring data integrity in EHR, disregarding the impact of single-visit data on recommendation results; not adequate in learning about multilevel dependencies; and ignoring the effect of asynchronous relationships in irregular time intervals on recommendation results. To solve the above limitations, the Multilevel Asynchronous Time Network for Medication Recommendation (MLATNet) model is proposed. MLATNet first enhances the embedding of the EHR data using graph attention networks. Secondly, we use a transformer global fusion module to learn patients' long-distance global information, and a multikernel CNN module to learn local time dependencies information, thus obtaining global-local multilevel dependency information. Then, we design an asynchronous time module to fuse irregular time series. Moreover, through a DDI loss, MLATNet effectively controlling DDI rate to achieve medication recommendation. MLATNet outperforms all baseline methods, achieving a Jaccard score of 52.96%, an F1-score of 68.93%, and a PR-AUC of 77.56% on the MIMIC-III test set.

Keywords: Multilevel dependencies · Asynchronous time · Multikernel CNN · Medication recommendation

1 Introduction

Medication recommendation [11–13] has attracted a lot of attention in recent years. Deep learning techniques have been successfully applied to medication recommendation. Some methods learn representations of medical entities (e.g., patients, diagnoses, medications) from patient EHR data and then use them to generate new representations to complete the healthcare recommendation task. To accurately learn the representations, To learn the characterization accurately, some methods are based on transformer for drug recommendation, such as, G-BERT [20], TAHDNet [15], COGNet [16]. These methods are generally used to capture information about a patient's global characteristics to enable more accurate drug prediction. In addition, some methods use the time

© The Author(s), under exclusive license to Springer Nature Singapore Pte Ltd. 2024
H. Xu et al. (Eds.): CHIP 2023, CCIS 1993, pp. 333–351, 2024.
https://doi.org/10.1007/978-981-99-9864-7_22

dependency between clinical events, e.g. [1, 2, 4].These methods make drug recommendations by learning the similarity of the patient's historical visit information. However, these deep learning based medication recommendation methods have the following three limitations:

- Discarding single-visit data in the training, disregarding the impact of single-visit data on recommendation results.
- Most methods are built on the assumption that visits occurring at the same time intervals exert an identical impact on the course of a disease, a premise that may occasionally contradict the actual progression of the disease [2, 5]. The asynchronous dependency of irregular time series in dynamic procedure history should be important, but most people don't consider it.
- Multilevel dependencies between global and local are not fully considered. Learning global information means learning the distant information of each visit to get the overall representation of the visit. Learning local information means learning the local representation between neighboring visit records [15]. Therefore, the multilevel dependencies are important for recommendation results, but most people ignore them. The multilevel dependency structure refers to the visit information in Fig. 1.

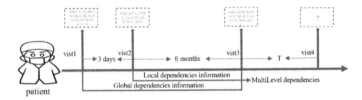

Fig. 1. This is a patient's visit information.

To reduce the above limitations, the MLATNet model is proposed. MLATNet is an end-to-end deep learning model for medication recommendation. The main contributions of MLATNet are summarized as follows:

- We propose MLATNet, a novel drug recommendation model that predicts accurate and safe drug recommendation by learning multilevel dependency and asynchronous time dependency.
- We design a multilevel dependency module. The goal of this module is to capture both global and local information. The module consists of a global transformer module and a multikernel CNN module. The global transformer module captures local information through a multihead self-attention mechanism and allows the model to establish distant relationships between different locations. The multikernel CNN module captures temporal correlations in irregular time intervals through different convolutional kernels for better extraction of local features.
- We propose an asynchronous time module for calculating the correlation between irregular time intervals and other data items so that the model can focus on asynchronous irregular time intervals.

2 Related Work

Existing methods for medication recommendation can be categorized into three main approaches: longitudinal-based methods, instance-based methods, and rule-based methods.

1. *Longitudinal-based methods.* Longitudinal approaches, as proposed by Choi et al., aim to leverage the time-dependent nature of clinical history. Among these approaches, RETAIN [1] employs a two-level Recurrent Neural Network (RNN) with inverse temporal attention to capture longitudinal information. GAMENet [13], on the other hand, utilizes a memory neural network to store historical medication data as a reference for predicting future procedures.

2. *Instance-based methods.* Instance-based methods mainly center on the patient's current health status. For instance, LEAP, which extracts feature data from the patient's present condition and utilizes a multi-instance multilabel (MIML) framework for its recommendation. LEAP formulates medication recommendation as a MIML task and utilizes a content attention mechanism.

3. *Rule-based methods.* Rule-based models typically rely on clinical guidelines designed by human experts, which often necessitate considerable input from clinicians. Despite the initial success of these approaches, they still have the following limitations: they ignoring the impact of asynchronous timing information on drug recommendation; and they inadequately model global- local multilevel dependencies.

In this paper, asynchronous time refers to temporal interactions between time intervals, especially for irregular time intervals. While most neural network approaches focus on modeling the sequential aspects of EHR data, it's crucial to recognize that EHR data possess both sequential and temporal attributes. Furthermore, due to the dynamic and irregular nature of each visit time, effectively utilizing irregular temporal information becomes a paramount concern. Existing solutions include RetainEX [7], which addresses irregular time intervals in longitudinal medical records by considering information decay in addition to traditional attention mechanisms.

The concept of multilevel dependency involves capturing interaction information from various perspectives within visit records to enhance data representativeness, thereby improving its utility in medical tasks. The incorporation of attention mechanisms [8] into neural networks has led to the development of several models that utilize attention to assign different weights to individual patient visits and produce weighted representations [9–13]. A global attention mechanism (GATT) was introduced by Zhou et al. They evaluate the importance of each input visit to the overall visit order reconstruction, with special emphasis on the local contribution of the recommendation task. RETAIN [1] trains two RNNs in reverse chronological order to effectively compute attention variables. It simulates physician behavior by attending to electronic medical records in reverse chronological order, thus assigning higher attention weights to recent clinical visits. On the other hand, INPREM takes a different approach by employing a transparent linear model. It encodes patient representations as learning weights using nonlinear connections to represent dependencies between local visits. It allows the model to derive the contribution matrix of input variables, serving as evidence for predicted outcomes.

In summary, existing approaches often ignore global-local dependency learning and asynchronous time-series information. Therefore, we propose a multilevel asynchronous time series network (MLATNet). It focuses on asynchronous interactions of irregular time series based on a new perspective on global and interlocal multilevel dependency learning for more accurate drug recommendations.

3   Methods

3.1   Problem Formalization

Definition 1 (EHR).
A patient's EHR data describe the patient's medical history in a longitudinal vector format of medical codes (e.g., diagnosis C_d, procedure C_p, and medication C_m). Formally, we denote that the EHR of patient P can be represented as a continuous multivariate sequence $x_P = [x_1^{(1)}, x_2^{(2)}, x_3^{(3)}, ... x_{t)}^{(i)}]$, where i denotes the total number of patients, and t denotes the number of visits of the t-th patient. To simplify the formula expression, for the same patient we use two primary medical codes (diagnosis code C_d (ICD-9) and medication code C_m (ATC)) to represent each visit of the patient, $x_P = C_d^P \cup C_m^P$. Where $C_d^P \cup C_m^P$ is the diagnosis code $C_d^P \in C_d$ and the concatenation of the medication code $C_m^P \in C_m$.

Definition 2 (Asynchronous Time Interval Sequence).
For a patient with multiple visits, we calculated the asynchronous time interval (in days) between two adjacent visits for that patient. The asynchronous irregular time interval sequence can be expressed as: $\delta^{(i)} = \left[\delta_{T(1)}^1, \delta_{T(2)}^2, \delta_{T(3)}^3 ... \delta_{T(i)}^i \right]$, where i denotes the total number of patients and $T(i)$ is the number of visits of the ith patient. To simplify the expression, in the same way as for describing EHR. The asynchronous time interval is expressed as $\delta_n = W_\delta(t_n - t_{n-1}) + b_\delta$, where δ_n denotes the embedded asynchronous time interval between the $n - th$ visit and the previous visit. Since there is no time interval for the first visit, we set $\delta_1 = 0$.

Definition 3 (Medication Recommendation Results).
For the same patient, given the diagnosis code C_d^t at visit time t, the patient's medical history, based on the patient's visits prior to time t, is represented as: $x_{1:t-1} = \{x_1, x_2, x_3...x_{t-1}\}$. In this paper, we recommend multiple medications by generating a multilabel output $y_p \in \{0, 1\}^{|C_m|}$.

The main notations used in this article are listed in Table 1.

3.2   Overview

In this section, we introduce the MLATNet model. Figure 2 is the overview of MLATNet. The MLATNet model includes three components: (1) **GAT Embedding module**, which filters the EHR data to reduce the data scale and uses a graph attention network to encode EHR data. (2) **Multilevel Dependency module**, which consists of Global Transformer module and MultiKernel CNN module. The goal of this module is to capture both global

Table 1. The main notations used in MLATNet

$x_t^{(i)}$	The clinical visit of the patient i at visit t
C_d, C_m, C_p	The diagnosis, drug and procedure code
$C_{ij}^d, C_{ij}^m, C_{ij}^p$	The diagnosis, drug and procedure similarity
$\alpha_{ij}^d, \alpha_{ij}^m, \alpha_{ij}^p$	The diagnosis, drug and procedure attention coefficient
X_p, t_p	The EHR data, irregular time interval sequence emdedding
e_p, δ_p	The EHR data, irregular time interval sequence linear vectors
z_i	The multi-head self-attention weights of global information
O_g	The global perceptual feature representation
$t'_{C3}, t'_{C5}, t'_{C7}$	The local features representations of different convolution kernels
O_m	The global-local multilevel dependency feature representation
$W_{(i,c)}$	The irregular time intervals sequence correlation weight matrix
O_t	The asynchronous time dependency feature representation

and local information. The **global transformer fusion module** captures local information through a multihead self-attention mechanism. The **multikernel CNN module** captures temporal correlations in irregular time intervals through different convolutional kernels. (3) **Asynchronous Time module**, which learn the correlation of asynchronous irregular time intervals. We input irregularly time data and the patient's EHR representation code. Then, by calculating the inner product, we obtain a correlation matrix, which is used as the weight matrix of the attention. Finally, we introduce a controlled loss function (DDI loss) to determine the drug recommendation results.

3.3 GAT Embedding Module

Inspired by G-BERT [20], for the GAT embedding module we use a similar approach to G- BERT. For EHR, diagnosis codes are coded using ICD-9, and drug codes are coded using ATC. We cleaned the data in the diagnosis records and procedure records, and performed deletion operations for duplicates, missing data, and unneeded data. This greatly reduces the data size and reduces the training time scale of the model.

GAT augmented embedding first calculates the similarity between neighboring data in diagnosis records, medication records, and procedure records, which is calculated as follows:

$$C_{ij}^d = a\left(\mathbf{w}\overrightarrow{C_{di}}, \mathbf{w}\overrightarrow{C_{dj}}\right) \tag{1}$$

$$C_{ij}^m = a\left(\mathbf{w}\overrightarrow{C_{pi}}, \mathbf{w}\overrightarrow{C_{pj}}\right) \tag{2}$$

$$C_{ij}^p = a\left(\mathbf{w}\overrightarrow{C_{mi}}, \mathbf{w}\overrightarrow{C_{mj}}\right) \tag{3}$$

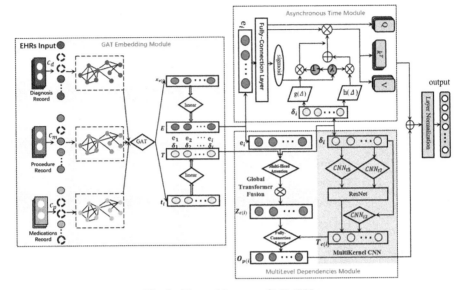

Fig. 2. The architecture of MLATNet.

where $\overrightarrow{C_{di}}$, $\overrightarrow{C_{dj}}$ represent the diagnosis vectors, $\overrightarrow{C_{di}}$, $\overrightarrow{C_{dj}} \in \mathbb{R}^{\tilde{h}}$, and $\tilde{h}$ is the hidden size. $\overrightarrow{C_{pi}}$, $\overrightarrow{C_{pj}}$ represent the direction vector, and $\overrightarrow{C_{mi}}$, $\overrightarrow{C_{mj}}$ represent the drug vector. $\mathbf{w}$ is the hyperparameter. The function a maps the spliced high-dimensional features to $\boldsymbol{a}$ numerical value.

Using Softmax function for C_{ij}^d, C_{ij}^m and C_{ij}^p to obtain the attention coefficient of EHR data,

$$\alpha_{ij}^d = \frac{exp(LeakyReLU(C_{ij}^d))}{\sum_{k\in\mathcal{N}d} exp(LeakyReLU(C_{ik}^d))} \tag{4}$$

$$\alpha_{ij}^m = \frac{exp\left(LeakyReLU\left(C_{ij}^m\right)\right)}{\sum_{k\in\mathcal{N}m} exp\left(LeakyReLU\left(C_{ik}^m\right)\right)} \tag{5}$$

$$\alpha_{ij}^p = \frac{exp(LeakyReLU(C_{ij}^p))}{\sum_{k\in\mathcal{N}p} exp(LeakyReLU(C_{ik}^p))} \tag{6}$$

where $\mathcal{N}$ is the number of vectors. α_{ij} is the attention coefficient.

Then, we use the GAT [16] to enhance the embedding of the EHR data to obtain the embedding X_p of EHR data. And we extracted the irregular time interval sequence data to obtain the embedding encoding t_p of the time series. The embedding process is as follows:

$$X_p = GAT(\alpha_{ij}^d, \alpha_{ij}^p, \alpha_{ij}^m) \tag{7}$$

$$t_p = select(X_p) = Select(GAT(\alpha_{ij}^d, \alpha_{ij}^p, \alpha_{ij}^m)) \tag{8}$$

3.4 Multilevel Dependency Module

EHR data contain multiple sequences, such as diagnosis records, procedure records, and medication records. Each of them contains multilevel structural information. Due to the multilevel structure of EHR data, we propose a multilevel dependency module based on global transformer and multikernel CNN to fully capture the multilevel relationships between global and local information.

Global Transformer Fusion Module
The transformer architecture has achieved much in medication recommendation, but existing transformer-based models do not adequately take into consideration the dependencies between multiple levels. Inspired by COGNet [16], we utilize the transformer architecture to capture the global information of patients and fuse the global information.

First, we convert the patient's electronic health records (EHR) into embedding vectors using the following linear function:

$$e_P = W_e X_p + b_e \tag{9}$$

where $e_p \in \mathbb{R}^{\tilde{h}}$, $\tilde{h}$ is the hidden size, $W_e \in \mathbb{R}^{\tilde{h} \times N}$ is the weighting matrix, and $b_e \in \mathbb{R}^{\tilde{h}}$ is the bias vector. In this way, the input data for each patient can be represented by $E = [e_1, e_2, \cdots, e_P]$.

The learning of the correlation between the input embedding vectors e_p, is calculated as follows:

$$Q_i = QW_i^Q, \ K_i = KW_i^K, \ V_i = VW_i^V, i = 1, 2, \ldots 8 \tag{10}$$

where $Q, K, V \in \mathbb{R}^{\tilde{h}}$, Q, K, V is the learning of the correlation between the input embedding vectors e_p. To learn Q, simultaneously multiply e_p by 8 different random matrices to obtain Q_i. Similarly, K_i, V_i can be obtained.

Then, we use the Transformer architecture with multi-head self-attention to learn the global information of the patient and compute the weights of each embedding vector. The computation process is shown in the following:

$$z_i = softmax\left(\frac{Q_i K_i^T}{\sqrt{d_k}}\right) V_i = \frac{exp(z_i)}{\sum_{i=1}^{8}\left(exp\left(\frac{Q_i K_i^T}{\sqrt{d_k}}\right)\right)}, i = 1, 2, \ldots 8 \tag{11}$$

where $\sqrt{d_k}$ is set to the default value of 64, which gives the model a more stable gradient.

Finally, these vectors are weighted and averaged by the weights to obtain the **global** perceptual feature representation O_g:

$$Z^C = concact(z_1, \ldots z_8) \tag{12}$$

$$O_g = Z^C \cdot W_O \tag{13}$$

where Z^C is the sum of each embedding vector weight z_i, W_O is the weight matrix, and Z is the product of the dot product of Z^C and W_O.

Multi-Kernel CNN Module

Currently, most drug recommendation models [17] are based on recurrent neural networks (e.g., RNN, LSTM, GRU, etc.) to capture and enhance interactions between time series, but ignore the local irregular time correlation problem. Instead, we choose to use multikernel CNN networks to capture local irregular time information of patients. Irregular time intervals between the current visit and previous visits can be modeled using multikernel CNN networks.

In this section, we draw on the work of TAHDNet [15] and make a few adjustments to its 1D-CNN structure: We change the input to irregular time interval sequences, which can better capture the dependencies between the patient's local information and the irregular time intervals. For irregular time interval sequences, different sizes of convolution kernels are applied to perform convolution operations to capture local features at different time scales. Then, we use ResNet to unify the dimensions of the features generated by different convolutional kernels.

First, the irregular time interval sequence is transformed into an embedding vector using the following linear function:

$$\delta_p = W_e t_p + b_e \tag{14}$$

where $\delta_p \in \mathbb{R}^{\tilde{h}}$, $\tilde{h}$ is the hide size, $W_e \in \mathbb{R}^{\tilde{h} \times N}$ is the weight matrix, and $b_e \in \mathbb{R}^{\tilde{h}}$ is the bias vector. In this way, the input data for each patient can be represented by T $= [\delta_1, \delta_2, \cdots, \delta_P]$.

Next, irregular time interval data are processed using convolutional operations. The embedding vectors are taken as input and use different sized convolution kernels to capture local features at different time scales. The computational procedure is as follows:

$$t'_{C3} = CNN_{T3}(\delta_1, \delta_2, \cdots, \delta_P) \tag{15}$$

$$t'_{C5} = CNN_{T5}(\delta_1, \delta_2, \cdots, \delta_P) \tag{16}$$

$$t'_{C7} = CNN_{T7}(\delta_1, \delta_2, \cdots, \delta_P) \tag{17}$$

where $t'_C \in \mathbb{R}^{\tilde{h} \times |C^*|}$ is the output of the hidden layer of the multikernel CNN network, while $\tilde{h}$ is a hyperparameter of the hidden size of the MLATNet.

Since different convolutional kernels produce different feature dimensions, we use ResNet to downscale the feature dimensions produced by 5*5 convolutional kernels as well as 7*7 convolutional kernels, so that the feature dimensions are consistent with those produced by 3*3 convolutional kernels. The calculation process is as follows:

$$T'_C = x_1 + \sum_{i=1}^{2} F(x_i, W_i) \tag{18}$$

where x_1 represents $t_{C5'}$, x_2 represents $t_{C7'}$, and x_1 represents the input to the residual unit, and F is the learned residual.

To avoid internal covariate shifts, we introduce layer normalization in the Multi-Kernel CNN block,

$$T_C = LayerNorm\left(h'_C\right) = \alpha \odot \frac{x - \mu}{\sqrt{\sigma^2 + \epsilon}} + \beta \tag{19}$$

where μ is the mean of the layer, σ^2 is the variance of the layer, and α and β denote the parameter vectors for scaling and translation.

Then, through the fully connected layer, we combine the transformer's global information with the multikernel CNN's local information to generate a **global-local multilevel** dependent feature representation O_m :

$$O_m = O_p W_o + T_C W_o \tag{20}$$

where O_p is the feature representation generated by the transformer-based global fusion module, T_C is the local feature representation generated by the multikernel CNN module, and W_o is the weight matrix.

3.5 Asynchronous Time Module

Traditional medication recommendation models [1, 6, 7] deal with time intervals with the assumption that the effect of past visits on current visits decays as the time interval increases. However, this assumption is not true. The progression of some diseases is cyclical, which results in cyclical diagnosis and medication. Therefore, it is important to learn the asynchronous interaction information between irregular time intervals by taking into account the correlation between irregular time interval sequences and patient medication information. We propose an asynchronous timing module to model irregular time intervals to generate better representations for prediction tasks. The module is implemented by means of an inner-attention mechanism.

First, we correlate the patient's electronic health records (EHR) embedding vector E with a sequence of irregular time intervals T to obtain a correlation matrix.

$$S_{(i,i)}(E, T) = \frac{\text{cov}(e_i, t_i)}{(\sigma e_i * \sigma t_i)}, \quad (i = 1, 2 \ldots p) \tag{21}$$

$$M_{(i,i)} = \begin{bmatrix} S_{(1,1)} & \cdots & S_{(1,i)} \\ \vdots & \ddots & \vdots \\ S_{(i,1)} & \cdots & S_{(i,i)} \end{bmatrix}, \quad (i = 1, 2 \ldots p) \tag{22}$$

where p is the number of visits per patient and $M_{(i,i)}$ is the obtained correlation matrix.

Apply Softmax function to the correlation matrix to obtain the correlation weight matrix $W_{(i,c)}$:

$$W_{(i,c)} = \frac{exp\left(M_{(i,c)}\right)}{\sum_{i=1}^{p} exp\left(M_{(i,c)}\right)} \tag{23}$$

The correlation between the patient's electronic health records (EHR) embedding vector E and the sequence of irregular time intervals T is learned and calculated as follows:

$$Q_i = QW_{(i,c)}, K_i = KW_{(i,c)}, V_i = VW_{(i,c)}, i = 1, 2, \ldots p \tag{24}$$

According to the internal attention mechanism, we compute the attention weights, generate the feature representation of asynchronous tensors, and normalize them to obtain the feature representation O_t of the dependencies between asynchronous time:

$$\phi_i = \boldsymbol{Attention}(Q, K, V) = \frac{Q_i K_i^T}{\sqrt{d_k}} V_i, i = 1, 2, \ldots p \tag{25}$$

$$O_t = \boldsymbol{LayerNorm}(\phi_1, \phi_2, \cdots, \phi_i), i = 1, 2, \ldots p \tag{26}$$

where Q, K, V $\in \mathbb{R}^{\tilde{h}}$, Q_i, K_i, V_i are the matrices generated by learning the correlation weight matrix.

3.6 Model Training and Inference

Based on the global-local multilevel dependency feature representation O_p obtained in 4.3 and the asynchronous time dependency feature representation O_l obtained in 4.4, we construct an MLP-based prediction layer to predict the recommended medication codes by stitching O_p and O_l:

$$O^{'} = \boldsymbol{Concat}(O_m, O_t) \tag{27}$$

$$y_p = \boldsymbol{Sigmoid}\big(W_p O\prime + b_p\big) \tag{28}$$

where $O^{'} \in \mathbb{R}^{5 \times \tilde{h}}$, $W_p \in \mathbb{R}^{|C^m| \times 5\tilde{h}}$, and $b_p \in \mathbb{R}^{|C^m|}$. W_p, b_p are hyperparameters.

In this paper, we formulate the medication recommendation task as multilabel binary classification. Assume that $|\mathcal{M}|$ is the total number of medications. We denote the target medication recommendation by $m^{(t)}$ and the output of the medication recommendation by $\hat{o}^{(t)}$. We treat the prediction of each medication as a subproblem and use binary cross entropy (BCE) as the loss:

$$L_{bce} = -\sum_{i=1}^{|\mathcal{M}|} m_i^{(t)} \boldsymbol{log}(\hat{o}_i^{(t)}) + (1 - m_i^{(t)}) \boldsymbol{log}(1 - \hat{o}_i^{(t)}) \tag{29}$$

where $m_i^{(t)}$ and $\hat{o}_i^{(t)}$ refer to the i-th term. To make the results more stable, we also employ a multilabel loss:

$$L_{multi} = \sum_{i,j:m_i^{(t)}=1, m_j^{(t)}=0} \frac{\boldsymbol{max}(0, 1-(\hat{o}_i^{(t)} - \hat{o}_j^{(t)}))}{|\mathcal{M}|} \tag{30}$$

Inspired by SafeDrug [18], we introduce a controlled loss function (incorporating the DDI loss) to control the level of DDI.

$$L_{ddi} = \sum_{i=1}^{|\mathcal{M}|} \sum_{j=1}^{|\mathcal{M}|} \boldsymbol{D}_{ij} \cdot \hat{\boldsymbol{o}}_i^{(t)} \cdot \hat{\boldsymbol{o}}_j^{(t)} \tag{31}$$

Ultimately, by incorporating the above losses to determine the outcome of the medication recommendation,

$$L = \beta(\alpha L_{bce} + (1 - \alpha)L_{multi}) + (1 - \beta)L_{ddi} \tag{32}$$

$$\beta = \begin{cases} 1, & DDI \leq \gamma \\ max\left\{0, 1 - \frac{DDI-\gamma}{K_p}\right\}, & DDI > \gamma \end{cases} \tag{33}$$

where α usually predefined hyperparameters, K_p is a correcting factor for the proportional signal and γ is the highest bound of the output DDI rate.

4 Experiment

4.1 Dataset

We used EHR data from MIMIC-III. MIMIC-III is a large and free dataset built by the MIT Computational Physiology Laboratory [19]. The dataset consists of health data information on more than 40,000 patients [17]. The dataset focuses on clinical diagnosis reports of patients hospitalized in ICUs since 2001. The report includes patient vital characteristic fluctuations, laboratory test results, treatments, medications, nursing staff work records, imaging reports, and death information notes.

4.2 Preprocessing

The diagnosis records of this dataset were coded using the ICD-9 coding system [14] and administered using the ATC system [15] coding medication records. We preprocessed the dataset to obtain single-visit data and multi-visit data. Among them, there are 30,744 single-visit data and 6,351 multi-visit data. Then, we randomly split the multiple access data in the ratio of $\frac{4}{5} : \frac{1}{10} : \frac{1}{10}$. $\frac{1}{10}$ of the single-visit data are randomly selected as the training set, and then $\frac{1}{100}$ of the remaining single-visit data are selected as the test set. The training set, evaluation set, and test set are finally constructed, and the model is tested according to the cross-validation method. The statistics of the postprocessed data are shown in Table 2.

Table 2. Statistics of the EHR (rc: medication code, dc: diagnosis code).

Stats	Multi-Visit	Single-Visit
# of patients	6,350	30,745
avg # of visits	2.36	1.00
avg # of dc	10.51	39
avg # of rc	8.80	52
# of unique dc	1,958	1,997
# of unique rc	145	323

4.3 HyperParameters

The model was trained on NVIDIA GeForce RTX 3090 GPUs. The configuration environment is NVIDIA CUDA 11.1.1, PyTorch 1.8.0.

The hyperparameters for MLATNet were configured to mirror the baseline of TAHD-Net [15], including a hidden layer dimension of 300, a location perspective network dimension of 300, 200 hidden layers, and 4 attention heads per layer. To establish initial parameter stability, we conducted pre-training for 100 epochs. For model evaluation, we trained MLATNet for an additional 100 epochs, using a batch size of 64. We opted for the Adam optimizer with a learning rate of 0.0006.

4.4 Baseline Methods

We compare the MLATNet model with the following advanced methods.

Leap [3] proposes the LEAP (learn to prescribing) algorithm, which decomposes treatment recommendations as continuous strategies and personalizes drug recommendations based on the patient's specific situation.

TAHDNet [15] proposed a dynamic time-aware hierarchical dependency network that senses global as well as local information.

SafeDrug [18] has introduced a drug recommendation model that is controlled by Drug-Drug Interaction (DDI) considerations and employs the molecular structure of the drugs as a foundational element in its construction. The model incorporates a novel Knowledge Propagation Neural Network in conjunction with localized molecular structures to enhance its recommendation capabilities.

G-BERT [20] proposed a new model that combines the capabilities of graph neural network (GNN) and BERT. G-BERT is the first model to introduce a pretraining paradigm for language models into the healthcare domain.

SARMR [21] introduced a self-supervised adversarial regularization model. It achieves this by deriving target distributions related to safe drug combinations directly from unprocessed patient records. Furthermore, it mitigates Drug-Drug Interactions (DDI) by molding the distribution of patient representations through a regularization process.

4.5 Evaluation Metrics

Based on previous work on drug recommendation [19–21], we used Jaccard similarity (Jaccard), F1 score and precision recall AUC (PR-AUC) as evaluation metrics [15]. What's more, inspired by Safedrug [18], we used the DDI rate to measure the safety of recommended drugs with the following formula.

$$\Delta \mathbf{DDI} = \frac{\sum_k^N \sum_i^{T_k} \sum_{i,j} \left| \left\{ \left(c_i, c_j \in \hat{Y}_i^k \right) \right\} \right| \left(c_i, c_j \in \varepsilon_d \right)}{\sum_k^N \sum_i^{T_k} \sum_{i,j} 1} \tag{34}$$

where each drug pair (c_i, c_j) counts if the drug pair $\widehat{Y}$ belongs to the side recommendation set ε_d. N is the number of patients, T_k visits for the test dataset.

5 Experimental Results

5.1 Overall Performance

In this section, we compare MLATNet's work with existing work on drug recommendation, and the results are shown in Table 3. By analyzing the results of the experiments,
we draw some conclusions.

Table 3. The performance of different medication recommendation networks.

Methods	ΔDDI	Jaccard	F1	PR-AUC
LEAP	0.0731 ± 0.0008	0.3921 ± 0.0006	0.5508 ± 0.0004	0.5855 ± 0.0004
SARMR	0.0627 ± 0.0011	0.5019 ± 0.0033	0.6654 ± 0.0031	0.7687 ± 0.0026
SafeDrug	0.0589 ± 0.0005	0.5193 ± 0.0030	0.6768 ± 0.0027	0.7647 ± 0.0025
G-BERT	–	0.4536 ± 0.0008	0.6144 ± 0.0008	0.6904 ± 0.0005
TAHDNet	–	0.4824 ± 0.0010	0.6411 ± 0.0017	0.7188 ± 0.0008
MLATNet	0.0595 ± 0.0004	0.5296 ± 0.0005	0.6893 ± 0.0008	0.7756 ± 0.0001

Based on the evaluation metrics, we propose that the MLATNet model outperforms
almost all other models. Among them, MLATNet ensures a low DDI rate while maintaining a high recommendation accuracy, and these metrics prove the effectiveness of
our model. The MLATNet model has a significant advantage over TAHDNet [15], with
increases of 4.72%, 4.82%, and 5.68% in Jaccard, F1, and PR-AUC, respectively.

Regarding recommendation safety, SafeDrug [18] is designed with controlled DDI
losses to ensure safer drug recommendations that keep DDI at lower levels. Compared to
SafeDrug, MLATNet further increased the Jaccard and F1 values by 1.03% and 1.25%,
respectively. This is because the asynchronous time module focuses on irregular time
interval sequences and calculates the correlation between irregular time intervals and
patient information.

Based on the model architecture, the SARMR [20] model has good results in the accuracy of drug recommendation and keeps the DDI at a low level. Compared to SARMR,
MLATNet also further reduced the DDI rate by 0.32%, increased the Jaccard and F1
values by 2.77% and 2.39%, respectively. This is due to the transformer global fusion
module as well as the multikernel CNN local time series module, which learns the multilevel dependencies between global and local, allowing for better learning of patient
representations.

In summary, the MLATNet model enhances the embedding of EHR data through
GAT. The patient's EHR representation is then encoded into embedded vectors using
the transformer global fusion module, and the vectors are weighted and averaged through
a multihead self-attention mechanism. Thereby, the long-distance dependencies between
different locations are captured to generate a globally-aware feature representation. Next,
a convolutional operation is employed to process irregularly spaced data through the multikernel CNN module. Different sizes of convolution kernels are used to capture local

features at different time scales. The irregular interval data and the patient's EHR representation code are then input the asynchronous time module to compute the correlation between the irregular time interval dependence on medication. Finally, a controlled loss function (DDI loss) is introduced to determine the drug recommendation outcome.

5.2 Ablation Experiment

In this section, to evaluate the effectiveness and necessity of each MLATNet component, we employed three different variants of MLATNet. Table 4 presents the performance results for these variants alongside the complete MLATNet. The experimental setup and metrics align with those detailed in Sect. 5.3.

Table 4. The performance of the variants and the full MLATNet.

Methods	ΔDDI	Jaccard	F1	PR-AUC
No-GAT	0.0628	0.4901	0.6703	0.738
No-GTF	0.0606	0.4879	0.6631	0.7235
No-AT	0.07	0.4564	0.6498	0.706
No-MKC	0.0731	0.4296	0.6356	0.6896
MLATNet	0.0595	0.5296	0.6893	0.7756

- **No-GAT (No-GAT Embedding):** MLATNet uses a graph neural network to learn to encode EHR. no-DG does not perform this learning, but simply encodes the EHR.
- **No-GTF (No-Global Transformer Fusion):** MLATNet weights and averages the vectors through a multihead self-attention mechanism to generate a globally-aware feature representation, which in turn captures the long-distance dependence between different locations. no-GTF does not learn the global information.
- **No-MKC (No-Multi-Kernel CNN):** To further investigate the correlation of irregular time interval dependence on medication, Multi-Kernel CNN networks with convolutional kernels of different sizes are used to capture local features at different time scales. The No-Multi-Kernel CNN does not focus on local irregular time interval features.
- **No-AT (No-Asynchronous Time):** Ignore the asynchronous time dependencies when recommending medications to patients.

The results in Table 4 show that MLATNet has the best performance. As shown in Fig. 3, No-MKC has the highest DDI rate, and No-MKC has the lowest Jac-card, F1, and PR-AUC. No-MKC performs worse than the other variants, demonstrating the importance of learning local time dependency information. No-AT performs worse than the other variants, demonstrating the importance of learning asynchronous time dependency information. The performance of No-GAT and No-GTF is also degraded compared to the full MLATNet, which verifies that learning global dependency information and GAT

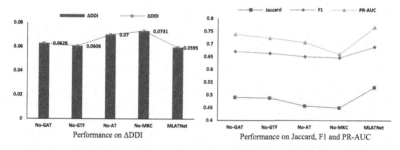

Fig. 3. The performance of the variants and MLATNet.

enhanced embedding is also crucial for the drug recommendation task. The results suggest that asynchronous time information in the diagnosis and procedure processes should be modeled separately, rather than being treated directly as a whole.

5.3 Parameter Influence

To study the effect of hyperparameter settings on the model and to explore the effect of different embedding dimensions on MLATNet, this section sets up different embedding dimensions for parameter search experiments. Figure 4 depicts the performance of different embedding dimensions on ΔDDI, Jaccard, F1 and PR-AUC. From the results in Fig. 4, it can be seen that the performance of the model reaches its maximum when the embedding dimension is 300. (Given that the DDI represents the side effects between drugs, the lower the ΔDDI the better.) Therefore, the embedding dimension is set to 300 in this paper [19].

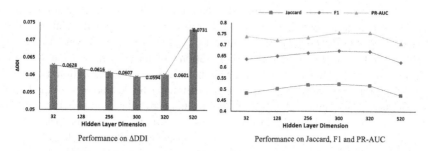

Fig. 4. The performance of different embedding dimensions.

In addition, we set up experiments with different learning rates to explore the effect of different learning rates on the model. Each learning rate was repeated five times and the average of the five tests was calculated. Figure 5 depicts the performance of different learning rates on ΔDDI, Jaccard, F1 and PR-AUC. From the results in Fig. 5, it can be seen that the performance of the model reaches its maximum when the learning rate is 0.0006. (Given that the DDI represents the side effects between drugs, the lower the ΔDDI the better.) Therefore, the learning rate is set to 0.0006 in this paper.

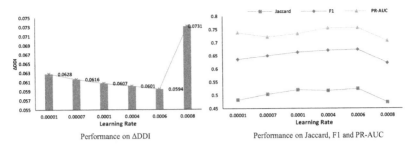

Fig. 5. The performance of different learning rates.

5.4 Case Study

As mentioned above, our proposed MLATNet outperforms all baseline models in medication recommendation. Therefore, in this section, we choose an example of a MIMIC-III patient to illustrate how MLATNet can improve medication recommendation through the asynchronous time module. We will use the asynchronous timing module as an example to further analyze how the components of MLATNet can make comprehensive decisions about medication.

First selecting a patient from the MIMIC-III dataset, we chose a complex case for comprehensive decision making. This case had a visit record involving multiple disease complications and treatment medications. This patient visited the hospital three times. The visit information is shown in Table 4. The patient's first visit was on May 8, 2015, and he was mainly treated with codes 4513, 9904, and 3893. Later, the patient visited once again, on May 14, 2015, where the patient developed some new illnesses in addition to the previously diagnosed illnesses and underwent treatment coded as 4444. The first two visits were three days apart and were strongly correlated, with a high rate of duplication among the recommended medications. Based on the first two visits we can see that the asynchronous time interval has a significant impact on drug recommendations. When the patient goes to the hospital for the third time, after a series of laboratory tests and diagnoses, and further learning from the correlation with the asynchronous time intervals of the first two visits, MLATNet model can predict in advance the medications that may be needed for this treatment, which can be used as a reference for the doctor's comprehensive decision. In this way, although the prediction results may not be completely correct, the prediction results can also help doctors improve the efficiency of decisions, especially for junior or inexperienced doctors, who can provide some reference value (Table 5).

As shown in Table 5, we can visualize the accuracy of medication recommendation after learning the asynchronous time interval correlation. At the third visit, our model learns the time correlation of the previous two visits to make medication recommendations. Visit3 (MLATNet) recommended a large number of medications that were present at the previous two visits, such as A06A, A12C, and N02A, and a larger number of medications were recommended. In contrast, when there was no asynchronous time module processing, significantly fewer medications were recommended and the correctness rate was reduced. The results are shown in Visit3 (No-AT) in Table 5. The above analysis shows that the asynchronous time module in the MLATNet model learns the relevance of the previous visit interval and makes recommendations with reference to the drugs

Table 5. The records of the patient's three visits.

	Vist Time	Diagnosis	Procedures	Medications
Visit 1	2015.05.08	530.7,344.00,285.1, 599.0, 577.1, V12.51, 907.2, 337.9, 442.84	4513, 9904, 3893	A06A,A12A,B05C,N02B, A12B,A12C, A02B,N05C, A04A,N05B,N02A,N05A, B02B, C05A
Visit 2	2015.05.14	442.884,578.1,344.0, 305.01,305.60,599.0, 305.1,305.20,V16.3, V12.51	4444, 3893, 9904	A06A,A07A,A12B,A1A, A12C,A02B,N05C,A0A, N02A, B03A
Visit 3 (MLATNet)	2015.11.20	442.84, 599.0, 285.1, 790.7, 9072, E9298, V12.51, 411.1, V09.0, 577.1	4444, 8847,9904	A06A,N02B,A12B,A02B, B02B,A12C,J01M, N02A, N05B,D04A, J01E
Visit 3 (No-AT)	2015.11.20	442.84, 599.0, 285.1, 790.7, 9072, E9298, V12.51, 411.1, V09.0, 577.1	4444, 8847,9904	A06A,A12B,B02B,A12C, J01M, N05B,D04A, J01E

used in the visit records with higher relevance. In addition, some new drugs such as D04A and J01E can be generated appropriately. This shows that MLATNet can not only learn historical drugs based on the correlation of time intervals, but also generate new drugs based on new diagnoses.

6 Conclusion

In this paper, we propose a multilevel asynchronous time network (MLATNet) for medication recommendation tasks. MLATNet better captures the changes in patient's condition by learning asynchronous time information of patient's visit and multilevel dependencies, thus giving more accurate and lower DDI drug combinations. We validated the performance of the model on the public dataset MIMIC-III. We conclude the article by demonstrating the effectiveness of each component in MLATNet through ablation experiments and parametric experiments. In the future, we will consider combined drug potentiation for more accurate drug recommendations with the lowest DDI.

Acknowledgment. This work is supported by grant from the Natural Science Foundation of China (No. 62072070).

References

1. Choi, E., Bahadori, M.T., Sun, J., Kulas, J., Schuetz, A., Stewart, W.F.: RETAIN: an interpretable predictive model for healthcare using reverse time attention mechanism. In: Advances in Neural Information Processing Systems 29: Annual Conference on Neural Information Processing Systems 2016, 5–10 December 2016, Barcelona, Spain, pp. 3504–3512 (2016)

2. Cheng, L., Shi, Y., Zhang, K.: Medical treatment migration behavior prediction and recommendation based on health insurance data. World Wide Web **23**(3), 2023–2042 (2020)
3. Zhang, Y., Chen, R., Tang, J., Stewart, W.F., Sun, J.: LEAP: learning to prescribe effective and safe treatment combinations for multimorbidity. In: Proceedings of the 23rd ACM SIGKDD International Conference on Knowledge Discovery and Data Mining, Halifax, NS, Canada, 13–17 August 2017, pp. 1315–1324. ACM (2017)
4. Baytas, I.M., Xiao, C., Zhang, X., Wang, F., Jain, A.K., Zhou, J.: Patient subtyping via time-aware LSTM networks. In: Proceedings of the 23rd ACM SIGKDD International Conference on Knowledge Discovery and Data Mining, Halifax, NS, Canada, 13–17 August 2017, pp. 65–74. ACM (2017)
5. Wang, D., Xu, D., Yu, D., Xu, G.: Time-aware sequence model for next-item recommendation. Appl. Intell. **51**(2), 906–920 (2021)
6. Wang, S., Ren, P., Chen, Z., Ren, Z., Ma, J., de Rijke, M.: Order-free medicine combination prediction with graph convolutional reinforcement learning. In: Zhu, W., et al. (eds.), Proceedings of the 28th ACM International Conference on Information and Knowledge Management, CIKM 2019, Beijing, China, 3–7 November 2019, pp. 1623–1632. ACM (2019)
7. Symeonidis, P., Chairistanidis, S., Zanker, M.: Recommending what drug to prescribe next for accurate and explainable medical decisions. In: Almeida, J.R., et al. (eds.), 4th IEEE International Symposium on Computer-Based Medical Systems, CBMS 2021, Aveiro, Portugal, 7–9 June 2021, pp. 213–218. IEEE (2021)
8. Luo, J., Ye, M., Xiao, C., Ma, F.: Hitanet: hierarchical time-aware attention networks for risk prediction on electronic health records. In: KDD '20: The 26th ACM SIGKDD Conference on Knowledge Discovery and Data Mining, Virtual Event, CA, USA, 23–27 August 2020, pp. 647–656. ACM (2020)
9. Kwon, B.C., et al.: Retainvis: visual analytics with interpretable and interactive recurrent neural networks on electronic medical records. IEEE Trans. Vis. Comput. Graph. **25**(1), 299–309 (2019)
10. Shang, J., Ma, T., Xiao, C., Sun, J.: Pre-training of graph augmented transformers for medication recommendation. In: Proceedings of the Twenty-Eighth International Joint Conference on Artificial Intelligence, IJCAI 2019, Macao, China, 10–16 August 2019, pp. 5953–5959 (2019). ijcai.org
11. Shang, J., Xiao, C., Ma, T., Li, H., Sun, J.: Gamenet: graph augmented memory networks for recommending medication combination. In: AAAI, vol. 33, pp. 1126–1133 (2019)
12. Shang, J., Xiao, C., Ma, T., Li, H., Sun, J.: Gamenet: graph augmented memory networks for recommending medication combination. In: Proceedings of the AAAI Conference on Artificial Intelligence, vol. 33, no. 01, pp. 1126–1133 (2019)
13. Chaoqi, Y., Cao, X., Fenglong, M., Lucas, G., Jimeng, S.: SafeDrug: dual molecular graph encoders for recommending effective and safe drug combinations. In: Zhou, Z.-H. (ed.), Proceedings of the Thirtieth International Joint Conference on Artificial Intelligence, IJCAI 2021, Virtual Event/Montreal, Canada, 19–27 August 2021, pp. 3735–3741 (2021). ijcai.org
14. An, Y., et al.: MeSIN: multilevel selective and interactive network for medication recommendation (2021)
15. Su, Y., et al.: TAHDNet: time-aware hierarchical dependency network for medication recommendation. J. Biomed. Inform. 104069 (2022)
16. Gunlicks-Stoessel, M., Mufson, L., Westervelt, A., Almirall, D., Murphy, S.: A pilot SMART for developing an adaptive treatment strategy for adolescent depression. J. Clin. Child Adolesc. Psychol. **45**(4), 480–494 (2016)
17. Wu, R., et al.: Conditional generation net for medication recommendation (2022)
18. Li, X., et al.: DGCL: distance-wise and graph contrastive learning for medication recommendation. J. Biomed. Inform. **139**, 104301 (2023). https://doi.org/10.1016/j.jbi.2023.104301

19. Yang, C., et al.: SafeDrug: dual molecular graph encoders for safe drug recommendations (2021)
20. Shang, J., et al.: Pre-training of Graph Augmented Transformers for Medication Recommendation (2019). https://doi.org/10.24963/ijcai.2019/825
21. Wang, Y., et al.: Self-supervised adversarial distribution regularization for medication recommendation. In: International Joint Conference on Artificial Intelligence (2021)

Semantic and Emotional Feature Fusion Model for Early Depressive Prediction

Weiwei Zhu[1], Yijia Zhang[1(✉)], Xingyu Yu[1], Mingyu Lu[2(✉)], and Hongfei Lin[3]

[1] Dalian Information Science and Technology College, Dalian Maritime University,
Dalian 116000, Liaoning, China
{zww126,zhangyijia,yuxy}@dlmu.edu.cn
[2] College of Artificial Intelligence, Dalian Maritime University, Dalian 116000, Liaoning, China
lumingyu@dlmu.edu.cn
[3] School of Computer Science and Technology, Dalian University of Technology,
Dalian 116000, Liaoning, China
hflin@dlut.edu.cn

Abstract. In recent years, depression has caused severe social and psychological problems. The purpose of the paper is to automatically identify users with depressive tendencies to facilitate early intervention and prevent the progression of depression into more severe consequences. The paper proposes a Depression Prediction model based on Multi-feature Fusion (DPMFF), which extracts contextual semantic features and deep emotional features from user documents to predict depression risk. The behavioral and linguistic features of depressed users were examined through statistical analysis. Experiments on micro-blog datasets demonstrate that DPMFF can effectively identify users with depressive tendencies and outperform other models. The data analysis found that compared with normal users, users with depressive tendencies were usually active on social networks late at night, and the proportion of content containing absolute words and negative words was significantly higher than average.

Keywords: Early depressive prediction · Feature Fusion · Attention mechanism
Introduction

1 Introduction

In recent years, mental health problems such as depression have been widely discussed by people. According to the World Mental Health Report released by the World Health Organization (WHO)[1] in 2022, as of 2019, about 1 billion people around the world are suffering from mental disorders, especially after the COVID-19 pandemic. The number of people suffering from significant depression and anxiety increased by 28% and 26%, respectively. Depression has become a major cause of death and disability worldwide. Therefore, it is vital to detect and intervene in the early stage of depression.

---

[1] https://www.who.int/publications/i/item/9789240049338.

H. Xu et al. (Eds.): CHIP 2023, CCIS 1993, pp. 352–368, 2024.
https://doi.org/10.1007/978-981-99-9864-7_23

The traditional intervention for depression is through a mental health questionnaire combined with a professional doctor's diagnosis. Because patients are required to disclose negative psychology, this method has subjective bias and requires a lot of manpower and material resources. With the development of the internet, social media has become universal and diversified. The number of netizens is increasing, and the public is more willing to share their feelings and emotions on social media [1]. The advantages of openness and low cost of social platforms overcome the limitations of traditional depression detection methods, and there is a link between users' online behavior and depression. Studies have shown that social media can provide meaningful data to infer the mental health status of the public [2]. The latest Micro-blog financial report[2] shows that Weibo currently has more than 250 million daily active users and more than 590 million monthly active users, which provides data support for early depression tendency prediction research based on Micro-blog.

Table 1 is an example of user posts obtained from Microblog. It can be seen that the posts of users with depressive tendencies contain negative words such as "death", "pain" and "tired". On the contrary, such words are obviously absent from normal users' posts, which makes it possible to automatically identify users with depressive tendencies from online posts.

Table 1. Comparison between posts with depression and normal posts

Post Category	Text Content
Normal Post	My daughter's painting tonight, although not a dragon, is perfect, and she has to borrow my phone to take a selfie. Wishing everyone a happy New Year!
Posts with Depressive Tendencies	I'm speechless and don't want to live at all. Breathing is tiring. Once you die, you will be forgotten, and you won't have to think so much. I am in great pain

Recent studies have shown that negative emotions do not form in a short period of time, and this time span can be as long as several months or even years [3]. Historical content posted by Micro-blog users can help identify depressive tendencies. An example of a user post with a depressive tendency is shown in Fig. 1.

From the examples, it can be observed that the user did not exhibit significant depressive tendencies in the latest posts. Without a complete analysis of historical texts, it is difficult to identify the user's potential depressive tendencies, indicating that time cues play an important role in modeling the user's psychological state. Unlike extracting features from a single post, this article extracts features from all posts posted by a user within a specific time interval to predict whether the user has a depressive tendency, which is more practical.

In previous studies, Sawhney et al. used a time-aware transformer model to model user tweets for preliminary screening of suicide risk [4]. Ren et al.'s experiment showed

---

[2] http://ir.weibo.com.

that increasing emotional information is beneficial for predicting depressive tendencies [5]. Although the previous methods achieved good results, they did not fully interact with semantic features and emotional features, neglecting the role of deep emotional semantic information in identifying changes in user psychological states. Based on this, on the basis of the hierarchical structure of user documents, this article uses hierarchical attention networks to fully capture the contextual semantic information of users, which solves the problem of incomplete feature extraction of historical information in previous text structures and shows promising results in long text classification work; At the same time, the advanced emotional semantic perception module is used to obtain deep emotional semantic features to identify user emotional change points and different features are extracted from users' open Micro-blog accounts for the past year to construct user document representations, providing a methodological basis for early prediction of depression tendency based on user documents.

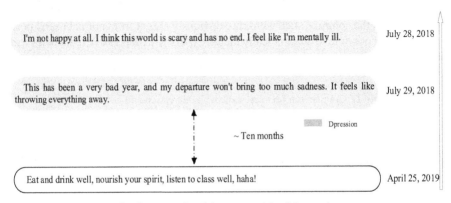

Fig. 1. Example of the user at risk of depression

2   Related Work

In the field of predicting depression propensity, commonly used methods include questionnaire-based methods and social media-based methods. The method based on questionnaire surveys has apparent drawbacks; the subjectivity of emotions and experiences increases the variability of conclusions. With the development of the internet, the anonymity of social media has made people more willing to express emotions on social platforms. Research has shown that users tend to use mass social media for mental health information exchange activities [12], which provides theoretical support for predicting depression propensity based on social media.

2.1   Traditional Questionnaire-Based Depression Detection

Research has shown that predicting depression propensity based on psychological measurement self-report has high effectiveness and credibility [6]. Early clinical methods used various questionnaires for scoring. For example, Beck Depression Scale II (BDI-II) [7], Hamilton Depression Scale (HRSD) [8], Self-Rating Depression Scale (SDS) [9], etc. They can intuitively reflect the mental state of patients with depression and are professional and effective. However, questionnaires rely on the subjective will of a person and are often unreliable, and when faced with large-scale groups, they can incur significant human and time costs [10]. Research has shown that conducting suicide assessments may have negative effects on people with depressive symptoms [11].

2.2 Depression Detection from Social Media

Recently, significant progress has been made in using social media for depression screening, mainly by identifying users' risk of depression tendencies based on their language content and online behavior on social media.

Dictionary-Based Vocabulary Method. Determine the user's depression tendency based on whether depression-related words appear in the text. The Internet Early Risk Detection eRisk Challenge aims to locate depressed users by searching for specific expressions such as' I have been diagnosed with depression' [14]. Alternatively, use a LIWC dictionary to analyze posts on social media based on language features such as part of speech and tense [13]. However, with the increasing number of people suffering from depression, it is unrealistic to use dictionary-based vocabulary methods to identify social media data in Shanghai. It is not only time-consuming and labor-intensive but also unable to accurately identify potential users with depression tendencies solely through simple language expression.

Machine Learning-Based Methods. The rise of machine learning has brought new methods for researchers to conduct quantitative analysis. Using machine learning methods to predict early depression tendencies can improve work efficiency and accuracy. At present, traditional machine learning algorithms widely used in the field of predicting depression propensity include logistic regression (LR) [15], K Nearest Neighbors (KNN) [16], Naive Bayes (NB) [17], Support Vector Machine (SVM) [18], etc. Although applying traditional machine learning methods to social media-based depression tendency prediction can perform automated, objective, and effective assessments, its performance often depends on feature selection and construction, which not only requires the knowledge and experience of domain experts but also requires a lot of manpower.

Deep Learning-Based Methods. With the development of deep learning in natural language processing, more and more methods for predicting depression tendencies based on deep learning have been proposed. Compared to traditional machine learning, deep learning has stronger stability and generalization due to its ability to extract features automatically and can achieve more outstanding detection performance [19]. At present, deep learning architectures such as Convolutional Neural Networks (CNN) [20], Recurrent Neural Networks (RNNs) [21], Attention Mechanism (AM) algorithms [22], and Transformer based BERT [23] have been widely used in the field of depression detection. For example, Cao et al. used suicide-oriented word embedding technology combined with Long Short Term Memory (LSTM) and Attention mechanism to detect users with suicidal ideation on Micro-blog datasets [24]. Senn et al. integrated multiple BERT models and adopted an integration strategy to improve the classification performance of depression on 12 thematic datasets [25].

3 Methods

The main goal of the model method depression tendency recognition task is to analyze user $U_l \in \{U_1, U_2, ..., U_L\}$ posted on social media by $p_i \in \{p_1, p_2, ..., p_N\}$ to predict users' depressive tendencies $Y \in \{0, 1\}$, where L is the number of users and N is the number of posts posted by the user, where 0 indicates that the user has a depressive tendency and 1 indicates a normal user. The paper abstracts the work of predicting depression propensity as a binary classification task.

The overall architecture of the DPMFF model is shown in Fig. 2, which mainly consists of two parts. The first part uses the Context Semantic Understanding Module (CSU) to extract the historical contextual semantic features of a given user. In order to accurately identify users with depressive tendencies in social media, attention mechanisms are used to capture keywords and sentences related to depression. The second part extracts deep emotional semantic features through the Advanced Emotional Semantic Perception Module (AESP) to enhance the model's ability to identify depression risk. Finally, the two features are fused and fed into the classifier to predict whether the user is at risk of depression.

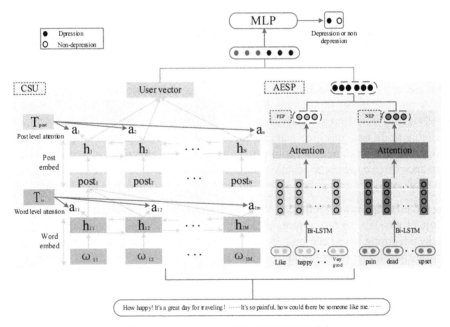

Fig. 2. Architecture of the DPMFF Model

3.1 Context Semantic Understanding Module

Based on the hierarchical structure of user documents, this section uses the CSU module to capture contextual semantic information of user documents. The CSU module includes a word-level encoding layer, a word-level attention layer, a post-level encoding layer, and a post-level attention layer.

Word-Level Encoding Layer. For user posts $p_i = \{\omega_{i1}, \omega_{i2}, \ldots\ldots, \omega_{iM}\}$, first apply the pre-trained word vector through $x_{im} = W_e\omega_{im}$ embeds words into a vector and obtains a sequence representation of $X = \{x_{i1}, x_{i2}, \ldots\ldots, x_{iM}\} \in R^{M \times d_e}$, where W_e is the embedding matrix, M is the number of words in the post, and d_e is the embedded dimension. Then, input X into the bidirectional GRU to summarize the information of words from the front and back directions to obtain word annotations, thereby obtaining the contextual information of the post. Bidirectional GRU includes forward $\overrightarrow{GRU}$ and backward $\overleftarrow{GRU}$, and the former will post p_i from ω_{i1} read ω_{iM}, and the latter will post p_i from ω_{iM} read ω_{i1}. The specific calculation formula is as follows:

$$x_{im} = W_e\omega_{im}, m\epsilon[1, M] \tag{1}$$

$$\overrightarrow{h_{im}} = \overrightarrow{GRU}(x_{im}, \overrightarrow{h_{im-1}}), m\epsilon[1, M] \tag{2}$$

$$\overleftarrow{h_{im}} = \overleftarrow{GRU}(x_{im}, \overleftarrow{h_{im+1}}), m\epsilon[M, 1] \tag{3}$$

Splicing Forward Hidden State $\overrightarrow{h_{im}}$ and Backward Hidden State $\overleftarrow{h_{im}}$ to Obtain Words ω_{im} Comment $h_{im} = [\overrightarrow{h_{im}}, \overleftarrow{h_{im}}]$, thus obtaining the hidden layer output $H_i = [h_{i1}, h_{i2}, ..., h_{iM}]$ of the post.

Word-Level Attention Layer. Not all words in a post have the same effect on identifying users' depressive tendencies. In order to accurately capture keyword information, attention mechanisms are used to learn the weights of each word in the post. Aggregating the expressions of words that have significant meaning to a post into a post vector, the specific calculation formula is as follows:

$$u_{im} = \tanh(W_\omega h_{im} + b_\omega) \tag{4}$$

$$a_{im} = \frac{\exp(u_{im}{}^T u_\omega)}{\sum_t \exp(u_{im}{}^T u_\omega)} \tag{5}$$

$$p_i = \sum_t a_{im} h_{im} \tag{6}$$

Among them, u_{im} is the hidden representation vector of word annotation h_{im}, W_ω, b_ω is the model parameter, and u_ω is the word context vector that is randomly initialized and jointly learned during the training process.

Post-level Encoding Layer. Given the post vector p_i, A similar method can be used to obtain the user's document vector representation. Use bidirectional GRU to encode each post of user U_1, and the specific calculation formula is as follows:

$$\overrightarrow{h_i} = \overrightarrow{GRU}(p_i, \overrightarrow{h_{i-1}}), i\epsilon[1, N] \tag{7}$$

$$\overleftarrow{h_i} = \overleftarrow{GRU}(p_i, \overleftarrow{h_{i+1}}, i \epsilon[N, 1]) \tag{8}$$

By concatenating $\overrightarrow{h_i}$ and $\overleftarrow{h_i}$, the vector representation $h_i = [\overrightarrow{h_i}, \overleftarrow{h_i}]$ of post p_i is obtained. h_i represents the contextual semantic feature information of post p_i.

Post-level Attention Layer. The time span of user posts is large, containing rich semantic information, and not every post shows a tendency towards depression. Generally speaking, among the large number of posts posted by users, only a few posts indicate that the user is at risk of depression. Therefore, this section uses the attention mechanism to introduce the post-level context vector u_p. And use this vector to measure the importance of different posts. The specific calculation formula is as follows:

$$u_i = \tanh(W_i h_i + b_i) \tag{9}$$

$$a_i = \frac{\exp(u_i{}^T u_p)}{\sum_i \exp(u_i{}^T u_p)} \tag{10}$$

$$v = \sum_i a_i h_i \tag{11}$$

Among them, v represents the document vector, which summarizes the contextual semantic feature information of all posts in the user, and the post-level context vector u_p is randomly initialized and jointly learned during the training process.

3.2   Advanced Emotional Semantic Perception Module

This section constructs a deep emotional semantic representation of user documents based on the AESP module for predicting depression tendency. The AESP module includes a feature extraction layer and a feature fusion layer.

Emotional Feature Extraction Layer. The emotion feature extraction layer includes two parts: Negative Emotion Perception (NEP) and Positive Emotion Perception (PEP), which are used to capture negative and positive emotion information, respectively. Firstly, based on the Chinese suicide dictionary, the user document is divided into the negative word set $NEG = \{n_1, n_2, ..., n_k\}$ and the positive word sets $POS = \{n_1, n_2, ..., n_r\}$, and mapped to the word vector matrix to obtain the word vector representations R_{pos} and R_{neg}, respectively.

Bidirectional Long Short Term Memory Network (Bi-LSTM) is widely used in NLP tasks to capture contextual information, including forward $\overrightarrow{LSTM}$ and reverse $\overleftarrow{LSTM}$. The paper uses R_{pos} and R_{neg} as inputs to the Bi-LSTM network to capture emotional information in posts and obtain negative emotion hidden layer output $h_{neg} = [\overrightarrow{h_{neg}}, \overleftarrow{h_{neg}}]$ and positive emotion hidden layer output $h_{pos} = [\overrightarrow{h_{pos}}, \overleftarrow{h_{pos}}]$. In order to further capture important emotions in the two-unit texts, an attention mechanism is applied, which operates the same as the CSU module. Add h_{pos} and h_{neg}, as the input of the attention network, assigns different weights to words, and ultimately obtains the negative word emotional feature representation $Att_{neg(i)}$ from the negative emotion perception unit and the positive word emotional feature representation $Att_{pos(i)}$ from the positive emotion perception unit.

Emotional Feature Fusion Layer. The fusion of negative and positive emotional information in the emotional feature fusion layer is used to improve the performance of depression tendency prediction. The deep emotion feature vectors $\text{Att}_{\text{pos(i)}}$ and $\text{Att}_{\text{neg(i)}}$ can be learned during the training process, and these two parts can be fused to obtain the final deep emotion semantic feature representation s. The specific calculation process is as follows:

$$s = \text{add}\left[\text{Att}_{\text{pos(i)}}, \text{Att}_{\text{neg(i)}}\right] \tag{12}$$

3.3 Depression Prediction

In this section, the contextual semantic feature representation v obtained in the CSU module and the advanced emotional feature representation s obtained in the AESP module will be fused to obtain the final user document feature representation f_{end}. The cross-entropy loss function will be used for predicting depression tendency to minimize model loss as much as possible. The final classification strategy for predicting user depression propensity is achieved through the softmax function. The specific calculation formula is as follows:

$$f_{end} = \text{Add}[v, s] \tag{13}$$

$$\hat{y}_i = \text{softmax}(w \cdot f_{end} + b) \tag{14}$$

$$\text{Loss} = \frac{1}{L}\sum\nolimits_{i=1}^{L}[-\sum\nolimits_{j=1}^{2} y_i^x \log \hat{y}_i^x] \tag{15}$$

Among them, L represents the size of the training sample. $\hat{y}_i$ represents the predicted category label of sample i, x represents the predicted category of user depression tendency risk, and y_i^x represents the true category label of sample i.

4 Experiments

4.1 Depression Datasets

The experimental data in this article comes from the *Sina-Weibo-Dataset*[3] released by Tsinghua University, which includes 744, 031 posts from May 1, 2018 to April 30, 2019. The data is randomly divided into training, validation, and testing sets, and the average F1 value is selected as the evaluation indicator. The specific distribution of dataset categories is shown in Table 2.

Weibo text has the characteristics of colloquialism, free formatting, and a large amount of dirty data. In order to reduce the impact of noisy data on experimental results, this article implements the following data preprocessing program. 1) Use regularization expressions to remove website-related content and meaningless characters such as # and &. 2) Excluding stop words and English text, this experiment only focuses on Chinese. 3) All posts have the word "<PAD>" filled in with a fixed length of n and a fixed number of m. 4) Using a Chinese suicide dictionary to assist in word segmentation using the Jieba tool.

---

[3] https://github.com/bryant03/Sina-Weibo-Dataset.

Table 2. Sina weibo dataset

Category	Users	Posts
Depression	3,652	252,901
No-depression	3,677	491,130

4.2 Experimental Setup

All experiments in this article were written and run using Python 3.6, using a deep learning framework of Python 1.0.0. During the training process, the optimizer adopts the Stochastic Gradient Descent (SGD), with the loss function set as the Cross-Entropy Loss function. The word embedding layer uses a pre-trained word vector Word2vec[4] based on the Weibo corpus. Some other important neural network parameters are shown in Table 3 and determined through experimental debugging.

Table 3. Parameter settings

Parameter Description	Value
Learning Rate	0.001
Bach	10
Word Embed	300
Epoch	200
Word-hidden-embed	50
Post-hidden-embed	50
Post Length	60
Number of Posts	60

4.3 Baseline

This article selects the following baseline methods to compare and verify their effectiveness with the DPMFF model.

(1) Support Vector Machine (SVM), Logistic Regression (LR), K Nearest Neighbors (KNN), Naive Bayes (NB): Four representative machine learning methods, with classifiers accepting text features for predicting users' depressive tendencies.

(2) TextCNN: Kim's CNN-based text classification model extracts text features through convolutional kernels of different sizes for depression tendency prediction.

(3) TextRCNN: Using Bi-LSTM instead of convolutional layers to extract contextual features as a new word embedding representation, then concatenating the hidden

---

[4] https://github.com/Embedding/Chinese-Word-Vectors.

layer output with the original word embedding to form a new word embedding and introducing maximum pooling for depression tendency prediction.

(4) TextRNN: Using Bi LSTM to extract features can capture contextual information between depression-related words and other words.

(5) TextRNN+Attention: Add an attention mechanism on the basis of Bi-LSTM to give different weights to words in the text in order to improve the recognition ability of the model.

(6) DPCNN: Deep pyramid convolutional network, which mainly obtains long-distance relationship dependencies of text by stacking convolutional layers.

(7) FastText: A fast text classifier and representation learning model based on randomly generated vectors and layered softmax published by Facebook, which predicts depression tendency based on three different word embeddings: unigram, bigram, and trigram

(8) Transformer: A sequence model based on a self-attention mechanism consisting of an encoder and a decoder. It is used to automatically model text sequences, extract text features, and then use fully connected layers to predict users' depression tendencies.

4.4 Results and Discussion

The comparative experimental results of various benchmark models and the DPMFF method in the prediction task of depression propensity are shown in Table 4.

Table 4. Comparison of experimental results

Model	F1 (%)
SVM	71.00
LR	73.00
KNN	60.70
NB	58.50
Text-CNN	81.60
Text-RCNN	86.10
Text-RNN	69.50
Text-RNN+Attention	87.10
Fast-Text	85.00
DPCNN	67.50
Transformer	75.10
DPMFF (Ours)	**92.50**

The experimental results show that the proposed model method has the best performance indicators among all comparative models, and the specific analysis is as follows:

Deep learning methods are significantly superior to machine learning models that manually construct features and have advantages in predicting depression tendencies. The reason is that the accuracy of machine learning methods relies on manually constructed features for classification and recognition, and the selection of features is achieved through manual construction for classification and recognition. Deep learning models can automatically learn features from data to improve classification performance.

Therefore, the effectiveness of the TextRCNN method is superior to the TextCNN and TextRNN. In the TextRCNN method, Bi-LSTM is used to replace the convolutional layer to capture contextual information, which learns more sequence information than the TextCNN method. The pooling layer can obtain critical features of the text, making up for the shortcomings of the TextRNN method. The TextRNN+Attention model outperforms the TextRNN method in F1 values, as the attention machine focuses on crucial information in posts and documents, which can accurately express text semantics.

Extracting multi-feature information from text is effective. The FastText method achieved good results in tasks because it obtained rich word embedding information. Due to the limitation of text length in the Transformer method, the features of Weibo user documents are missing, resulting in a decrease in model performance. Compared with all baseline methods, the model proposed in this paper exhibits the best performance, indicating that the depression tendency prediction model based on multi-feature fusion can effectively mine the global information of users.

4.5   Ablation Experiment

The paper further designed several variants of DPMFF for ablation experiments to analyze the impact of different components on the model. This section takes DPMFF as the benchmark, removing the contextual semantic understanding module ("w/o CSU") and the advanced emotional semantic perception module ("w/o AESP"), respectively. The F1 score report is shown in Table 5. The experimental results showed that removing the emotional semantic extraction module ("w/o AESP") significantly reduced the performance of the model, indicating that emotional features contain more information that helps distinguish depressed users. When two modules are combined, the model achieves optimal performance due to the total fusion and interaction of contextual semantic features and deep emotional semantic features, mining the rich feature information of users, thereby improving classification performance.

Table 5. Effectiveness experiments of different modules

Model	F1 (%)
w/o AESP	89.90
w/o CSU	90.50
DPMFF	92.50

In addition, this section takes the Semantic Understanding Module (CSU) as a benchmark to explore the impact of different categories of emotional perception units on the

Table 6. Effectiveness experiments of different emotional units

Model	F1 (%)
CSU	89.90
w/o PEP	86.70
w/o NEP	90.90

model. Among them, "w/o PEP" and "w/o NEP" respectively represent the removal of positive and negative emotion perception units. The F1 scores of their ablation studies are reported in Table 6. The experimental results indicate that the performance of the experiment with the addition of positive emotional units (PEP) is better than that with the addition of negative emotional units (NEP), as positive words contain more key information that helps predict depression propensity. Adding both PEP and NEP units at the same time constitutes the model in this paper. The optimal performance indicates that mining different categories of emotional features can help predict user depression tendencies.

4.6 Analysis of Factors Affecting Prediction Effectiveness

The number of posts (n-post) and the length of posts (n-post length) are two key parameters that affect the effectiveness of the experiment. Statistics have found that the number and length of posts in different user documents vary greatly, and the degree of textual information they contain varies. Therefore, this section explores the impact of the number and length of posts on the predictive performance of the model.

a) The impact of post length on experimental results

According to the statistics of all user documents, it was found that the maximum length of posts is 212. Based on the DPMFF model, keeping the number of posts at 60 and changing the length of posts, the experimental results are shown in Fig. 3. From the figure, it can be seen that the F1 value gradually increases with the decrease of post length. When the post length is reduced to 60, the performance is best. At this time, as the post length decreases, the F1 value shows a downward trend. This is because when the length of the post is set too large, it will cause too much noise data to be added when aligning the text during the experiment, thereby affecting the predictive performance of the model. When the length is set too short, it will also discard some important feature information in the text, leading to a decrease in the model's classification ability. Based on the results obtained from this experiment, set the post length to 60.

b) The impact of the number of posts on experimental results

Statistics have found that among all users, the maximum number of posts in the document is 100. Maintain a post length of 60 and continuously change the number of posts during the experiment. The experimental results are shown in Fig. 4. From it, it can be observed that as the number of posts continues to decrease, the F1 value shows

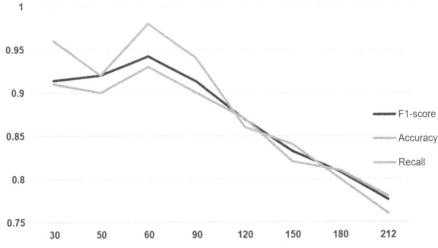

Fig. 3. The impact of post length on model performance

an upward trend. When the number of posts decreases to 60, the F1 value of the model reaches its highest, and then, as the number of posts continues to decrease, the F1 value gradually decreases. This is similar to the reason why the F1 value changes with the length of posts. Setting the number of posts too high will increase noise data, while setting the number of posts too low will discard important information. Based on the results obtained from this experiment, set the number of posts to 60.

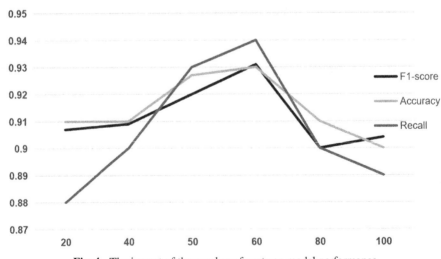

Fig. 4. The impact of the number of posts on model performance

4.7 Analysis of Internet Behavior of Users with Depression

Research has found that users' online behavior contains psychological health information. Analyzing the behavior of individuals at risk of depression on the internet can help to understand the characteristics and preferences of depressed individuals from different perspectives, providing support for accurately identifying depression-prone patients from online communities.

The network behavior data of users mainly refers to the characteristics that can represent the content of user interaction behavior. This includes gender, username, number of posts, followers, number of images, time of posting, etc.

The paper divides all user data containing such features into depressed user groups and normal user groups, resulting in 3,453 normal users and 1,357 users with depressive tendencies. After a series of statistical analyses, the online behavioral characteristics of users with depressive tendencies were obtained, and the differences in behavioral characteristics between them and normal users are shown in Table 7.

Table 7. Statistical results of network behavior characteristics

Characteristic	Depression User Group	Normal User Group
Followers (>100)	53.5%	84.1%
Fans (>100)	41.2%	89.57%
Per capita daily Post volume	1.94	2.92
Male users	22%	54.5%
Female users	78%	45.5%
Posting time (0:00–5:59)	7.8%	2.0%

From the table, it can be seen that 78% of users with depressive tendencies are women, and compared to men, women are more likely to suffer from depression. There are two main reasons: firstly, biological factors. Changes in progesterone and estrogen can directly affect women's mood, especially during the menstrual cycle, menopause, pregnancy, and before and after childbirth, which is also an important reason for the high incidence of postpartum depression in women. The second is social environmental factors, where women are naturally disadvantaged in terms of physical strength and are more susceptible to sexual abuse and domestic violence.

By dividing the daily interval of six hours into four time periods and analyzing the posting behavior of two groups of users at different times, it was found that users with depression tendencies have a clear pattern of active time on Weibo. Users with depressive tendencies posted significantly more posts than normal users between 0:00 and 5:59, indicating that users with mental health issues mostly engage in late-night activities, which is related to the prevalence of insomnia or sleep disorders in patients with depression.

Pay attention to the average daily number of posts posted by users, and it can be seen that the average number of posts posted by depressed users is significantly lower than that of normal users. Users with depressive tendencies usually have fewer followers than normal users, indicating that they have fewer friends. The attention level of depressed users is significantly lower than that of normal users, and their social participation ability is relatively low.

4.8 Analysis of Language Characteristics of Weibo Users with Depressive Tendencies

A searching analysis of posts published by users with depressive tendencies found that posts with depressive tendencies had a higher frequency of negative related words such as insults, irritability, terror, pain, and depression compared to normal users, indicating that depressed users often experience emotional distress. Compared with normal users, users with depressive tendencies usually prefer to use personal pronouns and use first-person pronouns more, such as "me" and "myself". This phenomenon indicates that users with depressive tendencies are more concerned about themselves, have stronger self-awareness, and have less contact with others. Researchers report that pronouns are actually more reliable than negative words in identifying depressive tendencies.

From the perspective of language style, depressed users prefer to use vocabulary that expresses absolute concepts, such as "always" and "never". There is an experimental inference that the world in the eyes of depression patients is either black or white, which is prone to extreme thinking patterns. In this way, these words are more suitable as markers for identifying depression tendencies than pronouns or negative words. Compared to normal users, posts posted by users at risk of depression are usually shorter, simpler in form, lacking flexibility, and using more simple vocabulary.

4.9 The Risk of Depression Caused by Public Health Emergencies

In recent years, public health emergencies have brought great changes to people's lives around the world. The epidemic has increased the number of depression and anxiety patients worldwide by 160 million, and the number of insomnia patients has also doubled. During the outbreak of COVID-19, the detection rate of people's anxiety increased significantly, which is related to people's fear that they or their families are in danger of being infected. In addition, paying more attention to negative information can activate users' unreasonable health beliefs, prompting them to overly focus on their physical feelings and triggering anxiety and panic about their own health. Therefore, when facing sudden public health events, the public should avoid paying too much attention to negative information, participate more in sports, and release psychological pressure.

People with mental health problems may face discrimination, leading to a decrease in public productivity and tension in social relations, thus hindering development. Therefore, the mental health status of the public should be given attention by society. Social institutions have the responsibility and obligation to make depression more widely recognized by the public, popularize psychological disease education, provide professional assistance and standardized treatment for depression patients, and improve the convenience and effectiveness of medical treatment. In the post-pandemic era, active response strategies should be adopted to provide psychological counseling, training, and intervention to populations experiencing sudden public health and safety incidents.

5   Conclusion

Using text published on social media to predict the risk of depression has the advantages of real-time and convenience, making it easy to carry out on a large scale. Accurate identification of early depression patients can provide timely assistance to prevent the worsening of depression and its serious consequences. Based on this, this article proposes a depression propensity prediction model based on multi-feature fusion (DPMFF), which extracts complete contextual semantic features and deep emotional semantic features from online users' posts in the past year for predicting depression propensity. The experiment shows that the performance of the model proposed in this article has significantly improved compared to other existing models. A series of ablation experiments have verified the effectiveness of each part of the model. In addition, research and analysis have found that users with depressive tendencies on social media have differences in behavioral and linguistic characteristics compared to normal users, which helps in the early identification and intervention of depressed users.

Depression is seriously affecting people's normal lives and even endangering their lives. Early identification is important, but more importantly, it can reduce the occurrence of depression from its root. Future work will explore the underlying causes of mental health problems by accurately identifying implicit data using more modal features based on the behavioral language characteristics of individuals with depression and combining them with clinical questionnaires. There are many online behaviors on social media that are almost indistinguishable from normal users but are deeply troubled by depression. What methods to use to identify such populations will also be a focus of future work.

Acknowledgment. This work is supported by a grant from the Social and Science Foundation of Liaoning Province (No. L20BTQ008).

References

1. Braithwaite, S.R., Giraud-Carrier, C., West, J., Barnes, M.D., Hanson, C.L.: Validating machine learning algorithms for Twitter data against established measures of suicidality. JMIR Mental Health 3(2), e21 (2016)
2. Chancellor, S., Birnbaum, M.L., Caine, E.D., et al.: A taxonomy of ethical tensions in inferring mental health states from social media. In: Proceedings of the Conference on Fairness, Accountability, and Transparency, New York, NY, USA, pp. 79–88. Association for Computing Machinery (2019)
3. Ben-Porath, E.N., Shaker, L.: News images, race, and attribution in the wake of Hurricane Katrina. J. Commun. 60, 466–490 (2010)
4. Sawhney, R., Joshi, H., Gandhi, S., et al.: A time-aware transformer based model for suicide ideation detection on social media. In: Proceedings of the 2020 Conference on Empirical Methods in Natural Language Processing (EMNLP), pp. 7685–7697. Association for Computational Linguistics (2020)
5. Ren, L., Lin, H., Xu, B., et al.: Depression detection on reddit with an emotion-based attention network: algorithm development and validation. JMIR Med. Inform. 9(7), e28754 (2021)
6. Lowe, B., Kroenke, K., Herzoge, W., et al.: Measuring depression outcome with a brief self-report instrument: sensitivity to change of the Patient Health Questionnaire (PHQ-9). J. Affect. Disord. 81(1), 61–66 (2004)

7. McPherson, A., Martin, C.R.: A narrative review of the Beck Depression Inventory (BDI) and implications for its use in an alcohol-dependent population. J. Psychiatr. Ment. Health Nurs. **17**(1), 19–30 (2010)

8. Hamilton, M.: A rating scale for depression. J. Neurol. Neurosurg. Psychiatry **23**(1), 56–62 (1960)

9. Zung, W.W.: A self-rating depression scale. Arch. Gen. Psychiatry **12**(1), 63–70 (1965)

10. Xezonaki, D., Paraskevopoulos, G., Potamianos, A., et al.: Affective conditioning on hierarchical attention networks applied to depression detection from transcribed clinical interviews. In: INTERSPEECH 2020, pp. 4556–4560 (2020)

11. Harris, K.M., Goh, M.T.: Is suicide assessment harmful to participants? Findings from a randomized controlled trial. Int. J. Ment. Health Nurs. **26**(2), 181–190 (2017)

12. Shen, Y., Yang, H., Lin, L.: Automatic depression detection: an emotional audio-textual corpus and a GRU/BiLSTM-based model. In: 2022 IEEE International Conference on Acoustics, Speech and Signal Processing (ICASSP), ICASSP 2022, Singapore, Singapore, pp. 6247–6251 (2022)

13. Johnson Viouls, M., Moulahi, B., Az, J., Bringay, S.: Detection of suicide-related posts in twitter data streams. IBM J. Res. Dev. **62**(1), 7:1–7:12 (2018)

14. Losada, D.E., Crestani, F., Parapar, J.: Overview of eRisk: early risk prediction on the internet. In: Bellot, P., et al. (eds.) CLEF 2018. LNCS, vol. 11018, pp. 343–361. Springer, Cham (2018). https://doi.org/10.1007/978-3-319-98932-7_30

15. Chiong, R., Budhi, G.S., Dhakal, S., et al.: A textual-based featuring approach for depression detection using machine learning classifiers and social media texts. Computs Biol. Med. **135**, 104499 (2021)

16. Islam, M.R., Kamal, A.R., Sutana, N., et al.: Detecting depression using K-Nearest Neighbors (KNN) classification technique. In: 2018 International Conference on Computer, Communication, Chemical, Material and Electronic (IC4ME2), pp. 1–4 (2018)

17. Chatterjee, R., Gupta, R.K., Gupta, B.: Depression detection from social media posts using multinomial naive theorem. In: IOP Conference Series: Materials Science and Engineering, p. 1022 (2021)

18. Peng, Z., Hu, Q., Dang, J.: Multi-kernel SVM based depression recognition using social media data. Int. J. Mach. Learn. Cybern. **10**(1), 43–57 (2019)

19. Lee, A., Kummerfeld, J.K., An, L., et al.: Micromodels for efficient, explainable, and reusable systems: a case study on mental health. In: Findings of the Association for Computational Linguistics: EMNLP 2021, Punta Cana, Dominican Republic, pp. 4257–4272. Association for Computational Linguistics (2021)

20. Kim, J., Lee, J., Park, E., et al.: A deep learning model for detecting mental illness from user content on social media. Sci. Rep. **10**(1), 1–6 (2020)

21. Amanat, A., Rizwan, M., Javed, A.R., et al.: Deep learning for depression detection from textual data. Electronics **11**(5), 676 (2022)

22. Zhang, D., Shi, N., Peng, C., Aziz, A., Zhao, W., Xia, F.: MAM: a metaphor-based approach for mental illness detection. In: Paszynski, M., Kranzlmüller, D., Krzhizhanovskaya, V.V., Dongarra, J.J., Sloot, P.M.A. (eds.) ICCS 2021. LNCS, vol. 12744, pp. 570–583. Springer, Cham (2021). https://doi.org/10.1007/978-3-030-77967-2_47

23. Wang, X., Chen, S., Li, T., et al.: Depression risk prediction for Chinese microblogs via deep-learning methods: content analysis. JMIR Med. Inform. **8**(7), e17958 (2020)

24. Cao, L., Zhang, H., Feng, L., et al.: Latent suicide risk detection on microblog via suicide-oriented word embeddings and layered attention. In: Conference on Empirical Methods in Natural Language Processing, pp. 1718–1728 (2019)

25. Senn, S., Tlachac, M.L., Flores, R., et al.: Ensembles of BERT for depression classification. In: 2022 44th Annual International Conference of the IEEE Engineering in Medicine and Biology Society (EMBC), pp. 4691–4694 (2022)

Automatic Prediction of Multiple Associated Diseases Using a Dual-Attention Neural Network Model

Yafeng Ren[1,2,3]($\boxtimes$), Zilin Wang[3], and Wei Tong[3]

[1] School and Interpreting and Translation Studies, Guangdong University of Foreign Studies, Guangzhou, China
[2] Laboratory of Language and Artificial Intelligence, Center for Linguistics and Applied Linguistics, Guangdong University of Foreign Studies, Guangzhou, China
[3] School and Information Science and Technology, Guangdong University of Foreign Studies, Guangzhou, China
{renyafeng,20221050025,20211050020}@gdufs.edu.cn

Abstract. In recent years, disease prediction based on electronic health records (EHR) has attracted extensive attention in the field of biomedical text mining. However, the existing work has two issues. First, most of the existing methods focus on the prediction of a single disease and little attention is paid to the prediction of multiple associated diseases. Second, these methods usually use simple feature modeling, and fail to fully capture and mine the information from EHR, which usually contains two main information: the textual description and physical indicators. To address these issues, we design a dual-attention neural network model to predict the probability of coronary heart disease and kidney disease in hypertension patients. Specifically, the proposed model consists of three main parts: a textual module, a numerical module and a global BiLSTM. Given one piece of EHR, the textual module is utilized for encoding the textual information, such as diagnosis texts. The numerical module handles the numerical indicators, such as physical indicators. The dual-attention mechanism enables the model to better capture the intrinsic and implicit semantic features behind the clinic texts and numerical indicators, respectively. The experimental results on the datasets show the effectiveness of the proposed model, and our model outperforms previous methods and strong neural baselines by a large margin. Meanwhile, the attention mechanism can capture the risk factors between the associated diseases.

Keywords: Disease prediction · Attention mechanism · Electronic health records · Neural networks

1 Introduction

Disease prediction is one of the important studies in biomedical text mining, and has attracted extensive attention from researchers [5,17,27,63]. The existing

H. Xu et al. (Eds.): CHIP 2023, CCIS 1993, pp. 369–391, 2024.
https://doi.org/10.1007/978-981-99-9864-7_24

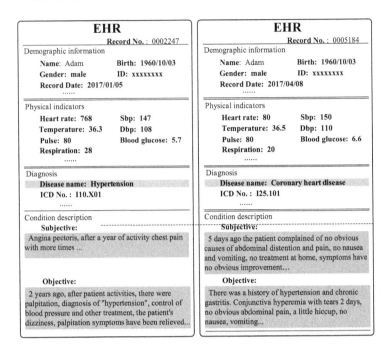

Fig. 1. Two pieces of EHRs for one patient.

work can be divided into two main directions. First, a line of work focuses on the prediction of single target disease [1,6,30,37]. For instance, Jabbar et al. (2016) use random forest and chi square to predict heart disease [30]. Liu et al. (2018) apply deep neural network for predicting chronic disease by modeling the EHR data [37]. Second, several efforts try to explore the molecular mechanism of diseases [2,35,42,59]. For example, Le and Dang (2016) investigate an ontology-based similarity network for disease gene prediction [35]. However, less attention is paid for the associated prediction of multiple diseases.

In recent years, an increasing number of people has suffering from various diseases such as hypertension, coronary heart disease, kidney disease and diabetes, etc. Unfortunately, some people are attacked by multiple diseases at the same time, and these diseases are closely interrelated that one disease is likely to trigger another. Taking coronary heart disease as example, many studies analyze the risk of coronary heart disease and it is generally accepted that hypertension is closely associated with the development of coronary heart disease [3,15,62]. For kidney disease, it is widely believed that hypertension can lead to the development of kidney disease under certain conditions [11,14,29,36,39,43].

Two real EHRs are shown in Fig. 1. We can observe that the patient *Adam* was diagnosed with hypertension on January 5, 2017. Three months later, he was diagnosed with coronary heart disease (CHD). For this patient, it can be inferred that the occurrence of coronary heart disease is strongly associated with previous hypertension, which has been confirmed by a large number of previous studies [3,15,62]. If we can design models that accurately predict the probability of developing coronary heart disease or other complications based on his EHRs, and capture risk factors and indicators among these associated diseases. Based on these warning information, the patient can receive timely treatment and even avoid these complications. Therefore, it is particularly important to design models for predicting the associated diseases.

Multiple diseases associated prediction (MDAP) is an important research topic, which aims to predict the probability of a target disease in the case of another specific disease that has been diagnosed. Chen et al. (2017) first evaluate risk factors for the development of coronary heart disease in hypertension patients using a logistic regression model [11], while they adopt traditional statistical model that requires a number of hand-designed features. More recently, Ren et al. (2019) predict kidney disease in hypertension patients using a hybrid neural model by integrating BiLSTM and autoencoder [47]. However, this model fails to take into account multiple EHRs of one patient in different times, limiting the performance of the task.

Given a hypertension patient, this paper aims to predict the probability of the patient developing coronary heart disease and kidney disease. Inspired by the success of neural networks in various text mining tasks [31,32,49,50,54,55,61], we propose a dual-attention neural network model for predicting coronary heart disease and kidney disease in hypertension patients, and capturing the risk factors of multiple associated diseases. Specifically, we first construct two datasets based on a large amount of raw EHR data. Then we build a dual-attention neural network model by incorporating a bi-directional long short-term memory (BiLSTM) and convolutional neural network (CNN). Here, BiLSTM is used to process the textual information in EHR for learning the textual representation, and CNN uses the physical indicators as input to represent the numerical features. To handle multiple time-ordered EHRs of a patient, we employ another BiLSTM to globally encode the EHR representation. Finally, we use a softmax classifier to make prediction.

The experimental results on the datasets show that our model achieves the competitive performance, outperforming previous methods and strong baseline systems by a large margin. Meanwhile, the proposed dual-attention mechanism captures the risk factors that uncover the association from hypertension to coronary heart disease and kidney disease.

2   Related Work

Disease prediction, especially chronic disease such as coronary heart disease and hypertension, is becoming a heated research topic in the field of biomedical text mining [8,13,20,22,23,57]. Early studies aim at making predictions with various numerical indicators, such as laboratory test characteristics, physical examination factors, demographic information, etc. For example, Wilson et al. (1998) predict coronary heart disease using a logistic regression model combined with discrete features [58]. Subsequent researchers exploit more non-traditional risk factors to predict coronary heart disease for achieving better results [44,57]. Another a line of work tries to predict the disease risk from genetic perspective and attempts to look for underlying molecular mechanism of diseases [16,26,35]. For example, Wray et al. (2007) present the dense genome-wide single-nucleotide polymorphism (SNP) panels to assess the genetic risk of diseases [59]. Recently, some studies also investigate the genes associated with diseases to better understand the genetic mechanisms of these diseases [2,42]. However, the existing studies have two limitations. First, these work mainly focuses on the prediction of a single disease, and less attention is paid to the prediction of multiple associated diseases. Second, most of the existing work uses traditional statistical models with hand-designed discrete features, and fails to fully capture the information in EHRs. Note that recent studies for disease prediction on EHR has investigated neural models [37], while unfortunately we find that no efforts are paid for the direction of multiple association diseases prediction.

More recently, some preliminary work is proposed for the prediction of multiple association diseases based on electronic health records [11,47]. Typically, Chen et al. (2017) first evaluate risk factors for the development of coronary heart disease in hypertension patients using a logistic regression model [11], while they adopt traditional statistical model with a number of hand-designed features. Furthermore, Ren et al. (2019) predict kidney disease in hypertension patients using a hybrid neural network model, which integrates bidirectional long short-term memory and autoencoder [47], while this model fails to fully capture the information in the EHRs. For example, they do not consider multiple EHRs for one patient in different times.

With the success of deep learning, neural network models such as CNN, RNN, and LSTM, are widely used in various text mining tasks, achieving competitive results [18,19,46,51,52,60,61,64]. Recently, neural network models have been gradually applied to various tasks in biomedical text mining [4,9,38,48,65]. For instance, Zhao et al. (2016) investigate a deep multi-layer neural network model to extract the information of protein-protein interaction from the biomedical literature [65]. More recently, neural networks have been successfully utilized for representing the EHR data for predicting disease risks or medical events. For example, Cheng et al. (2016) propose a CNN approach to represent EHR as a temporal matrix for disease risk prediction [12]. Rajkomar et al. (2018) explore a representation of patients' entire raw EHR using a deep learning method [45]. Different from the above methods, we explore an dual-attention neural network model for the prediction of coronary heart disease and kidney disease in hypertension patients.

3   Task Modeling and Dataset Construction

3.1   Task Modeling

Given a hypertension patient, this paper aims to predict the probability of the patient to meanwhile suffer from coronary heart disease or kidney disease. We denote hypertension as source disease (s), and coronary heart disease or kidney disease as target disease (t). However, we cannot directly predict whether the target disease is positive or negative for one patient based on one raw EHR record. The reason can be three-fold. 1) One single record is insufficient to carry the association clues of the source and target disease, which means that it is not reasonable to make analysis based on one single EHR. 2) The diagnosis information in EHR data for one patient scales over time. If we make prediction directly for each EHR record, we may separate the underlying connection between multiple diseases and the time-variant factors behind clinical diagnosis results. 3) The goal of multiple association diseases prediction is individual-level, which means that our research objective is an individual, instead of one EHR.

We consider a constructed collection of samples as our dataset:

$$D_{(s \to t)} = \{d^1, \cdots, d^p, \cdots, d^P\} \quad (p = [1, \cdots, P]), \tag{1}$$

where P is the total number of the patients, and also the dataset size. $s \to t$ denotes from the source disease s to the target disease t, and each sample is denoted as d^p for the patient p. Specifically, each sample of the patient p contains a time-ordered EHR sequence, which is denoted as

$$d^p = \{(E_1^p, L_1), \cdots, (E_K^p, L_K)\}, \tag{2}$$

where E_k^p denotes the k-th EHR and K is the total number of EHR, with its label $L_i \in \{l^+, l^-\}$. For each sample d^p, more than one EHR E_k^p of patient p should be diagnosed and recorded in the source disease. The reason is that, we want to predict the likelihood of a patient to further suffer from a target disease in the condition of the source disease, so the source disease should be definitely diagnosed as the precondition. In other words, we can formulate the process as a conditioned probability prediction:

$$y^p(t|s) = y^p(E_1^p(\mathbb{1}_s, L_1), \cdots, E_1^K(\mathbb{1}_s, L_K)), \tag{3}$$

where $y^p(t|s)$ is the goal conditioned probability for the patient p to be a positive source disease t when p has already caught source disease s, denoted as $\mathbb{1}_s$. Furthermore, the target disease maybe or maybe not exists in the patient p's k-th EHR E_k^p. If a patient p is further diagnosed with the target disease, the label L_k of EHR E_k^p is denoted as l^+, a positive sample; if not, $L_k = l^-$, a negative sample. That's it, we model the prediction as a binary classification task, where our system first is trained based on the dataset $D_{(s \to t)}$, and then to make prediction of the label for a cohort of EHR.

3.2   Dataset Construction

Preprocessing. We first collect large amounts of EHR data, which contains raw records from hospitals in China. As shown in Fig. 1, one EHR contains overall clinical information about a diagnosis, including textual information and numerical information. Since the raw EHR contains personal privacy, such as patient's name, resident ID number and institute number, etc., which are irrelevant to our research. In addition, there are some noises or errors in the records that may have negative impact on our experiments. Moreover, some features, such as gender and disease name, are presented as non-numerical form, which can be better functioned if they are converted into numerical continuous values. Finally, as mentioned above, our target is the prediction from the source disease to the target disease, therefore we only keep those records where the observed diseases (hypertension, coronary heart disease and kidney disease) are occurred. So we conduct the following preprocessing steps for each record. We denote the EHR data after preprocessing as $D^\dagger$.

- Filter out those records of the patients who are not involved in the source disease.
- Remove the irrelevant fields of records, including name, resident ID, institute number and inpatient number, etc.
- Assign 1 as male, 2 as female.
- Compute the age by the birth date and recording date.
- Replace the disease name by looking up the 10th International Classification of Diseases (ICD-10) tables.
- Drop the wrong character in the textual fields and merge the textual description of subjective and objective into one.
- Drop those records where some numerical values are out of rational range.

Construction. Here, we elaborate the construction of datasets $D_{(s \to t)}$ based on $D^\dagger$, where $(s \to t)$ are (hypertension $\to$ coronary heart disease) and (hypertension $\to$ kidney disease), respectively. As emphasized previously, the basic unit of our goal is a patient. Thus, we first sort from EHR records $D^\dagger$ into just one sample d^p belonging to same patient p. Also, the EHRs in d^p is time-sequentially ordered. We then assign the label for each sample d^p, under the following criteria:

- For d^p, at leat one EHR record E_k^p is recorded with target disease: $L_p = l^+$.
- For d^p, no EHR record is involved in target disease: $L_p = l^-$.

We keep such steps for each sample d^p, until we obtain two datasets D (hypertension $\to$ coronary heart disease, hypertension $\to$ kidney disease). The constructed dataset (hypertension $\to$ coronary heart disease) is illustrated in Fig. 2.

In the dataset of predicting hypertension to coronary heart disease, we obtain 40,039 samples, of which 36,352 are recorded as negative and 3,687 as positive. For the dataset of predicting hypertension to kidney disease, we obtain 40,097 samples, of which 34,232 are negative and 5,865 are positive. We can find that two datasets are highly imbalanced, which is problematic for direct experiments. To solve this problem, we use an undersampling approach to balance classes [7]. Taking the prediction of coronary heart disease as example, we reduce the sample size of the large number category by randomly selecting 3,687 samples from 36,352. This reduces the sample size of the dataset to 7,374, thus making

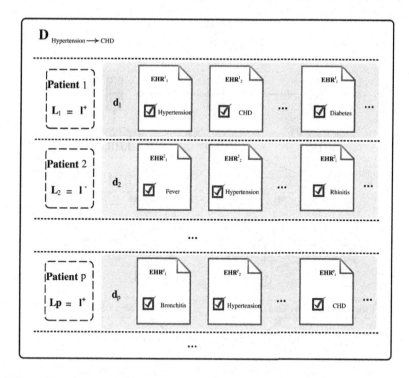

Fig. 2. The construction illustration of the dataset (hypertension → CHD).

the dataset balanced. To make the result more credible, the undersampling is repeated ten times. The final result is the average of the algorithms over all ten experiments. Similarly, the same method is conducted for the prediction of kidney disease.

4 Method

Figure 3 shows the overall framework of the proposed dual-attention neural network model, which consists of three main parts: a textual module, a numerical module and a global BiLSTM. Given one piece of EHR, the textual module is utilized for encoding the textual information, such as diagnosis texts. The numerical module handles the numerical indicators, such as physical indicators. The dual-attention mechanism enables the model to better capture the intrinsic and implicit semantic features behind the clinic texts and numerical indicators, respectively. Since one patient usually contains a list of EHRs ordered time-sequentially. Finally, the global BiLSTM, on the top of the above two modules, is used to integrate multiple EHRs representations.

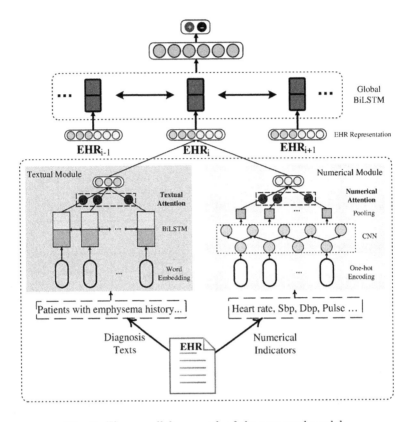

Fig. 3. The overall framework of the proposed model.

4.1 Textual Module

The textual information in the EHR describes the underlying disease symptoms, in which may imply useful clues, either explicit or implicit. We first use the embedding layer to take the textual data as input. For each word w_i, a look-up table E is used to obtain its embedding $e(w_i) \in \mathbb{R}^L$, where $E \in \mathbb{R}^{L \times V}$ (L is the dimension of embedding vector and V represents the vocabulary size).

BiLSTM is then used to learn the representation of textual description. Basically, LSTM represents each time step with an input, a memory and an output gate. BiLSTM has two parallel layers in both forward and backward directions. Here, $\boldsymbol{h}_{f_t}$ and $\boldsymbol{h}_{b_t}$ denote the output of LSTM unit in forward layer and backward layer, respectively. We then concatenate these two hidden outputs as the words representation:

$$\boldsymbol{h}_t^{(T)} = [\boldsymbol{h}_{f_t}; \boldsymbol{h}_{b_t}], \tag{4}$$

Textual Attention. Not all words or phrases in a text are equally important for predicting the target disease. To capture the most task-relevant elements of a sentence, we employ the self-attention mechanism, which has significant effect on textual modeling. We use an alignment function to aggregate the representation of the salient words to form an attention vector $\boldsymbol{v}^{(Ti)}$. Specific formula are as follows:

$$u_t^{(Ti)} = tanh(\boldsymbol{W}^{(Ti)} h_t^{(Ti)} + b^{(Ti)}),$$

$$\alpha_t^{(Ti)} = \frac{exp(u_t^{(Ti)T} u_t^{(Ti)})}{\sum_t exp(u_t^{(Ti)T} u_t^{(Ti)})}, \tag{5}$$

$$\boldsymbol{v}^{(Ti)} = \sum_t \alpha_t^{(Ti)} \boldsymbol{h}_t^{(bi)}.$$

We first feed the word representation $\boldsymbol{h}_t^{(T)}$ by a linear transformation to obtain $u_t^{(Ti)}$. Then we measure the importance of the word by computing the relatedness of $u_t^{(Ti)}$ with a word-level context vector $u^{(Ti)}$ to obtain a normalized importance weight $\alpha_t^{(Ti)}$. Thereafter, we compute the attention vector $\boldsymbol{v}^{(Ti)}$ as a weighted sum based on the weight, which is the final representation of the textual module.

4.2 Numerical Module

In clinical data, numerical features usually suffer from temporality, sparsity, noisiness and bias, etc. Therefore, we employ a CNN to learn the representation of numerical features. We first convert all numerical values into one-hot representation. Then, CNN takes temporal matrix of numerical features as input.

CNN has strong ability on learning feature locality by its filters, and can capture the important features with the highest value for each feature mapping. Here, $\boldsymbol{x}_i \in \mathbb{R}^d$ denotes the d-dimensional numerical feature vector corresponding to the i-th one-hot representation of numerical features from a piece of EHR. Then $\boldsymbol{x}_i$ can be represented as:

$$\boldsymbol{x}_{1:n} = \boldsymbol{x}_1 \oplus \boldsymbol{x}_2 \oplus \cdots \oplus \boldsymbol{x}_n, \tag{6}$$

where $\oplus$ denotes the concatenation operator. $\boldsymbol{x}_{i:i+j}$ refers to the concatenation of numerical feature vector $\boldsymbol{x}_i, \boldsymbol{x}_{i+1}, \cdots, \boldsymbol{x}_{i+j}$. A one-side convolution operation involves a filter $\boldsymbol{w} \in \mathbb{R}^{d \times h}$, which is applied to a window of h features to generate a new feature. The feature $\boldsymbol{c}_i$ is generated from $\boldsymbol{x}_{i:i+h-1}$ by

$$\boldsymbol{c}_i = f(\boldsymbol{w} \cdot \boldsymbol{x}_{i:i+h-1} + b). \tag{7}$$

The filters are applied to each possible window of each element $\boldsymbol{x}_{1:n}$ to produce a feature mapping:

$$\boldsymbol{c} = [\boldsymbol{c}_1; \boldsymbol{c}_2; \cdots ; \boldsymbol{c}_{n-h+1}], \tag{8}$$

where $\boldsymbol{c} \in \mathbb{R}^{n-h+1}$. Then, we apply a max pooling over the feature mapping and take the maximum value:

$$\boldsymbol{h}^{(d)} = max\{\boldsymbol{c}\}. \tag{9}$$

By this, we obtain the raw discrete representation for numerical values.

Numerical Attention. To explore the most relevant factors from the physical indicators, we also employ an attention layer. Different from the self-attention mechanism in textual attention, we use an alignment function to measure the word representation $h_t^{(T)}$ from textual module and discrete representation $h^{(d)}$ from numerical module. Specifically,

$$
\begin{aligned}
u_t^{(Ni)} &= tanh(W_N^{(Ni)} h_t^{(di)} + W_T^{(Ni)} h_t^{(Ti)} + b^{(Bi)}), \\
\alpha_t^{(Ni)} &= \frac{exp(u_t^{(Ni)T} u_t^{(Ni)})}{\sum_t exp(u_t^{(Ni)T} u_t^{(Ni)})}, \\
v^{(Ni)} &= \sum_t \alpha_t^{(Ni)} h_t^{(di)},
\end{aligned}
\tag{10}
$$

where $W_N^{(Ni)}$ and $W_T^{(Ni)}$ are weight matrices for words representation $h_t^{(T)}$ and discrete representation $h^{(d)}$, respectively. After the numerical attention layer, we output the representation from numerical module.

4.3   Global Fusion

After encoding the textual and numerical parts of the i-th EHR in the sample d^p, we obtain the representation $v^{(Ti)}$ and $v^{(Ni)}$. We need to make comprehensive learning for multiple time-sequential EHRs of the patient p. Therefore, we first concatenate the above two representation of the i-th EHR:

$$
EHR_i = [v^{(Ti)}; v^{(Ni)}].
\tag{11}
$$

Then, we use another BiLSTM to globally encode EHR_i $(i = [0, \cdots, K])$ for each EHR at each timestamp. Afterwards, we can obtain the final representation of d^p for the overall EHR sequence. Finally, we employ the *softmax* function as a classifier to make final prediction based on the output representation.

5   Experiments Settings

5.1   Evaluation Settings

We conduct experiments on two datasets (hypertension $\rightarrow$ coronary heart disease, hypertension $\rightarrow$ kidney disease). In our experiments, ten-fold cross-validation settings are used to report the overall performance. Each dataset is divided into ten equal sections, each decoded by the model trained from the remaining nine sections. We randomly select one of the nine training sections as the validating set to adjust hyper-parameters. The performance of all models is measured by F1 score.

Table 1. Parameter settings.

Parameter	Value	Parameter	Value
max seq len	128	$H_{globalBiLSTM}$	400
max EHR num	50	λ	0.001
L	200	dropout	0.3
$H_{textBiLSTM}$	200	batch size	32
F_{CNN}	[2, 3, 4, 5]	epoch	15

5.2 Parameter Settings

We set the dimension of hidden representation of textual BiLSTM and all embedding dimensions as 200, and the hidden size of global BiLSTM is 400. Besides, L denotes the dimension of the word vectors and F_{CNN} represents the number of filters of CNN layer. The sequence length is limited to 128, and the max number of EHRs of one patient is limited to 50. We use Adam [33] to optimize the training with an initial learning rate λ of 0.001. Dropout is adopted for the attention network with a 0.7 keeping rate. We initialize all matrices and vector parameters with Xavier methods [25]. The dropout rate is 0.3. All experiments are conducted by using a GTX1080Ti GPU with 8 GB memory. Specific parameters are shown in Table 1.

5.3 Baselines

To show the effectiveness of our model, we compare our model with multiple baseline systems, which include two classes: discrete models (All discrete models are implemented with sklean 0.21 toolkit.) and neural models (All neural models are coded with keras 2.0 framework.).

Discrete Models. The representative discrete model includes Support Vector Machine (SVM), Naive Bayes (NB) and Gradient Boosting Decision Tree (GBDT), which have been extensively utilized for text classification tasks, achieving competitive results [40,41,56]. Besides, Chen et al. (2017) predict coronary heart disease in hypertension patients by using a LR model with physical indicators [10].

For discrete models, they can only take the discrete features as input. Therefore, we represent the sentences with one-hot vectors, while keeping raw numerical values as input features, and then we concatenate them as the input of models. Moreover, discrete models cannot directly decode one cohort of EHRs time-sequentially for a patient, so we concatenate all the one-hot vectors of each EHR as the overall input of models.

Neural Models. We use two representative models as neural baselines including CNN and BiLSTM, both of which are extensively employed in many NLP tasks. Our proposed model also employs these two basic models, where BiL-STM encodes textual information and CNN encodes numerical values. For neural baselines, we additionally make CNN encode a text, or make BiLSTM encode numerical values, or let them encode the concatenation of both textual information and discrete values. Ren et al. (2019) predict kidney disease in hypertension patients using a hybrid neural network model, which integrates BiLSTM and autoencoder [47]. Besides, we also use a hybrid model of CNN+BiLSTM (CBiL-STM) [34], which only takes as input the concatenation of textual information and discrete values. Note that all these neural baselines only encode one piece of EHR, so we use an additional BiLSTM for them to fusing the time-sequential EHR representation, as our model does.

5.4   Feature Settings

In a EHR, there are two types of information: textual and numerical features. In our experiments, we study the ablation by using different combinations of two types of features for each model: 1) textual input only, note as Textual; 2) numerical input only, note as Numerical; 3) textual input and numerical input, note as Textual+Numerical.

To investigate the effectiveness of the dual-attention mechanism in our model, we conduct ablation by removing the textual attention layer from textual module, or removing the numerical attention layer from numerical module, or deleting both the textual attention layer and numerical attention layer, respectively.

6   Experimental Results

6.1   Main Results

Table 2 shows the results of discrete models. Taking the prediction of coronary heart disease as example, we can observe that the model LR proposed by Chen et al. (2017) gives only 58.5% F1 score. The reason is that their model only uses numerical physical indicators as input, and ignores the textual information of the EHR, which is crucial for the final prediction. Furthermore, the performance can be improved to 74.1% by integrating the textual description information. Among all discrete models, GBDT achieves the best result (80.6% F1 score), based on Textual+Numerical features. This is because GBDT contains multiple meta-classifiers, which make the GBDT model more powerful. Similar to coronary heart disease, the same trend can be found in the prediction of kidney disease.

Table 2. Experimental results of discrete models, CHD denotes coronary heart disease.

Model	Features	CHD F1 score (%)	Kidney F1 score (%)
LR	Numerical	58.5	60.6
	Textual	70.3	68.5
	Textual+Numerical	74.1	70.0
NB	Numerical	52.6	61.6
	Textual	68.6	66.0
	Textual+Numerical	69.7	67.2
SVM	Numerical	60.7	65.4
	Textual	72.1	71.3
	Textual+Numerical	74.6	71.8
GBDT	Numerical	67.3	65.3
	Textual	78.9	74.8
	Textual+Numerical	**80.6**	**76.5**

Table 3. Results of different neural models. Original represents the original version of our model. w/o T-Att denotes without textual attention, w/o N-Att denotes removing numerical attention, w/o T&N-Att denotes without both textual and numerical attention. w/o Global means replacing the upper global BiLSTM encoder as a linear transformation layer.

Model	Features	CHD F1 score (%)	Kidney F1 score (%)
CNN	Numerical	70.5	72.6
	Textual	83.6	82.7
	Textual+Numerical	84.2	86.5
BiLSTM	Numerical	72.6	71.0
	Textual	82.3	81.3
	Textual+Numerical	85.7	86.3
CBiLSTM	Textual+Numerical	86.8	87.2
BiLSTM+AE	Textual+Numerical	87.5	88.4
Original	Textual+Numerical	**91.9**	**90.6**
w/o N-Att	Numerical	77.7	75.4
	Textual	86.1	84.3
	Textual+Numerical	88.6	87.8
w/o T-Att	Numerical	76.3	74.3
	Textual	85.9	83.8
	Textual+Numerical	87.6	86.5
w/o T&N-Att	Textual+Numerical	87.5	88.5
w/o Global	Textual+Numerical	80.4	74.2

Table 3 shows the results of different neural models. Taking the prediction of coronary heart disease as example, CNN gives 84.2% F1 score and BiLSTM gives 85.7% F1 score, respectively, based on Textual+Numerical features. These two simple neural models outperform traditional discrete models, even the best discrete model GBDT. This shows the strong ability of neural models for the task. By integrating BiLSTM, CBiLSTM achieves 86.8% F1 score with Textual+Numerical features, and gives a comparative result with the current best model proposed by Ren et al. (2019), which investigate a hybrid neural model by integrating BiLSTM and autoencoder [47]. This shows that the neural models have a powerful ability to capture the intrinsic features from EHRs. Finally, the proposed model gives the highest F1 score (91.9%) on Textual+Numerical features. The same trend can be found in the prediction of kidney disease, and the best result can be obtained (90.6% F1) by our model, outperforming the current best model by a large margin. We also find that the performance of the model slightly declines without textual attention or numerical attention. This indicates that dual-attention module exerts the role in improving the performance. Furthermore, we can observe that when replacing the global encoder layer with a linear transformation layer based on the concatenation of time-series of EHRs representation, the performances on two tasks drop a lot. This indicates the effectiveness of the proposed global encoder for modeling the time-sequential EHRs. The above analysis shows the effectiveness of the proposed model.

Besides, we can find that all model can achieve better performance based on a combination of textual and numerical features compared with the only textual features or numerical features. This is reasonable, since different types of features in EHR can make different contributions. Moreover, we find that the models with textual features can obtain better performance than those with numerical features, demonstrating the usefulness of the diagnosis texts or descriptions in clinic EHR. The main reason is that the textual data intuitively carry strong cues for indicating the diseases association. For example, the most important risk factors (e.g., the disease symptoms, and disease conditions), often are contained in the textual description of a EHR. The neural model can effectively capture such features and connections.

6.2   Effect of Word Embedding

Previous work shows that word representation is highly important to a neural network model [21,53]. So we study the influences of word vector initialization, by comparing pre-trained embedding Word2vec, pre-trained embedding Glove, pre-trained embedding from bio&clinical corpus, and stochastically initialized embedding. Specifically, for GloVe, we use Stanford publicly available embedding trained on 6 billion words from Wikipedia and web text. For Word2vec, we train a word embedding from Wikipedia corpus on 3.1 billion words using Google Word2vec toolkit. For the bio&clinical embedding, we train it from biomedical and clinical corpus: the PubMed Central Open Access subset (PMC) and the available PubMed abstracts, to bring the rich functional semantic biomedical and clinical knowledge for our model. The stochastically initialized embedding is initialized with uniform samples from $[-\sqrt{\frac{6}{r+c}}, +\sqrt{\frac{6}{r+c}}]$, where r and c are the number of rows and columns in the structure. All embedding parameters can be trained and updated during training.

Figure 4 shows the results of different embeddings. We can see that word embeddings with pre-trained initialization can improve the overall performance. Meanwhile, the pre-trained embeddings from bio&clinical corpus can achieve better performance, thanks to the additional transferred knowledge.

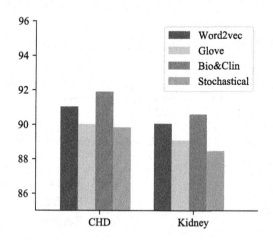

Fig. 4. Results of different word embeddings.

6.3 Impact of EHR Cohorts

Impact of Numbers of EHRs. For a patient p, one sample d^p may contain a list of EHRs. We now investigate the impact of the association prediction over varying number of EHRs for a patient. We make statistics on the F1 score over different number of EHRs on each patient's sample based on the development sets. The results are shown in Fig. 5, we can find that the model can obtain better performance with more EHR numbers in the sample. Intuitively, this is reasonable, because more sufficient information from EHRs can provide useful clues or risk factors.

Impact of the Order of EHR Sequence. We further explore the impact of different order for a EHR sequence. We first keep the original time-sequential order, then we reverse the sequential order. We also shuffle the order of a sequence. The results are displayed in Fig. 6. As what we exactly assumed, the EHR sequences after shuffling cause negative influence on the performances of two datasets. This indicates that some of the information behind the time-order is useful for the association prediction. We also find the scores on the reversed EHR sequences is slightly dropped, with an acceptable numbers. This owes to

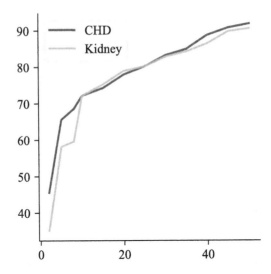

Fig. 5. F1 scores on different numbers of EHRs.

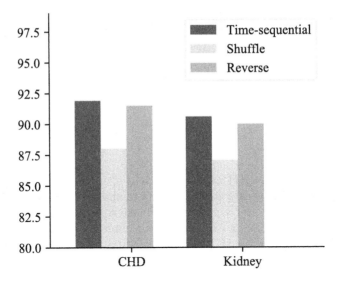

Fig. 6. Performances in different orders of EHR sequences.

the global bi-directional LSTM model, which encodes the EHR representation from two directions, and makes it compatible with the reversed sequence.

6.4 Case Study

In order to validate the effectiveness of the proposed dual-attention mechanism, we visualize the attention weights on two positive examples, which can illustrate the risk factors for leading to coronary heart disease or kidney disease in hypertension patients. The visualization is illustrated in Fig. 7.

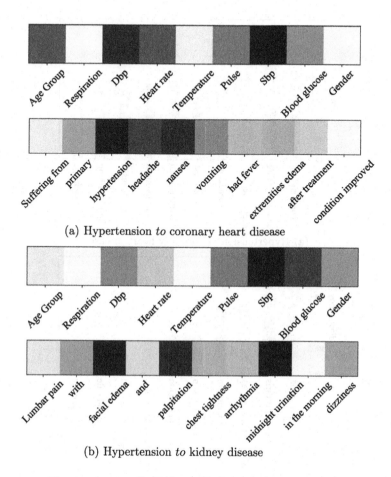

(a) Hypertension *to* coronary heart disease

(b) Hypertension *to* kidney disease

Fig. 7. Visualization of textual and numerical attention.

For each example pair, the upper represents the numerical physical indicators, and the lower represents the words or phrases in the textual description. The color depth represents the weight. In the first example (hypertension → coronary heart disease), the textual attention assigns larger weights for words *"hypertension"*, *"nausea"*, and *"headache"*, and the numerical attention gives higher weights on *"Dbp"*, *"Pulse"*. For the second example (hypertension → kidney disease), the numerical attention gives higher weights on *"Dbp"*, *"Blood glucose"*, and *"Sbp"*. The textual attention gives higher weights on *"facial edema"*, *"palpitation"*, *"arrhythmia"*, and *"urination"*. The words with high attention weights represent possible risk factors that leads to this type of disease.

6.5   Risk Factors

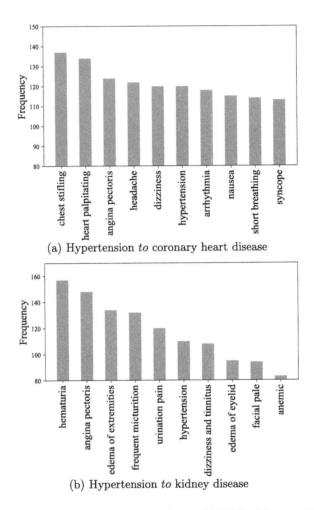

(a) Hypertension *to* coronary heart disease

(b) Hypertension *to* kidney disease

Fig. 8. Statistics of top 10 words/phrases highlighted by attention.

We further make statistics on the words or phrases to explore which factors in the texts exactly are key for developing into coronary heart disease or kidney disease in hypertension patients. Specifically, we first gather the top three words or phrases which have higher attention weights in the textual description information, and then show the top ten from all of them, as shown in Fig. 8. We can find, for leading to coronary heart disease, the phrases *"chest stifling"*, *"heart palpitating"*, *"angina pectoris"* and *"headache"*, etc., are the top ten keywords for indicating the patient condition. These symptoms can be regarded as risk factors for leading to coronary heart disease in hypertension patients. Note that these symptoms discovered by our system are much restricted by our used dataset, and do not form any clinical or medical suggestions.

For leading to kidney disease, the words *"hematuria"*, *"angina pectoris"*, *"edema of extremities"* and *"frequent micturition"*, etc., are the top ten keywords describing the corresponding patient condition. Intuitively, we can draw a conclusion that a hypertension patient involves multiple symptoms of Fig. 8(a) at the same time, and he or she is very likely to have coronary heart disease. If this patient involves multiple symptoms of Fig. 8(b), he or she is very likely to have kidney disease.

Table 4. Results from coronary heart disease and kidney disease to hypertension. Δ means the difference between the score in this table and the score in reversed dataset at Table 3. Note that we use both textual and numerical features for all models.

Model	CHD		Kidney	
	F1 score (%)	Δ	F1 score (%)	Δ
CNN	85.6	1.4	84.2	-2.3
BiLSTM	87.8	2.1	83.4	-2.9
CBiLSTM	89.6	2.8	85.1	-2.1
Ours	93.5	1.6	89.4	-1.2

6.6 Diseases Association

In this paper, we aim to study multiple diseases association from hypertension to coronary heart disease and kidney disease. A question can be naturally thrown: can CHD or kidney disease directly lead to hypertension? Therefore, we construct the datasets of (CHD → hypertension) and (kidney disease → hypertension), following the previous construction process, and conduct experiments based on the two reversed pairs of datasets.

The results are shown in Table 4 on both (kidney disease → hypertension, CHD → hypertension) datasets, we can find that F1 scores are as significant as that in Table 3. So we can say that the underlying association from kidney disease to hypertension and from CHD to hypertension are both sufficient. The observations coincide with the medical and clinical findings [24,28] that the associations between hypertension and coronary heart disease, or the hypertension and kidney disease are mutual and entangled.

7 Conclusion

We propose a dual-attention neural network model by integrating BiLSTM and CNN for the prediction of coronary heart disease and kidney disease in hypertension patients. Based on the constructed dataset from raw EHR data, the proposed model outperforms traditional statistical models and neural baseline systems by a large margin. Meanwhile, the attention mechanism captures risk factors that lead to coronary heart disease and kidney disease in hypertension patients. In future, we will explore the associated prediction from coronary heart disease and kidney disease to hypertension.

Acknowledgements. This work is supported by the National Natural Science Foundation of China (No. 61702121) and a research grant (No. LAI202301) from the Laboratory of Language and Artificial Intelligence, Center for Linguistics and Applied Linguistics, Guangdong University of Foreign Studies.

References

1. Agarwal, S., Ghanty, P., Pal, N.R.: Identification of a small set of plasma signalling proteins using neural network for prediction of Alzheimer's disease. Bioinformatics **31**(15), 2505–2513 (2015)
2. Akram, P., Li, L.: Prediction of missing common genes for disease pairs using network based module separation. In: Proceedings of IEEE International Conference on Computational Advances in Bio and Medical Sciences, p. 1 (2017)
3. Aspelund, T., Thorgeirsson, G., Sigurdsson, G., Gudnason, V.: Estimation of 10-year risk of fatal cardiovascular disease and coronary heart disease in Iceland with results comparable with those of the systematic coronary risk evaluation project. Eur. J. Cardiovasc. Prevent. Rehabil. **14**(6), 761–768 (2007)
4. Bahdanau, D., Cho, K., Bengio, Y.: Neural machine translation by jointly learning to align and translate. arXiv:1409.0473 (2014)
5. Beunza, J., et al.: Comparison of machine learning algorithms for clinical event prediction (risk of coronary heart disease). J. Biomed. Inform. **97**, 99217 (2019)
6. Chambless, L.E., et al.: Coronary heart disease risk prediction in the atherosclerosis risk in communities (ARIC) study. J. Clin. Epidemiol. **56**(9), 880–890 (2003)
7. Chawla, N.V.: Data mining for imbalanced datasets: an overview. In: Maimon, O., Rokach, L. (eds.) Data Mining and Knowledge Discovery Handbook, pp. 853–867. Springer, Boston (2005). https://doi.org/10.1007/0-387-25465-X_40
8. Chen, G.B., et al.: Performance of risk prediction for inflammatory bowel disease based on genotyping platform and genomic risk score method. BMC Med. Genet. **18**(1), 94 (2017)
9. Chen, L., Chen, B., Ren, Y., Ji, D.: Long short-term memory RNN for biomedical named entity recognition. BMC Bioinform. **18**(1), 462 (2017)
10. Chen, R., et al.: 3-year risk prediction of coronary heart disease in hypertension patients: a preliminary study. In: Proceedings of International Conference of the IEEE Engineering in Medicine and Biology Society, pp. 1182–1185 (2017)
11. Chen, W.W., et al.: China cardiovascular diseases report 2015: a summary. J. Geriatr. Cardiol. JGC **14**(1), 1–10 (2017)
12. Cheng, Y., Wang, F., Zhang, P., Hu, J.: Risk prediction with electronic health records: a deep learning approach. In: Proceedings of the 2016 SIAM International Conference on Data Mining, pp. 432–440 (2016)
13. Chiuve, S.E., et al.: Alternative dietary indices both strongly predict risk of chronic disease. J. Nutr. **142**(6), 1009–1018 (2012)
14. Collins, G.S., Altman, D.G.: An independent external validation and evaluation of QRISK cardiovascular risk prediction: a prospective open cohort study. BMJ **339**(7713), 144–147 (2009)

15. Conglong, W., et al.: Occupational physical activity and coronary heart disease in women's health initiative observational study. J. Gerontol.: Ser. A (12), 12 (2018)
16. Cullen, P., Funke, H.: Implications of the human genome project for the identification of genetic risk of coronary heart disease and its prevention in children. Nutr. Metab. Cardiovasc. Dis. 11(5), 45–51 (2001)
17. Fan, X., Zhang, S., Zhang, S., Zhu, K., Lu, S.: Prediction of LncRNA-disease associations by integrating diverse heterogeneous information sources with RWR algorithm and positive pointwise mutual information. BMC Bioinform. 20(1), 87:1–87:12 (2019)
18. Fei, H., Chua, T., Li, C., Ji, D., Zhang, M., Ren, Y.: On the robustness of aspect-based sentiment analysis: rethinking model, data, and training. ACM Trans. Inf. Syst. 41(2), 50:1–50:32 (2023)
19. Fei, H., Ji, D., Zhang, Y., Ren, Y.: Topic-enhanced capsule network for multi-label emotion classification. IEEE/ACM Trans. Audio Speech Lang. Process. 28, 1839–1848 (2020)
20. Fei, H., Ren, Y., Ji, D.: A tree-based neural network model for biomedical event trigger detection. Inf. Sci. 512, 175–185 (2020)
21. Fei, H., Ren, Y., Zhang, Y., Ji, D., Liang, X.: Enriching contextualized language model from knowledge graph for biomedical information extraction. Brief. Bioinform. (2020)
22. Fei, H., Zhang, Y., Ren, Y., Ji, D.: A span-graph neural model for overlapping entity relation extraction in biomedical texts. Bioinformatics 374, 222–231 (2020)
23. Flynt, A., Daepp, M.I.: Diet-related chronic disease in the northeastern united states: a model-based clustering approach. Int. J. Health Geogr. 14(1), 25 (2015)
24. Frohlich, E.D.: Uric acid: a risk factor for coronary heart disease. JAMA 270(3), 378–379 (1993)
25. Glorot, X., Bengio, Y.: Understanding the difficulty of training deep feedforward neural networks. In: Proceedings of the Thirteenth International Conference on Artificial Intelligence and Statistics, pp. 249–256 (2010)
26. Guglielmelli, P., et al.: Molecular profiling of CD34 + cells in idiopathic myelofibrosis identifies a set of disease-associated genes and reveals the clinical significance of Wilms' tumor gene 1 (WT1). Stem Cells 25(1), 165–173 (2007)
27. Ha, J., Park, C., Park, C., Park, S.: IMIPMF: inferring miRNA-disease interactions using probabilistic matrix factorization. J. Biomed. Inform. 102, 103358 (2020)
28. Hall, M.E., do Carmo, J.M., da Silva, A.A., Juncos, L.A., Wang, Z., Hall, J.E.: Obesity, hypertension, and chronic kidney disease. Int. J. Nephrol. Renovasc. Dis. 7, 75 (2014)
29. Hippisleycox, J., et al.: Predicting cardiovascular risk in England and wales: prospective derivation and validation of qrisk2. BMJ 336(7659), 1475–1482 (2008)
30. Jabbar, M.A., Deekshatulu, B.L., Chandra, P.: Prediction of heart disease using random forest and feature subset selection. In: Snášel, V., Abraham, A., Krömer, P., Pant, M., Muda, A.K. (eds.) Innovations in Bio-Inspired Computing and Applications. AISC, vol. 424, pp. 187–196. Springer, Cham (2016). https://doi.org/10.1007/978-3-319-28031-8_16
31. Ji, D., Gao, J., Fei, H., Teng, C., Ren, Y.: A deep neural network model for speakers coreference resolution in legal texts. Inf. Process. Manage. 57(6), 102365 (2020)
32. Ji, D., Tao, P., Fei, H., Ren, Y.: An end-to-end joint model for evidence information extraction from court record document. Inf. Process. Manage. 57(6), 102305 (2020)
33. Kingma, D.P., Ba, J.: Adam: a method for stochastic optimization. arXiv preprint arXiv:1412.6980 (2014)

34. Lai, S., Xu, L., Liu, K., Zhao, J.: Recurrent convolutional neural networks for text classification. In: Proceedings of the Twenty-Ninth AAAI Conference on Artificial Intelligence, pp. 2267–2273 (2015)
35. Le, D.H., Dang, V.T.: Ontology-based disease similarity network for disease gene prediction. Viet. J. Comput. Sci. **3**(3), 1–9 (2016)
36. Liang, M., Qian, L., Jiang, Y., Zhao, H., Niu, W.: Genetically elevated circulating homocysteine concentrations increase the risk of diabetic kidney disease in Chinese diabetic patients. J. Cell Mol. Med. **23**(4), 2794–2800 (2019)
37. Liu, J., Zhang, Z., Razavian, N.: Deep EHR: chronic disease prediction using medical notes. In: Proceedings of the Machine Learning for Healthcare Conference, pp. 440–464 (2018)
38. Liu, Z., et al.: Entity recognition from clinical texts via recurrent neural network. BMC Med. Inform. Decis. Mak. **17**(2), 67 (2017)
39. Luyckx, V.A., et al.: A developmental approach to the prevention of hypertension and kidney disease: a report from the low birth weight and nephron number working group. Lancet **390**(10092), 424–428 (2017)
40. Mason, L., Baxter, J., Bartlett, P.L., Frean, M.R.: Boosting algorithms as gradient descent. In: Proceedings of Advances in Neural Information Processing Systems, pp. 512–518 (2000)
41. McCallum, A., Nigam, K., et al.: A comparison of event models for naive bayes text classification. In: Proceedings of AAAI-98 Workshop on Learning for Text Categorization, pp. 41–48 (1998)
42. Meng, X., Zou, Q., Rodriguez-Paton, A., Zeng, X.: Iteratively collective prediction of disease-gene associations through the incomplete network. In: Proceedings of IEEE International Conference on Bioinformatics and Biomedicine, pp. 1324–1330 (2017)
43. Misghina, W., Margaret, S., Herrington, W.G., Clare, B., Mark, W.: Socioeconomic disadvantage and the risk of advanced chronic kidney disease: results from a cohort study with 1.4 million participants. Nephrol. Dialysis Transpl. **35**, 1562–1570 (2019)
44. Polonsky, T.S., et al.: Coronary artery calcium score and risk classification for coronary heart disease prediction: the multi-ethnic study of atherosclerosis. JAMA **303**(16), 1610–1616 (2010)
45. Rajkomar, A., et al.: Scalable and accurate deep learning with electronic health records. NPJ Digit. Med. **1**(1), 18 (2018)
46. Ren, Y., Fei, H., Ji, D.: Drug-drug interaction extraction using a span-based neural network model. In: Proceedings of the 2019 IEEE International Conference on Bioinformatics and Biomedicine, pp. 1237–1239 (2019)
47. Ren, Y., Fei, H., Liang, X., Ji, D., Cheng, M.: A hybrid neural network model for predicting kidney disease in hypertension patients based on electronic health records. BMC Med. Inform. Decis. Mak. **19**(2), 51 (2019)
48. Ren, Y., Fei, H., Peng, Q.: Detecting the scope of negation and speculation in biomedical texts by using recursive neural network. In: 2018 IEEE International Conference on Bioinformatics and Biomedicine, pp. 739–742 (2018)
49. Ren, Y., Ji, D.: Neural networks for deceptive opinion spam detection: an empirical study. Inf. Sci. **385–386**, 213–224 (2017)
50. Ren, Y., Ji, D., Ren, H.: Context-augmented convolutional neural networks for twitter sarcasm detection. Neurocomputing **308**, 1–7 (2018)
51. Ren, Y., Wang, Z., Peng, Q., Ji, D.: A knowledge-augmented neural network model for sarcasm detection. Inf. Process. Manage. **60**(6), 103521 (2023)

52. Ren, Y., Yan, M., Ji, D.: A hierarchical neural network model with user and product attention for deceptive reviews detection. Inf. Sci. **604**, 1–10 (2022)
53. Ren, Y., Zhang, Y., Zhang, M., Ji, D.: Context-sensitive twitter sentiment classification using neural network. In: Proceedings of the Thirtieth AAAI Conference on Artificial Intelligence, pp. 215–221 (2016)
54. Ren, Y., Zhang, Y., Zhang, M., Ji, D.: Improving twitter sentiment classification using topic-enriched multi-prototype word embeddings. In: Proceedings of the Thirtieth AAAI Conference on Artificial Intelligence, pp. 3038–3044 (2016)
55. Tang, D., Qin, B., Liu, T.: Document modeling with gated recurrent neural network for sentiment classification. In: Proceedings of Conference on Empirical Methods in Natural Language Processing, pp. 1422–1432 (2015)
56. Wang, Z., Wu, Z., Wang, R., Ren, Y.: Twitter sarcasm detection exploiting a context-based model. In: Wang, J., et al. (eds.) WISE 2015. LNCS, vol. 9418, pp. 77–91. Springer, Cham (2015). https://doi.org/10.1007/978-3-319-26190-4_6
57. Weedon, M.N., et al.: Combining information from common type 2 diabetes risk polymorphisms improves disease prediction. PLoS Med. **3**(10), 374 (2006)
58. Wilson, P.W., D'Agostino, R.B., Levy, D., Belanger, A.M., Silbershatz, H., Kannel, W.B.: Prediction of coronary heart disease using risk factor categories. Circulation **97**(18), 1837–1847 (1998)
59. Wray, N.R., Goddard, M.E., Visscher, P.M.: Prediction of individual genetic risk to disease from genome-wide association studies. Genome Res. **17**(10), 1520–1528 (2007)
60. Yang, Z., Yang, D., Dyer, C., He, X., Smola, A., Hovy, E.: Hierarchical attention networks for document classification. In: Proceedings of Conference of the North American Chapter of the Association for Computational Linguistics, pp. 1480–1489 (2017)
61. Zeng, D., Sun, C., Lin, L., Liu, B.: LSTM-CRF for drug-named entity recognition. Entropy **19**(6), 283 (2017)
62. Zhang, Q., Ai, Y., Dong, H., Wang, J., Xu, L.: Circulating oxidized low-density lipoprotein is a strong risk factor for the early stage of coronary heart disease. IUBMB Life **71**(2), 277–282 (2019)
63. Zhang, Y., Ibaraki, M., Schwartz, F.W.: Disease surveillance using online news: dengue and zika in tropical countries. J. Biomed. Inform. **102**, 103374 (2020)
64. Zhao, K., Ji, D., He, F., Liu, Y., Ren, Y.: Document-level event causality identification via graph inference mechanism. Inf. Sci. **561**, 115–129 (2021)
65. Zhao, Z., Yang, Z., Lin, H., Wang, J., Gao, S.: A protein-protein interaction extraction approach based on deep neural network. Int. J. Data Min. Bioinform. **15**(2), 145–164 (2016)

Constructing a Multi-scale Medical Knowledge Graph from Electronic Medical Records

Yikai Zhou, Ziyi Wang, Miao Li$^{(\boxtimes)}$, and Ji Wu

Department of Electronic Engineering, Tsinghua University, Beijing 100084, China
{zyj21,wangziyi21}@mails.tsinghua.edu.cn,
{miao-li,wuji_ee}@mail.tsinghua.edu.cn

Abstract. Knowledge graphs play a crucial role in the medical field. Most existing knowledge graphs are manually created by experts or extracted from medical encyclopedias, resulting in the omission of valuable knowledge from medical clinical practice. Entities like diseases and symptoms in medicine exist at different levels, but current knowledge graphs fail to handle the induction and integration of this multi-scale information effectively. In our study, we constructed a knowledge graph that better aligns with real clinical data and effectively integrates multi-scale medical information by performing data preparation, medical entity extraction, negation handling, relation extraction, and graph cleaning. The reliability and rationality of the knowledge graph have been verified through subjective and objective assessments.

Keywords: multi-scale knowledge · medical knowledge graph · knowledge graph construction

1 Introduction

Knowledge graphs express and store a large number of knowledge elements such as entities, concepts, properties, and relationships in a structured way, forming a knowledge network with associative relationships. It is widely used in various fields such as healthcare [9], military [8], and finance [2]. With the development of neural networks, knowledge graphs can provide support for other deep learning tasks more effectively [11] and can also expand the scale of knowledge graphs through deep learning [16], by which research on knowledge graphs is receiving more and more attention from researchers.

Unlike other fields, medical knowledge has stronger specialization and higher complexity. As shown in Fig. 1, this complexity is reflected in the multi-scale characteristics of various types of medical knowledge such as symptoms, diseases, signs, and locations, for example, "high fever" and "low fever" are both finer-scale symptoms of "fever". In many tasks in the medical field, such as assisted diagnosis, medical Q&A, and ICD coding, information at different scales plays an important role in refining task results and improving method robustness.

H. Xu et al. (Eds.): CHIP 2023, CCIS 1993, pp. 392–404, 2024.
https://doi.org/10.1007/978-981-99-9864-7_25

For example, in an intelligent assisted diagnosis task, if an intelligent diagnosis system diagnoses a patient with "acute pharyngitis" as "acute upper respiratory infection", it may seem like an incorrect diagnosis. However, in reality, "acute pharyngitis" is a subclass of "acute upper respiratory infection", so such an error may not be strictly considered a mistake. Perhaps if the patient provides more detailed information at a finer scale, the model can correct the result to "acute pharyngitis". However, current medical knowledge graphs generally ignore the multi-scale characteristics of medical knowledge and do not effectively integrate the hierarchical relationships between multi-scale medical knowledge into the knowledge graph.

In terms of knowledge storage, most knowledge graphs store knowledge in the form of triples (head entity, relationship, tail entity). The medical knowledge described by each triplet is absolutely relevant (it can be understood that the confidence level of each triplet is 1). However, in clinical practice, diseases are often not absolutely related to other medical entities. For a certain disease, some symptoms may occur in almost all patients with the disease, while others may only appear in some patients. Whether the symptom appears in the patient will be affected by other symptoms and signs of the patient. In knowledge graphs stored in triple form, the relationships between these symptoms and diseases are often blurred into the deterministic relationship of "disease-related symptoms", ignoring the modeling of the degree of correlation between diseases and symptoms, resulting in information loss.

For medical knowledge, many connections between medical entities exist implicitly in clinical text data, rather than explicitly in the cognition of medical experts or medical encyclopedias. Currently, some researchers are constructing medical knowledge graphs based on electronic medical record data [5,6,12,18]. However, in the process of extracting knowledge, they overlook the negation expressions in medical record texts. For a patient, the descriptions of "having a fever" and "not having a fever" have completely different meanings. If the content related to negation words such as "no" and "deny" is not handled separately, it will inevitably lead to errors in the information contained in the constructed knowledge graph.

To address the shortcomings of current medical knowledge graphs, we have constructed a knowledge graph that is more in line with real clinical data and incorporates hierarchical relationships between multi-scale knowledge based on electronic medical record data, using a combination of manual construction and automatic construction. We have verified the reliability of the constructed knowledge graph and the rationality of the graph construction method through subjective evaluation by medical experts and objective evaluation through experiments.

The main contributions of this article are as follows: 1. Believing that information at different scales is crucial for various applications in the medical field, we effectively organize and integrate the hierarchical relationships between medical entities of different scales into the constructed knowledge graph. These entities with hierarchical relationships include diseases, symptoms, signs, and locations. 2. In the process of mining implicit connections between medical entities from electronic medical record data, this paper proposes a new method to model the correlation degree between medical entities, which ensures the rationality and reliability of the medical knowledge graph. 3. When mining the relationships between medical entities through electronic medical record texts, we handle the entities related to negation words in the medical record texts separately, further improving the quality of the knowledge graph. This is a feature that other related works do not possess.

The remaining parts of the article will be presented in the following order. In Sect. 2, we will review related work on the construction of medical knowledge graphs. Section 3 will introduce the methods used to construct the knowledge graph in this article. Section 4 will describe how we evaluate the quality of the constructed knowledge graph. Section 5 will provide a summary of the work done in this article.

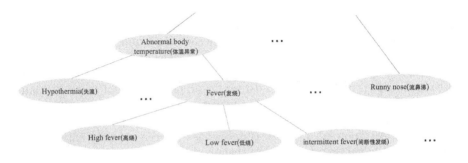

Fig. 1. In the medical field, entities have multi-scale characteristics.

2   Related Work

With the advancement of technology in the field of knowledge graphs, the construction of specialized and comprehensive medical knowledge graphs has become a hot research topic. The construction of medical knowledge graphs is driven by both medical knowledge resources from professional institutions or open-source, such as UMLS [1] and SNOMED CT [3], and real world clinical medical data.

There are some works constructing graphs based on co-occurrence relationships between entities. Finlayson et al. [4]analyzed and merged medical terms using over 20 million clinical medical data spanning over 19 years, constructing a co-occurrence matrix of 1 million medical clinical concepts to quantify the relationships between medical terms. Some works focus on designing a knowledge graph construction system for specific data, which are mainly based on rules. Lin et al. [7] proposed the MEDLedge model, which employs a hierarchical segmentation approach and a voting algorithm to extract entities and relationships from clinical data and construct a knowledge graph. Shi et al. [13] utilized data from the Health Information System from Zhejiang, China, to propose a medical information integration model that standardizes heterogeneous medical information into a shareable and consistent format. Additionally, some constructed knowledge bases are disease-centered, without relation exploitation between other types of entities. Rotmensch et al. [10]extracted medical concepts from over 270 thousand patient records, utilizing probability models like Bayesian models to automatically construct a knowledge graph that links diseases and symptoms, creating a high-quality knowledge base from medical records. Zhao et al. [18] sampled 992 medical records, representing medical entities as nodes and co-occurrence relationships as edges, to establish an EMR-based medical knowledge network (EMKN). Furthermore, Zhao et al. [17] integrated EMKN with Markov Random Fields (MRF) for general medical knowledge representation, including five types of medical entities, and designed different energy functions based on inference scenarios. Li et al. [6] constructed a knowledge graph from 16 million clinical records and comprehensively described the entire graph construction process. In contrast to traditional triplets, they proposed a new quadruplet structure that leverages some attributes, including co-occurrence probability, reliability, and specificity, to better express the relationship between entities. However, their approach to constructing knowledge graphs only considers the relationships between diseases and other types of medical entities, while neglecting the interconnections between entities beyond diseases. Considering the large-scale knowledge graph, Yu et al. [15] built the first large-scale publicly available biomedical knowledge graph, containing millions of bilingual concepts and terms and 7.3 million relation triplets, which are all generated algorithmically without human participation.

To the best of our knowledge, there is no work that has taken advantage of the multi-scale hierarchical relationships between entities in building a knowledge graph based on electronic medical record texts. Additionally, most of them only consider the correlation information between diseases and other types of entities, while ignoring the correlation information between entities other than diseases. Furthermore, no researchers have performed additional effective handling of negative expressions in the process of constructing knowledge graphs from electronic medical records, which greatly affects the quality of the knowledge graphs.

3   Method

In this study, we comprehensively consider the professionalism of medical knowledge and the authenticity of clinical knowledge. We determine the scale information of medical entities based on expert experience and obtain the entity relationships from medical records through automated methods. After five steps including data preparation, medical entity extraction, negation handling, relationship extraction, and graph cleaning, we construct a high-quality multi-scale medical knowledge graph. The overall construction process is shown in Fig. 2.

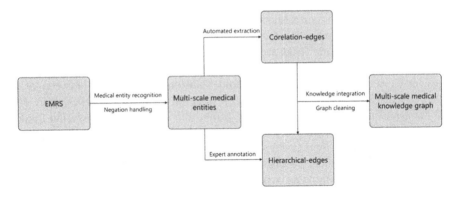

Fig. 2. Framework of our method to build a multi-scale medical knowledge graph.

3.1 Data Preparation

We aimed to construct a knowledge graph focused on lung diseases with a hierarchical structure. For these lung diseases, we sampled some medical records from the electronic medical record database, ensuring the distribution of medical records related to different diagnoses was as uniform as possible. These records will be used for both the construction of a multi-scale medical knowledge graph and as a dataset for subsequent validation of the quality of the knowledge graph.

Each medical record includes multiple sections such as "admission record", "initial course record", "examination report", and "discharge record". Each section contains multiple fields. To ensure comprehensive coverage of knowledge, we will use a total of 7 sections including "admission record", "examination report", and "discharge record", and 24 fields including "chief complaint", "present illness history", and "main symptoms" for the construction of this knowledge graph.

In addition to medical record data, the hierarchical relationships between diseases, symptoms, signs, and locations are essential for constructing a multi-scale medical knowledge graph. They organize the hierarchical information between medical entities and establish connections between the information hierarchy and diagnostic hierarchy. This hierarchical knowledge is annotated by medical experts.

3.2 Medical Entity Extraction

After obtaining the medical records required to construct the knowledge graph, we need to extract medical entities of different scales from the unstructured medical record texts. In the medical record texts, there are medical entities such as diseases, symptoms, signs, and medicine which are important for accurate diagnosis. It is crucial to extract these entities effectively, accurately, and comprehensively for the high-quality construction of the knowledge graph.

First, we remove irrelevant information such as symbols and stop words from the medical record texts. Then we perform medical entity recognition. Regarding the methods for entity recognition, we compared statistical-based recognition methods with dictionary-based bidirectional maximum matching recognition methods. It was observed that the statistical-based recognition method tends to identify entities at a very rough level. Entities with finer granularity often have longer text representations, and the statistical-based method often recognizes a fine-grained entity as multiple coarse-grained entities. For instance, the term "ANCA-associated vasculitis" is identified as three separate entities: "ANCA", "associated", and "vasculitis". "Chronic kidney disease stage 5" is recognized as "chronic" and "kidney disease". Obviously, this is very disadvantageous for constructing a medical knowledge graph with multiple scales of information. In contrast, the dictionary-based bidirectional maximum matching method effectively resolves this issue. Consequently, the dictionary-based bidirectional maximum matching algorithm is employed in this study for extracting medical entities.

3.3   Negation Handling

During the entity extraction process, we have observed a significant presence of disease denials and negative symptoms in the medical records. For instance, in the phrase "no fever symptoms, without vomiting", both "fever" and "vomiting" are negative symptoms. If these negative symptoms are not appropriately addressed, they may be mistakenly identified as positive symptoms, leading to confusion and compromising the quality of the knowledge graph.

To mitigate this issue, we employ text understanding techniques to identify entities associated with disease denials and negative symptoms in the medical records. Subsequently, we process these entities separately and incorporate the negation semantic information into the knowledge graph.

3.4   Relation Extraction

Furthermore, we need to extract the relationships between entities from medical records. Unlike conventional knowledge graphs that store entity relationships using triplets, we calculate a weight for each possible triplet to measure its confidence.

We refer to the graph construction method of TextGCN [14] and model the medical record text as a disease document node. By calculating the TF-IDF weights between the document node and various medical entities in the medical record, we model the relevance between disease and non-disease entities. For the relevance between non-disease medical entities in the medical record text, we use PMI weights for modeling.

When calculating the weights between nodes in the knowledge graph, we take into account that the number of medical records for each diagnosis varies and the length of each medical record text is also different. Therefore, we consider both factors and normalize the weights to a range between 0 and 1.

In addition, for entities with hierarchical relationships in the hierarchy system, considering that the weight reflects the relevance between two entities and the hierarchical relationship is annotated by medical experts, we believe that medical entities with hierarchical relationships have a strong correlation, so we directly set their weight to 1.

3.5   Graph Cleaning

After completing the preliminary construction of the knowledge graph, there remains a significant amount of redundant information that needs to be processed. Whether it is introducing the relationship between disease and non-disease entities through TF-IDF or introducing the relationship between non-disease entities through PMI, a considerable amount of noise is introduced into the constructed knowledge graph. The abundance of noise makes the connection between different diseases relatively similar and difficult to distinguish.

Therefore, to enhance the diversity of connections between different diseases in the graph, we undertake a cleaning process on the preliminary constructed knowledge graph. Since the weights between entities directly reflect their relevance, we establish thresholds for both PMI weights and TF-IDF weights. By setting these thresholds, we delete edges with lower relevance, thereby further improving the quality of the knowledge graph.

4   Knowledge Graph Quality Assessment

In order to validate our method, we selected 28 lung diseases that have hierarchical relationships with each other as the disease system within the knowledge graph. We sampled a total of 4548 medical records with main diagnoses that fall within the aforementioned 28 diseases from a large electronic medical record database; and ensured that the distribution of medical records related to different diagnoses was as uniform as possible. Based on the above process, we constructed a multi-scale medical knowledge graph containing 21,950 entities and 1,540,375 edges, in which 3346 multi-scale entities are included, while the numbers of each type of edge are illustrated in Table 1. The quality of this knowledge graph was then verified through subjective and objective evaluations.

During the subjective evaluation, we primarily focused on two questions: 1. For sibling disease pairs, whether the differences reflected in the knowledge graph support the differentiation of the two diseases? 2. For parent-child disease pairs, whether there is consistency at the scale level between the hierarchy of diseases and the hierarchy of related entities? In objective evaluation, we verified the quality of the constructed knowledge graph and the effectiveness of the knowledge graph construction method through a disease classification task.

4.1   Subjective Assessment

After completing the construction of the knowledge graph, we conducted a preliminary evaluation to assess the quality of the knowledge graph, verifying

Table 1. Number of Different Types of Edges in our Knowledge Graph.

hierarchical edge	TF-IDF edge	PMI edge
3346	127403	1409626

whether the information reflected by different diseases in the knowledge graph
has discriminative significance. We selected some representative sibling disease
pairs and parent-child disease pairs from the disease tree, extracted disease subgraphs from the knowledge graph, compared the disease subgraphs, and counted
the discriminative entities between disease pairs. Medical experts then evaluated the discriminative entities extracted from the knowledge graph to verify
whether they conform to the clinical significance of discrimination. Our method
for extracting discriminative entities is illustrated in Fig. 3.

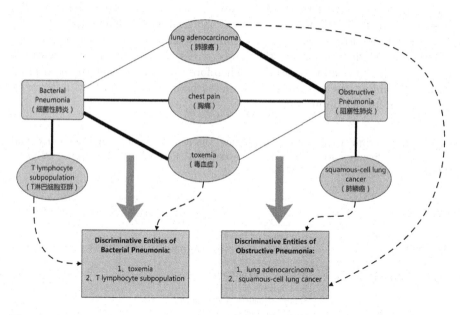

Fig. 3. This figure illustrates our method for extracting discriminative entities. The
thickness of the lines connecting diseases and their related entities represents the degree
of correlation between them. In two scenarios, the associated entities of a disease are
extracted as discriminative entities. 1) The entity is only associated with that disease
and not with its sibling diseases. 2) The degree of correlation between the entity and
the disease is much higher compared to its sibling diseases (shown as a significant
difference in line thickness in the figure).

When verifying the information difference between sibling disease pairs, we
took "obstructive pneumonia" and "bacterial pneumonia" as examples. We
sorted the discriminative entities reflected by these two diseases in the knowledge

graph based on their weights. We found that in the knowledge graph, the discriminative entities of "obstructive pneumonia" include "pulmonary squamous cell carcinoma", "malignant tumor immunotherapy", "small cell lung cancer", etc., while the discriminative entities of "bacterial pneumonia" include "T lymphocyte subset", "acid-fast staining", "serum myoglobin", etc. We asked doctors to label these high-confidence discriminating entities extracted from the knowledge graph. The results of the doctor's labeling are shown in Table 2. (where ✓ represents approval, × represents objection, ⋆ represents uncertainty), it is evident that doctors also believe these entities have significant discriminatory value for these two diseases in clinical practice. In addition, relevant medical knowledge further demonstrates the reliability of the knowledge graph. Medical knowledge shows that the cause of bacterial pneumonia is bacterial infection, and common pathogens include Streptococcus pneumoniae, Haemophilus influenzae, Staphylococcus aureus, etc.; while the cause of obstructive pneumonia is chronic obstructive pulmonary disease (COPD) and other respiratory system diseases, leading to airway narrowing, gas exchange disorders, etc. We observed that the discriminative entities of bacterial pneumonia primarily consist of examination entities, while the discriminative entities of obstructive pneumonia mainly include some obstructive lung diseases, which are consistent with the clinical etiology of the two diseases. Therefore, we believe that the associated entities of sibling diseases in the constructed knowledge graph have differential information for discrimination.

Table 2. Discriminative Entities of Sibling Disease Pair(Bacterial Pneumonia and Obstructive Pneumonia), in which ✓ represents APPROVAL, × represents OBJECTION, ⋆ represents UNCERTAINTY.

Disease	Discriminative Entities from Knowledge Graph	Expert Annotation
Bacterial Pneumonia (细菌性肺炎)	T lymphocyte subpopulation(T淋巴细胞亚群)	✓
	acid-fast stain(抗酸染色)	✓
	acute upper respiratory tract infection(急性上呼吸道感染)	✓
	absolute count(绝对计数)	⋆
	serum myoglobin(血清肌红蛋白)	✓
	vena epigastrica(腹壁静脉)	×
	Serum troponin T(血清肌钙蛋白T)	⋆
	gram stain(革兰染色)	✓
Obstructive Pneumonia (阻塞性肺炎)	squamous-cell lung cancer(肺鳞癌)	✓
	Castleman disease(castleman病)	✓
	aversion to cold with fever(恶寒发热)	⋆
	immunotherapy for malignant tumors(恶性肿瘤免疫治疗)	✓
	lung-distension(肺胀)	⋆
	lung adenocarcinoma(肺腺癌)	✓
	small cell lung cancer(小细胞肺癌)	✓
	liver puncture(肝脏穿刺)	×

In addition, we also observed the consistency of discriminative entities between parent-child disease pairs, confirming the consistency of the scale level between superordinate and subordinate disease entities and other types of superordinate and subordinate entities. We took the three diseases "respiratory tract infection", "acute upper respiratory tract infection" and "pulmonary infection" as examples. "Acute upper respiratory tract infection" and "pulmonary infection" are both sub-disease nodes of "respiratory tract infection". We found that in the knowledge graph, "neck" is the discriminative entity for "respiratory tract infection", while the sub-entities "pharynx" and "tonsil" of "neck" are the discriminative entities for "acute upper respiratory tract infection". "Pain" and "enlargement" are the discriminative entities for "respiratory tract infection", while the sub-entities "chest pain" and "enlarged cardiac silhouette" of "pain" and "enlargement" are the discriminative entities for "pulmonary infection". Figure 4 shows the consistency of diseases and symptoms in terms of scale in the knowledge graph. It can be seen that the constructed knowledge graph not only reflects the differences in related entities between sibling diseases but also the associated entities of parent-child diseases have consistency at the scale level, which basically meets our expectations for the quality of the knowledge graph.

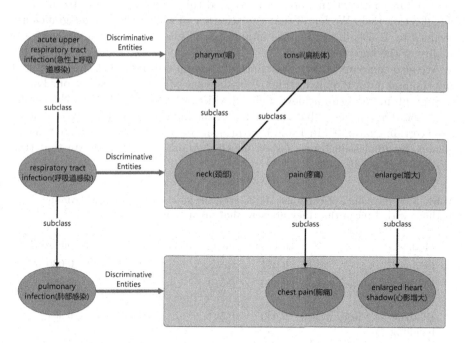

Fig. 4. For parent-child disease pairs (take "Respiratory Tract Infection", "Acute Upper Respiratory Tract Infection" and "Pulmonary Infection" as examples), there is consistency at the scale level between the hierarchy of diseases and the hierarchy of related entities.

4.2 Objective Assessment

In order to further verify the quality of the constructed knowledge graph, we designed a simple disease classification task. We used medical records as input, extracted all medical entities from the records, and connected them to the knowledge graph. Based on these entities, we extracted a subgraph from the knowledge graph and directly classified it into 28 disease categories.

It is worth mentioning that in this validation task, we did not have any model training process. For each subgraph of medical records, we set the node features as 28 dimensions, with each dimension representing the TF-IDF weight value of the node with respect to the 28 diseases. The PMI weights between nodes in the subgraph were stored using an adjacency matrix. Then, we read out each subgraph node into a 1*28 dimensional vector, and after applying softmax operation, we unexpectedly achieved 44.0% accuracy in the 28-class classification of the medical records. It should be noted that if these test data are randomly classified into 28 categories, the performance can only achieve an accuracy of 5.1%. Based on this, we constructed a knowledge graph without considering the handling of negation words; and applied this knowledge graph to the same classification task. We found that the accuracy of the classification significantly declined to 41.5%, indicating the importance of negation word handling for the quality of the knowledge graph.

We also compared the performance of Bert on our dataset. Clearly, without any training data, Bert is unable to classify these diseases. However, our knowledge graph method can achieve a classification accuracy of 44.0% in the case of zero-shot. This suggests that the quality of the knowledge graph we constructed has a certain guarantee. In Table 3, we present the performance of different methods on the 28-classification task, in which methods with "(*)" mean that they are zero-shot predictions.

Table 3. Performance of Different Methods on the 28-classification Task(Among them, methods with * mean that they are zero-shot predictions.)

Method	accuracy	macro-precision	macro-recall	macro-f1
random(*)	0.051	0.028	0.033	0.030
KG-based w/o negation handling(*)	0.415	0.519	0.419	0.464
KG-based w/ negation handling(*)	0.440	0.541	0.443	0.487
Bert	0.521	0.492	0.510	0.501

5 Conclusion

In this paper, we constructed a multi-scale medical knowledge graph by mining the hidden connections between medical entities in electronic medical record data and introducing medical multi-scale information through expert annotation. It is worth noting that we also considered the impact of negation words in medical record texts on the quality of the knowledge graph and made additional processing during the construction of the knowledge graph. Subsequently, we preliminarily confirmed the quality of the constructed knowledge graph through subjective evaluation by medical experts, and further confirmed the effectiveness of our multi-scale knowledge graph construction method and the importance of handling negation through objective evaluation in experiments.

Acknowledgments. The work is supported by National Key R&D Program of China (2021ZD0113404).

References

1. Bodenreider, O.: The unified medical language system (UMLs): integrating biomedical terminology. Nucleic Acids Res. **32**(suppl_1), D267–D270 (2004)
2. Cheng, D., Yang, F., Wang, X., Zhang, Y., Zhang, L.: Knowledge graph-based event embedding framework for financial quantitative investments. In: Proceedings of the 43rd International ACM SIGIR Conference on Research and Development in Information Retrieval, pp. 2221–2230 (2020)
3. Donnelly, K., et al.: SNOMED-CT: the advanced terminology and coding system for ehealth. Stud. Health Technol. Inform. **121**, 279 (2006)
4. Finlayson, S.G., LePendu, P., Shah, N.H.: Building the graph of medicine from millions of clinical narratives. Sci. Data **1**(1), 1–9 (2014)
5. Li, L., et al.: A method to learn embedding of a probabilistic medical knowledge graph: algorithm development. JMIR Med. Inform. **8**(5), e17645 (2020)
6. Li, L., et al.: Real-world data medical knowledge graph: construction and applications. Artif. Intell. Med. **103**, 101817 (2020)
7. Lin, K., Wu, M., Wang, X., Pan, Y.: MEDLedge: a Q&A based system for constructing medical knowledge base. In: 2016 11th International Conference on Computer Science & Education (ICCSE), pp. 485–489. IEEE (2016)
8. Liu, C., Yu, Y., Li, X., Wang, P.: Application of entity relation extraction method under CRF and syntax analysis tree in the construction of military equipment knowledge graph. IEEE Access **8**, 200581–200588 (2020)
9. Liu, W., Yin, L., Wang, C., Liu, F., Ni, Z., et al.: Multitask healthcare management recommendation system leveraging knowledge graph. J. Healthcare Eng. **2021** (2021)
10. Rotmensch, M., Halpern, Y., Tlimat, A., Horng, S., Sontag, D.: Learning a health knowledge graph from electronic medical records. Sci. Rep. **7**(1), 5994 (2017)
11. Sang, L., Xu, M., Qian, S., Wu, X.: Knowledge graph enhanced neural collaborative recommendation. Expert Syst. Appl. **164**, 113992 (2021)
12. Shen, Y., et al.: CBN: constructing a clinical Bayesian network based on data from the electronic medical record. J. Biomed. Inform. **88**, 1–10 (2018)
13. Shi, L., et al.: Semantic health knowledge graph: semantic integration of heterogeneous medical knowledge and services. BioMed Res. Int. **2017** (2017)
14. Yao, L., Mao, C., Luo, Y.: Graph convolutional networks for text classification. In: Proceedings of the AAAI Conference on Artificial Intelligence, vol. 33, pp. 7370–7377 (2019)

15. Yu, S., et al.: Bios: an algorithmically generated biomedical knowledge graph. arXiv preprint arXiv:2203.09975 (2022)
16. Zhang, Z., Zhuang, F., Zhu, H., Shi, Z., Xiong, H., He, Q.: Relational graph neural network with hierarchical attention for knowledge graph completion. In: Proceedings of the AAAI Conference on Artificial Intelligence, vol. 34, pp. 9612–9619 (2020)
17. Zhao, C., Jiang, J., Guan, Y., Guo, X., He, B.: EMR-based medical knowledge representation and inference via Markov random fields and distributed representation learning. Artif. Intell. Med. **87**, 49–59 (2018)
18. Zhao, C., Jiang, J., Xu, Z., Guan, Y.: A study of EMR-based medical knowledge network and its applications. Comput. Methods Programs Biomed. **143**, 13–23 (2017)

Time Series Prediction Models for Assisting the Diagnosis and Treatment of Gouty Arthritis

Tao Chen[1], Weihan Qiu[1], Fangjie Zhu[2], Hengdong Zhu[1], Shunhao Li[1], Maojie Wang[2,3,4(✉)], and Tianyong Hao[1]

[1] School of Computer Science, South China Normal University, Guangzhou, China
{20182333059,2022010216,haoty}@m.scnu.edu.cn
[2] The Second Affiliated Hospital of Guangzhou University of Chinese Medicine (Guangdong Provincial Hospital of Chinese Medicine), Guangzhou, China
maojiewang@gzucm.edu.cn
[3] Guangdong Provincial Key Laboratory of Clinical Research on Traditional Chinese Medicine Syndrome, Guangzhou, China
[4] State Key Laboratory of Dampness, Syndrome of Chinese Medicine, The Second Affiliated Hospital of Guangzhou University of Chinese Medicine, Guangzhou, China

Abstract. Clinical gout arthritis data tracks changes as essential indicators and reflects the recurrence status of patients within several weeks after patients' medication. Although the data may contain rich patient information, it is difficult to be fully utilized due to clinical data quality issues such as various time lengths, data missing, irregular sampling, etc. Time series prediction models have the potential to deal with these data problems. This paper compares a list of time series prediction models on the indicators of patients with gouty arthritis. We collected real data from the Guangdong Provincial Traditional Chinese Medicine Hospital including 160 patients. The Bidirectional long short-term memory (Bi-LSTM) model and the Crossformer model are applied to predict future physiological indicators and the recurrence status of patients. According to the results of Bi-LSTM and Crossformer, time series prediction models demonstrate strong performance in forecasting physiological indicators and the recurrence status of patients.

Keywords: Gouty arthritis · Disease prediction · Multivariate Time series prediction · Bi-LSTM · Crossformer

1 Introduction

Gouty arthritis is a common inflammatory disease that is aroused by the sedimentation of Monosodium Urate (MSU) in joints or soft tissues, directly related to hyperuricemia caused by the disorders of purine metabolism [1]. Patients with gouty arthritis often suffer from severe arthritis pain, joint malformations and tophus, and have a high likelihood of developing various comorbidities due to hyperuricemia, mainly affecting the patient kidney and cardiovascular system [2]. The prevalence of gouty arthritis is 1% to 6.8% worldwide [3] and 1.1% in China [4]. Unfortunately, the current situation of gout disease

H. Xu et al. (Eds.): CHIP 2023, CCIS 1993, pp. 405–419, 2024.
https://doi.org/10.1007/978-981-99-9864-7_26

treatment is unsatisfactory. Many reasons are drawn out, for example, 22.7% of patients are unable to sustain their medication due to side effects such as gastric ulcers and allergic reactions [5]. Therefore, more therapeutic interventions are desperately needed to meet different requests of individuals. If a model exists for predicting disease recurrence and the alterations in physical indicators of patients with gouty arthritis in advance, based on the patient's time series data, it would be advantageous for physicians to proactively devise treatment plans and expedite the patient's recovery as swiftly as possible.

As a typical task for machine learning methods, time series prediction is mainly used to analyze ordered data and make predictions about future data based on the information hidden in the former. In recent years, with the development of artificial intelligence and machine learning technology, predictive models based on neural networks and deep learning have also attracted more and more attention. Therefore, an increasing number of neural networks are being used to learn representations of data sets that are more challenging to understand [6, 7]. Many neural network models have demonstrated excellent performance for tasks in the medical field. These successes have made researchers and scholars in the field of healthcare aware of the excellent performance of recurrent neural networks (RNN) in the representation and processing of patient data [8–14]. The time series prediction methods used in this paper are the Bi-LSTM based on improved recurrent neural network and Crossformer based on Transformer architecture.

Sequence models such as long short-term memory (LSTM) recurrent neural networks [15] have achieved advanced results in many time series prediction applications, including speech recognition [16] and myoelectric motion decoding [17]. In recent years, the application of LSTM in the biomedical field has become more and more frequent. The correlation of past events has been required taking into account among the task of making predictions in the field of medicine, where the LSTM's architecture is well suited [18]. LSTM is used to combine the analysis of episodic clinical events and continuous monitoring data in the ICU environment and to predict the deterioration of a patient's condition [19]. LSTM is used to model multivariate pediatric intensive care time series to predict diagnosis for children. Pham et al. [20] proposed an extension of the LSTM model that uses information about the patient's diagnosis to modulate the input gate of the LSTM. At the same time, the information about the patient's diagnosis and procedure or medication received is used to modulate the forgetting gate and output gate. Other studies on medication adherence have also confirmed a strong relationship between time series predictions and patients' clinical history events [21, 22].

In recent years, novel time series forecasting methods have emerged, outperforming traditional approaches across various domains. While research historically focused on univariate time series forecasting, which analyzes temporal dependencies in individual measurements, practical applications often involve multivariate time series forecasting, where interconnected variables are more prevalent. With the rapid growth of deep learning, researchers are increasingly turning to deep learning models to address time series forecasting challenges. Deep learning models excel at data modeling and representation, often yielding superior results compared to traditional models [23]. Presently, significant research efforts are directed towards Transformer models, which hold great promise [24, 30–33]. However, Transformer models [25], known for self-attention mechanism, excel at modeling autocorrelation within individual sequences but may overlook dependencies between variables in different dimensions. Unlike univariate time series forecasting, the complexity of multivariate time series forecasting arises from potential interactions among data features across different dimensions, rather than just focusing on autocorrelation within individual sequences.

To that end, this paper utilizes the Bi-LSTM model and Crossformer model to explore the use of time series prediction models to mine essential indicators of gout patients. The data is 896 real outpatient medical records of 160 patients from Guangdong Provincial Traditional Chinese Medicine Hospital. The models can effectively predict the interval period and acute phase of the patients, which have dramatic effects on patients' life quality and also serve as a certain reference for clinical medication arrangement and treatment.

The main contributions of this paper lie in the three aspects:

1) To the best of our knowledge, this is the first application of time series prediction models on forecasting recurrence and changes in physiological indicators among patients with gouty arthritis.
2) Through applying the Bi-LSTM model, the accuracy in predicting the recurrence status of patients with gouty arthritis reaches 87%. These results can assist healthcare professionals in devising proactive treatment plans for patients, offering valuable insights for clinical practice.
3) In comparison to the latest state-of-the-art models in recent years, the Crossformer model exhibits outstanding performance, showcasing an improvement ranging from 5% to 25% in predicting the physiological indicators of patients with gouty arthritis.

2 The Methodology

2.1 The Overall Framework

The overall framework of application of time series prediction model for the diagnosis and treatment of gouty arthritis is shown in Fig. 1. The clinical indicator data and patient recurrence status dataset are extracted from clinical electronic medical records (EMR) and patient tracking log first. Then the data pre-processing mainly aims at combining the indicator data and the recurrence status dataset. Each indicator data of the patients should be matched with the recurrence status of the specific patient at the specific time, to form the series data. Afterwards, the series data is sent to the models. Two models are applied, the Bi-LSTM model and the Crossformer model. Both models are time series prediction models trained for the prediction of certain time series data.

2.2 LSTM Model

Long Short-Term Memory recurrent neural network (LSTM) is a classical recurrent neural network (RNN) structure used to handle modeling and prediction tasks for sequence data. LSTM introduces a gating mechanism based on common RNN. Through these gating mechanisms, LSTM can better capture long-term dependencies, effectively avoid the problems of gradient disappearance and gradient explosion, and achieve better performance in sequence modeling tasks. The structure of a single LSTM unit is shown

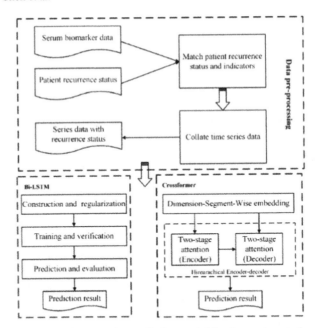

Fig. 1. The framework of time series prediction model for the treatment of gouty arthritis.

in Fig. 2. In the structure, b_f, b_i, b_o, and b_a respectively represent the bias weight of the forget gate, input gate, output gate and the feature extraction process; x_t represents the input of the moment t, $C(t-1)$ and $C(t)$ respectively represents the cell state of the moment $t-1$ and the moment t, h_{t-1} and h_t respectively represents the state of the hidden layer of the moment $t-1$ and t.

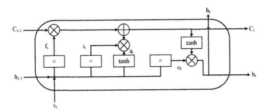

Fig. 2. The structure of a single LSTM unit.

The core idea of LSTM is to guide the flow of information and update memory through three gate control units (input gate, forget gate and output gate). Specifically, the LSTM contains the following key components:

(1) Cell State: The cell state is a memory unit in LSTM, a line running through the model that is mainly used to store and transmit information of hidden states. The cell state is updated at each time step according to the input gate, the forget gate and the extracted feature. The update of the cell state is shown in Eq. (1). $i(t), f(t)$ and

$a(t)$ respectively represent the computational content of the input gate, the forget gate, and the feature extraction.

$$C(t) = C(t-1) \odot f(t) + i(t) \odot a(t) \qquad (1)$$

(2) Input Gate: The updating of the neuron state is controlled by the input gate. A combination of the Sigmoid activation function and the tangent hyperbolic activation function is used to determine what information needs to be updated. As shown in Eq. (2), the tanh function is used to extract the valid information in the current input, while the Sigmoid function determines the information that needs to be added to the cell state through Eq. (3). Under the joint action of the two, the input gate of LSTM will screen and grade the extracted effective information component. The tangent hyperbolic function represented in Eq. (2) is shown in Eq. (4). The activation function Sigmoid represented in Eq. (3) is shown in Eq. (5). W_i and W_a represent the weight coefficients of h_{t-1} and x_t respectively of the input gate and feature extraction process.

$$a(t) = \tanh(W_a \cdot [h_{t-1}, x_t] + b_a) \qquad (2)$$

$$i(t) = \sigma(W_i \cdot [h_{t-1}, x_t] + b_i) \qquad (3)$$

$$\tanh(x) = \frac{1 - e^{-2x}}{1 + e^{-2x}} \qquad (4)$$

$$\sigma(x) = \frac{1}{1 + e^{-x}} \qquad (5)$$

(3) Forget Gate: The information that needs to be forgotten in the cell state at the previous moment is determined by the forget gate. It compresses the input to the interval of $(0,1)$ through the Sigmoid activation function, and forgets the information by judging the result of multiplying the cell state and the output of the forget gate at the previous time. The process of filtering using the Sigmoid function in the forgetting gate is described in Eq. (6). W_f represents the weight coefficient of h_{t-1} and x_t of the forget gate.

$$f(t) = \sigma(W_f \cdot [h_{t-1}, x_t] + b_f) \qquad (6)$$

(4) Output Gate: The information that needs to be output in the cell state at the current moment is determined by the output gate. This part of the information is determined by the Sigmoid activation function, and the cell state is multiplied by the output of the output gate to obtain the final output of LSTM. The calculation process of the output gate is described in Eq. (7). W_o represents the weight coefficient of h_{t-1} and x_t of the output gate. The final state of the hidden layer at the moment t is represented in Eq. (8), which is calculated from the output gate and the cell state at the current time. $\odot$ is the Hardmard Product.

$$o(t) = \sigma(W_o \cdot [h_{t-1}, x_t] + b_o) \qquad (7)$$

$$h(t) = o(t) \odot \tanh(C(t)) \qquad (8)$$

2.3 Bi-LSTM Model

Although the traditional LSTM has some improvement in solving the problems of gradient vanishing and gradient explosion, it still has some limitations, such as large number of parameters and high computational complexity. With the development of deep learning, some improved LSTM variants (such as Bidirectional LSTM, Gated Recurrent Unit, Mogrifier LSTM, etc.) have been proposed to further improve the performance of the model.

Bidirectional Long short-term memory recurrent neural network (Bi-LSTM) is an extended RNN structure used to handle modeling and prediction tasks of sequence data. Compared to traditional LSTM, Bi-LSTM [26] introduces an additional reverse LSTM layer, allowing information to be passed bi-directionally from the past to the future and from the future to the past at the same time. The double layers better fulfill the task of capturing contextual information.

Bi-LSTM has a good performance in sequence modeling tasks, especially for tasks that need to consider contextual information, such as language modeling, named entity recognition, sentiment analysis, etc. Bi-LSTM can capture dependencies and patterns in sequences more accurately. The input layer in Bi-LSTM indicates the input of each unit, and x_t is the input of the time. The output layer indicates the output of each unit, and o_t is the output of the time. The timing information t of the time is represented by h_t and $h_{t'}$. The unit structure of Bi-LSTM is shown in Fig. 3.

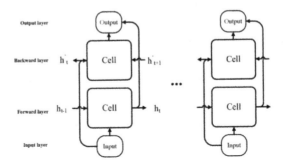

Fig. 3. The structure of a Bi-LSTM unit.

Compared with LSTM, Bi-LSTM has stronger modeling ability, but correspondingly has higher computational complexity. Several differences between LSTM and Bi-LSTM are as follows: information flow direction, parameter number, hidden states and output representation.

(1) Direction of information flow: In LSTM, information can only be transmitted one way from the past to the future in time series; An additional layer of reverse LSTM is introduced in Bi-LSTM, making it possible for information to be passed bi-directionally from past to future and from the future to the past at the same time, so that the model can take advantage of both the past and the future contextual information.

(2) Number of parameters: LSTM has only one layer in one direction, so the number of parameters is relatively small; Bi-LSTM contains a forward LSTM layer and a reverse LSTM layer, so the number of parameters is relatively large.

(3) Hidden states: The hidden states of LSTM only contain the information of the current time step; The hidden states of the Bi-LSTM are composed of the hidden states of the forward LSTM layer and reverse LSTM layer, with information of both the past and the future hidden states contained. Equation (9) and (10) show the use of the past and the future information by Bi-LSTM. h_{t-1}, h_t, h'_t and h'_{t+1} respectively represent the timing information of a time $t-1$ on the forward LSTM layer, the timing information of the time t on the forward LSTM layer, the timing information of the time t on the reverse LSTM layer, and the timing information of the next time $t+1$ on the reverse LSTM layer. ω_{if}, ω_f, ω_{ib} and ω_b respectively represent the weight coefficient of information from the input layer to the forward LSTM layer, the weight coefficient of the forward LSTM layer, the weight coefficient of the input layer to the reverse LSTM layer, and the weight coefficient of the reverse LSTM layer.

$$h_t = f(\omega_{if} x_t + \omega_f h_{t-1}) \tag{9}$$

$$h'_t = f(\omega_{ib} x_t + \omega_b h'_{t+1}) \tag{10}$$

(4) Output representation: The output of Bi-LSTM is a combination of forward LSTM layer and reverse LSTM layer outputs, with both the past and the future predictions contained. The output representation of Bi-LSTM is shown in Eq. (11). ω_{fo} and ω_{bo} respectively represents the weight coefficients from the forward LSTM layer to the output layer and the weight coefficients from the reverse LSTM layer to the output layer.

$$o_t = g(\omega_{fo} h_t + \omega_{bo} h'_t) \tag{11}$$

2.4 Crossformer Model

In multivariate time series forecasting, the goal is to predict future values of a time series at a specific time point $x_{T+1:T+\tau} \in \mathbb{R}^{\tau \times D}$ based on historical data $x_{1:T} \in \mathbb{R}^{T \times D}$, where the number of future and past time steps is denoted by τ and T, and D represents the number of variables. Improved predictive accuracy is often achieved when variables exhibit correlation. The Crossformer model [27] comprises three main components: the Dimension-Segment-Wise (DSW) embedding layer, the Two-Stage Attention (TSA) layer, and the Hierarchical Encoder-Decoder (HED) [28] architecture. The DSW embedding represents multivariate time series, the TSA layer captures dependencies among embedded segments, and the HED architecture combines these components to utilize information and features from various dimensions for the prediction task.

2.4.1 Dimension-Segment-Wise-Embedding

Traditional Transformer-based models for multivariate time series forecasting embedded data points into vectors to capture temporal dependencies, but failed to capture dependencies across variable dimensions, constraining predictive performance.

In Dimension-Segment-Wise (DSW), data within each dimension is divided into segments L_{seg} of a specific length L for embedding, resulting in a two-dimensional vector array $H = \left\{ h_{i,d} | 1 \le i \le \frac{T}{L_{seg}}, 1 \le d \le D \right\}$. Each vector $h_{i,d}$ in the array represents a univariate time series, created through operations like linear projection and positional embeddings. Notably, the projection matrix $E \in \mathbb{R}^{d \mod el \times L_{seg}}$ and positional embeddings $E_{i,d}^{(pos)} \in \mathbb{R}^{d \mod el}$ are trainable components.

$$x_{1:T} = \left\{ x_{i,d}^{(s)} | 1 \le i \le \frac{T}{seg}, 1 \le d \le D \right\} \tag{12}$$

$$x_{i,d}^{(s)} = \left\{ x_{t,d} | (i-1) \times L_{seg} < t \le i \times L_{seg} \right\} \tag{13}$$

$$h_{i,d} = E x_{i,d}^{(s)} + E_{i,d}^{(pos)} \tag{14}$$

2.4.2 Two-Stage Attention

Cross-Time Stage. The TSA layer accepts a 2D array labeled as $Z \in \mathbb{R}^{L \times D \times d \mod el}$, with dimensions L and D. Z can be acquired from DSW embedding or preceding TSA layers. For the sake of simplicity in notation, $Z_{i,:}$ signifies the vectors at the time step i, while $Z_{:,d}$ signifies those spanning all time steps in dimension d. Throughout the cross-time stage, multi-head self-attention is employed individually for each dimension. The calculation is shown in Eq. (15) and (16).

$$\hat{Z}_{:,d}^{time} = LayerNorm\left(Z_{i,:} + MSA^{time}(Z_{:,d}, Z_{:,d}, Z_{:,d}) \right) \tag{15}$$

$$Z^{time} = LayerNorm\left(\hat{Z}^{time} + MLP(\hat{Z}^{time}) \right) \tag{16}$$

LayerNorm is a commonly utilized layer normalization method. MLP stands for a multi-layer feedforward network (in this scenario, featuring two layers). MSA(Q, K, V) indicates the multi-head self-attention layer. All dimensions collectively employ a shared multi-head attention layer.

Cross-dimension Stage. A limited number of nodes are selected as routing nodes to gather information from dimensions before distribution, effectively reducing the complexity to $O(D * L)$, as calculated in Eq. (17), (18), and (19).

$$B_{i,:} = MSA_1^{dim}(R_{i,:}, Z_{i,:}^{time}, Z_{i,:}^{time}), 1 \le i \le L \tag{17}$$

$$\overline{Z}_{i,:}^{dim} = MSA_2^{dim}(Z_{i,:}^{time}, B_{i,:}, B_{i,:}), 1 \le i \le L \tag{18}$$

$$\hat{Z}^{dim} = LayerNorm(Z^{time} + \overline{Z}^{dim}) \tag{19}$$

$$Z^{dim} = LayerNorm\left((\hat{Z}^{dim} + MLP(\hat{Z}^{dim})) \right) \tag{20}$$

$R_{i,:} \in \mathbb{R}^{c \times d_{\text{model}}}$ functions as a learnable vector with the role of a router, serving as the query for the initial multi-head self-attention (MSA) module. In the subsequent MSA, $B_{i,:} \in \mathbb{R}^{c \times d_{\text{model}}}$ takes on the roles of both the key and value, effectively consolidating messages from all dimensions. Both MSA_1^{dim} and MSA_2^{dim} maintain consistency across all time steps, and the resulting output of the Cross-dimension Stage is labeled as Z^{dim}.

To achieve the ultimate TSA output, the results from both the Cross-time Stage and the Cross-dimension Stage are combined through summation, as outlined in Eq. (21). This integration ensures the capture of dependencies spanning across both time and dimensions.

$$Y = Z^{\text{dim}} = TSA(Z) \tag{21}$$

2.4.3   Hierarchical Encoder-Decoder

The Crossformer employs a Hierarchical architecture to handle multi-scale information, with lower layers processing smaller-scale vectors and upper layers handling larger-scale vectors. It integrates predictions from different scales to generate the final output. In the Encoder, starting from the second layer, adjacent vectors in the temporal domain are merged to create a coarse-level representation. The TSA (Two Stage Attention) layer captures dependencies at this scale, as shown in Eq. (22) and (23).

$$\begin{cases} \hat{Z}^{enc,l} = H & \text{if } l = 1 \\ \hat{Z}_{i,d}^{enc,l} = M\left[Z_{2i-1,d}^{enc,l-1} \cdot Z_{2i,d}^{enc,l-1}\right], \ 1 \le i \le \frac{L_{l-1}}{2}, \ 1 \le d \le D & \text{if } l > 1 \end{cases} \tag{22}$$

$$Z^{enc,l} = TSA(\hat{Z}^{enc,l}) \tag{23}$$

The Decoder employs $N + 1$ layers to process the $N + 1$ feature arrays generated by the Encoder. It assigns an index ranging from 0 to N, with each layer represented as l. Each layer takes the l-th encoding array as its input and produces a distinctive two-dimensional decoding array specific to that layer. This calculation process is elucidated in Eq. (24), (25), (26) and (27). Subsequently, the final result is output through a linear layer, as delineated in Eq. (28), (29) and (30).

$$\begin{cases} \tilde{Z}^{enc,l} = TSA(E^{(dec)}) & \text{if } l = 0 \\ \tilde{Z}^{dec,l} = TSA(Z^{dec,l-1}) & \text{if } l > 0 \end{cases} \tag{24}$$

$$\overline{Z}_{:,d}^{dec,l} = MSA(\tilde{Z}_{:,d}^{dec,l}, Z_{:,d}^{enc,l}, Z_{:,d}^{enc,l}), \ 1 \le d \le D \tag{25}$$

$$\hat{Z}^{dec,l} = LayerNorm(\tilde{Z}^{dec,l} + \overline{Z}^{dec,l}) \tag{26}$$

$$Z^{dec,l} = LayerNorm\left(\hat{Z}^{dec,l} + MLP(\hat{Z}^{dec,l})\right) \tag{27}$$

$$x_{i,d}^{(s),l} = W^l Z_{i,d}^{dec,l} \tag{28}$$

$$x_{T+1:T+\tau}^{pred,l} = \left\{ x_{i,d}^{(s),l} \big| 1 \le i \le \frac{\tau}{L_{seg}}, \ 1 \le d \le D \right\} \tag{29}$$

$$x^{pred}_{T+1:T+\tau} = \sum_{l=0}^{N} x^{pred,l}_{T+1:T+\tau} \tag{30}$$

3 Experiment Setups

Dataset. The dataset contains 896 valid data of serum biomarkers from 160 patients diagnosed with gouty arthritis from Guangdong Provincial Hospital of Chinese Medicine from 2020 to 2023. Data Masking (hiding the name and medical card number of the patients) was performed when the data was obtained, and the acquisition and processing of the data did not violate any ethical principles.

The dataset mainly consists of two parts. The first part is the masked serum biomarker data of patients at each examination. The serum biomarker data includes Fasting blood glucose (FBG), alanine aminotransferase (ALT), aspartate aminotransferase (AST), Urea, serum creatinine (Cr), uric acid (UA), Triglycerides, Total cholesterol, high density lipoprotein cholesterol (HDL-C), low density lipoprotein cholesterol (LDL-C), creatine kinase (CK), creatine kinase isoenzyme (CK-MB), lactate dehydrogenase (LDH), glomerular filtration rate (eGFR) and hypersensitive C-reactive protein (hCRP). The data for each patient were arranged chronologically, and each patient had at least two reviews to form the time series data. In the serum biomarker data of the patients, the distribution of patients with different data strips is shown in Fig. 4 below. From the figure, data distribution can be clearly observed where most patients have 7 or more records of the serum biomarker data to form the time series data. Adequate patient data can help improve the prediction effect of the model and reduce errors.

In addition to the serum biomarker data of patients, the second part of the dataset is the patient recurrence status data at the corresponding time period with labeled records. Two kinds of labels are displayed, "Interval Period" and "Acute Phase", and they are used as one of the prediction targets in this paper. The experiment data are the combination of these two original datasets, and pre-processed to time series data. All the time series data are used for the construction and prediction of the Bi-LSTM model and the Crossformer model.

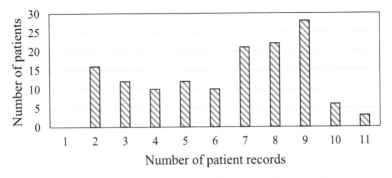

Fig. 4. Number of patient records of the serum biomarker data.

Evaluation Criteria. Mean Square Error (MSE) and Mean Absolute Error (MAE) are standard metrics for time series forecasting, with smaller values denoting closer predictions to the actual values [29].

Baseline Models. In order to assess the performance of the Crossformer model, the following models are compared as baseline methods, including seven of the latest state-of-the-art transformer-based models: Autoformer [30], Nonstationary_Transformer [31], LightTS [32], and Fedformer [33].

4 The Results

4.1 Results of the Bi-LSTM Model

Our results indicate that the Bi-LSTM model can successfully predict the recurrence status of pre-processed clinical time series data. The training effect on this dataset is shown in Fig. 5. The horizontal axis of both figures is the number of epochs, the vertical axis of the left figure is the loss, and the vertical axis of the right figure is the accuracy. The blue and red lines represent the performance of the training and validation sets, respectively. The figure on the left clearly shows that whether it is the training set or the validation set, the loss curve still fluctuates in a small range when the epoch is about 5, but tends to converge after the epoch reaches 10, and the loss is maintained at about 0.35. In the figure on the right, the prediction accuracy of the training set is maintained at about 0.894, while the prediction accuracy of the validation set is maintained at about 0.900.

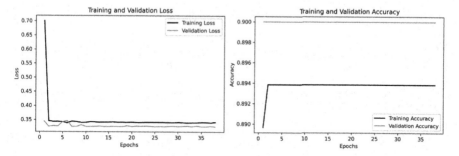

Fig. 5. Loss and accuracy of Bi-LSTM training set and validation set.

The result of the Bi-LSTM model plays an important role in predicting the recurrence status of patients. By introducing a reverse LSTM layer, the Bi-LSTM model can utilize both past and future information to capture context information in time series data. The recurrence status of gouty arthritis patients not only reflected the current physical condition, but also a long-term body state response which needs context information to predict more accurately.

While our data is of large scale by clinical standards of the follow-up of gouty arthritis patients, it is small relative to datasets in other deep learning tasks or prediction models. The discovery and sorting of time series data has always been a difficult point in the search for gouty arthritis patients. The low number of patients who are willing to provide indicator data and make complete records of serum biomarkers is one reason why models such as time series predicting are not best expressed in such data. Data integrity is also a concern. Although this kind of time series data has an insufficient quantity in clinic gouty arthritis, the time series prediction model can still reach good prediction results with more features and parameters that can be referred to. Time series predicting models may perform better in other clinical applications with longer patient data recording cycles.

4.2 Result of the Crossformer Model

The experiment conducted a comparative analysis of the effectiveness of multiple time series forecasting models, with MSE and MAE used as standards for time series prediction results. The experimental results are shown in Table 1. A smaller MSE and MAE indicate that the model's predictions are closer to the ground truth, indicating better prediction performance. The best experimental results for each metric are highlighted in bold.

Compared with other models, Crossformer achieved the top score in both metrics, surpassing the second-ranked LightTS by approximately 5%. Furthermore, compared to the lowest-performing models, Autoformer and Fedformer, it achieved an improvement of around 25%. Overall, the Crossformer model demonstrated excellent performance. The visualization of the data is depicted in Fig. 6. It can be observed that the model fits well in the early stages but gradually deviates in the later stages.

Table 1. Time series forecasting results of different models.

Model	MSE	MAE	Rank
Crossformer	**0.737**	**0.511**	1
Autoformer	0.976	0.633	4
Nonstationary_Transformer	0.870	0.552	3
LightTS	0.768	0.521	2
Fedformer	0.982	0.628	4

In the context of predicting physical detection indicators for gout patients, the Crossformer model, built upon an enhanced Transformer architecture, employs a two-stage attention mechanism. This approach effectively captures cross-temporal dimensions and dependencies among various variables, surpassing other models and providing a closer alignment with real patient scenarios. This predictive capability for gout disease serves as a valuable reference for clinicians in hospitals, aiding in formulating tailored treatment plans to alleviate patient discomfort and facilitate disease management.

Nevertheless, the Crossformer model does exhibit certain limitations. For instance, there is room for improvement in enhancing its capacity to capture trend information

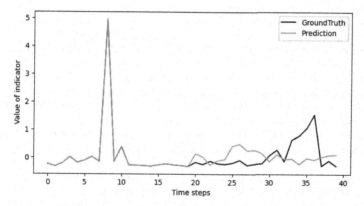

Fig. 6. The forecasting performance of Crossformer.

within the temporal dimension. Additionally, consideration could be given to streamlining the model structure to reduce training time and memory usage. These areas represent potential directions for future enhancements and refinements.

5 Conclusions

Two time series prediction models were used to mine the information from the indicators to predict recurrence status and changes in serum biomarkers from gouty arthritis patients. The displayed prediction results and evaluation of both Bi-LSTM and Crossformer models show the suitableness of time series prediction model for this dataset. The Bi-LSTM model shows that the accuracy of predicting the recurrence status of patients can reach 87%. The Crossformer model outperforms other models in gout prediction, demonstrating a notable improvement of 5% to 25% in both MSE and MAE evaluation metrics. Furthermore, the predicted results exhibit the highest level of consistency with real-world observations. Through the prediction results of the two models, reference can be provided for the clinical diagnosis and medication of gouty arthritis.

Acknowledgements. This work was supported by grants from National Natural Science Foundation of China (62372189) and the Key-Area Research and Development Program of Guangdong Province (2020B1111100010).

References

1. Chen, W., et al.: Discovering combination patterns of traditional chinese medicine for the treatment of gouty arthritis with renal dysfunction. In: Tang, B., et al. (eds.) Health Information Processing. CHIP 2022. Communications in Computer and Information Science, vol. 1772, pp. 170–183 (2022). https://doi.org/10.1007/978-981-19-9865-2_12
2. Kuo, C.F., Luo, S.F.: Risk of premature death in gout unchanged for years. Nat. Rev. Rheumatol. **13**(4), 200–201 (2017)

3. Dehlin, M., Jacobsson, L., Roddy, E.: Global epidemiology of gout: prevalence, incidence, treatment patterns and risk factors. Nat. Rev. Rheumatol. **16**(7), 380–390 (2020)
4. Liu, R., et al.: Prevalence of hyperuricemia and gout in mainland China from 2000 to 2014: a systematic review and meta-analysis. Biomed Res Int. 1–12 (2015)
5. Sheng. F., Fang, W., Zhang, B., Sha, Y., Zeng, X.: Adherence to gout management recommendations of Chinese patients. Medicine (Baltimore). e8532 (2017)
6. Krizhevsky, A., Sutskever, I., Hinton, G.E.: ImageNet classification with deep convolutional neural networks. Commun. ACM 84–90 (2017)
7. Sutskever, I., Vinyals, O., Le, Q.V.: Sequence to sequence learning with neural networks. In: Proceedings of the 27th International Conference on Neural Information Processing Systems, pp. 3104–3112 (2014)
8. Lipton, Z.C., Kale, D.C.: Modeling missing data in clinical time series with RNNs (2016)
9. Zheng, H., Shi, D.: Using a LSTM-RNN based deep learning framework for ICU mortality prediction. In: Meng, X., Li, R., Wang, K., Niu, B., Wang, X., Zhao, G. (eds.) WISA 2018. LNCS, vol. 11242, pp. 60–67. Springer, Cham (2018). https://doi.org/10.1007/978-3-030-02934-0_6
10. Rajkomar, A., et al.: Scalable and accurate deep learning with electronic health records. NPJ Digit Med. **1**, 18 (2018)
11. Suresh, H., Hunt, N., Johnson, A., Celi, L.A., Szolovits, P., Ghassemi, M.: Clinical intervention prediction and understanding with deep neural networks, pp. 332–337 (2017)
12. Aczon, M., Ledbetter, D., Ho, L., Gunny, A., Flynn, A., Williams, J.: Dynamic mortality risk predictions in pediatric critical care using recurrent neural networks, pp. 519–529 (2017)
13. Choi, E., Bahadori, M.T., Schuetz, A., Stewart, W.F., Sun, J.: Doctor AI: predicting clinical events via recurrent neural networks, pp. 301–318 (2015)
14. Harutyunyan, H., Khachatrian, H., Kale, D.C., Steeg, G.V., Galstyan, A.: Multitask learning and benchmarking with clinical time series data. Sci. Data. **6**, 96 (2019)
15. Hochreiter, S., Schmidhuber, J.: Long short-term memory. Neural Comput. **9**, 1735–1780 (1997)
16. Graves, A., Schmidhuber, J.: Framewise phoneme classification with bidirectional LSTM and other neural network architectures. Neural Netw. **18**(5–6), 602–610 (2005)
17. Xia, P., Hu, J., Peng, Y.: EMG-based estimation of limb movement using deep learning with recurrent convolutional neural networks. Artif. Organs **42**(5), E67–E77 (2018)
18. Xu, Y., Biswal, S., Deshpande, S.R., Maher, K.O.: RAIM: recurrent attentive and intensive model of multimodal patient monitoring data. In: KDD 2018-Proceedings of the 24th ACM SIGKDD International Conference on Knowledge Discovery and Data Mining, pp. 2565–2573 (2018)
19. Lipton, Z.C., Kale, D.C., Elkan, C., Wetzel, R.: Learning to diagnose with LSTM recurrent neural networks. Compu. Sci. (2017)
20. Pham, T., Tran, T., Phung, D., Venkatesh, S.: DeepCare: a deep dynamic memory model for predictive medicine. In: Bailey, J., Khan, L., Washio, T., Dobbie, G., Huang, J.Z., Wang, R. (eds.) PAKDD 2016. LNCS (LNAI), vol. 9652, pp. 30–41. Springer, Cham (2016). https://doi.org/10.1007/978-3-319-31750-2_3
21. Hu, F., Warren, J., Exeter, D.J.: Interrupted time series analysis on first cardiovascular disease hospitalization for adherence to lipid-lowering therapy. Pharmacoepidemiol. Drug Safety **29**(2), 150–160 (2020)
22. Pietrzykowski, Ł., et al.: Medication adherence and its determinants in patients after myocardial infarction. Sci. Rep. **10**(1), 12028 (2020)
23. Ruan T., et al.: Representation learning for clinical time series prediction tasks in electronic health records. BMC Med. Inform. Decis. Making 259 (2019)
24. Wen, Q., et al.: Transformers in time series: a survey. In: International Joint Conference on Artificial Intelligence (2022)

25. Vaswani, A., et al.: Attention is all you need, pp. 6000–6010 (2023)
26. Tan, Y., Huang, J., Zhuang, J., Huang, H., Liu, Y., Yu, X.: Identification of sepsis subpheno-types based on bi-directional long short-term memory auto-encoder using real-time laboratory data collected from intensive care units. In: Tang, B., et al. Health information processing. CHIP 2022. Communications in Computer and Information Science, vol. 1772, pp. 124–134. Springer, Cham (2023). https://doi.org/10.1007/978-981-19-9865-2_9
27. Zhang, Y., Yan, J.: Crossformer: transformer utilizing cross-dimension dependency for mul-tivariate time series forecasting. In: International Conference on Learning Representations (2023)
28. Tong, J., Xie, L., Yang, W., Zhang, K., Zhao, J.: Enhancing time series forecasting: a hier-archical transformer with probabilistic decomposition representation. Inf. Sci. **647**, 119410 (2023)
29. Zhou, H., et al.: Informer: beyond efficient transformer for long sequence time-series fore-casting. In: Proceedings of the AAAI Conference on Artificial Intelligence, pp. 11106–11115 (2021)
30. Wu, H., Xu, J., Wang, J., Long, M.: Autoformer: decomposition transformers with auto-correlation for long-term series forecasting. In: Advances in Neural Information Processing Systems, pp. 22419–22430 (2021)
31. Liu, Y., Wu, H., Wang, J., Long, M.: Non-stationary transformers: exploring the stationarity in time series forecasting. In: Advances in Neural Information Processing Systems, pp. 9881–9893 (2022)
32. Zhang, T., et al.: Less is more: fast multivariate time series forecasting with light sampling-oriented MLP structures (2023)
33. Zhou, T., Ma, Z., Wen, Q., Wang, X., Sun, L., Jin, R.: FEDformer: frequency enhanced decomposed transformer for long-term series forecasting. In: International Conference on Machine Learning. PMLR, pp. 27268–27286 (2022)

Asymptomatic Carriers are Associated with Shorter Negative Conversion Time in Children with Omicron Infections

Jianzhi Yan[2,3], Yang Xiang[2], Yang Zhou[1], Sicen Liu[3], Jinghua Wang[1,4], Fang Li[5], Siyuan Wang[1], Man Rao[1], Chuanchuan Yang[1], Buzhou Tang[2,3], and Hongzhou Lu[1(✉)]

[1] Shenzhen Third People's Hospital, Shenzhen, Guangdong, China
yangzhou@szsy.sustech.edu.cn, luhongzhou@fudan.edu.cn
[2] Peng Cheng Laboratory, Shenzhen, China
{yanjzh,xiangy}@pcl.ac.cn
[3] Harbin Institute of Technology at Shenzhen, Shenzhen, Guangdong, China
18b951039@stu.hit.edu.cn
[4] Tianjin Medical University General Hospital, Tianjin, China
jwang3@tmu.edu.cn
[5] University of Texas Health Science Center at Houston, Houston, TX, USA
fang.li@uth.tmc.edu

Abstract. Objective: Among the Omicron carriers, asymptomatic ones should be paid close attention to due to their silence in clinical symptoms and uncertainty in secondary transmission. The clinical characteristics associated with viral shedding of asymptomatic patients need to be carefully investigated especially for children. Methods: We revisited the clinical data from 471 pediatric patients who have been infected with the SARS-CoV-2 Omicron variant in 2022. The cases were divided into symptomatic and asymptomatic groups according to clinical manifestations. Descriptive analysis and survival analysis were applied for the comparison between the groups. Results: A total number of 333 patients were selected out of the original 471 children according to certain eligibility criteria, which resulted in 192 (57.7%) symptomatic and 141 (42.3%) asymptomatic cases. According to the univariate analysis, we discovered that the asymptomatic carriers had significantly shorter negative conversion time (NCT) (10 ± 8 days) compared with the symptomatic ones (14 ± 7 days) ($p < 0.001$). Conclusion: The NCT of asymptomatic patients, is shorter than the symptomatic ones, signifying that the asymptomatic patients may be equipped with shorter periods of self- or centralized isolation. These results could provide important implications for future policy-making or anti-virus treatment to lower the overall transmission risk to society.

Keywords: Omicron · Asymptomatic · Negative Conversion · Survival Analysis · Children

---

J. Yan, Y. Xiang, Y. Zhou and S. Liu—These authors share the first authorship.

H. Xu et al. (Eds.): CHIP 2023, CCIS 1993, pp. 420–430, 2024.
https://doi.org/10.1007/978-981-99-9864-7_27

1 Introduction

Starting from the end of 2021, Omicron has become one of the predominated variants of severe acute respiratory syndrome coronavirus-2 (SARS-CoV-2) and the infections have exploded worldwide [1]. A study from Shanghai, China shows that in the last year's largest Omicron wave in Shanghai (April-June, 2022), 94.3% of cases were asymptomatic [2]. Researchers found that the incidence rate of Omicron was 6 to 8 times that of the Delta variant in children younger than 5 years old [3]. Accelerating the negative conversion of SARS-CoV-2 for patients is beneficial in reducing the risk of secondary viral transmission [4]. However, systematic research on asymptomatic pediatric patients infected with Omicron remains lacking, and the corresponding information regarding the clinical manifestations and outcomes is still limited. Clinicians usually evaluate the virus infectivity for rapid antigen testing by RT-PCR cycle threshold (Ct) of nucleocapsid protein (N gene) and open reading frame 1ab (ORF1ab) values [5]. The corresponding Ct values and negative conversion time (NCT) of N genes and ORF1ab are significant indicators in determining the discharge criteria during hospitalization or centralized quarantine [6, 7]. Therefore, we carefully considered the aforementioned immunologic factors during our analyses.

In this study, we carried out a retrospective study to analyze the clinical characteristics of a pediatric cohort aged between 1 and 12 years. Attention was especially paid to the asymptomatic cases who were diagnosed with SARS-CoV-2, and Omicron but without any relevant clinical symptoms before hospitalization. Univariate and multivariate analyses were conducted to investigate the clinical outcomes among different groups to benefit the understanding of NCT and reduce the transmission risk of asymptomatic pediatric patients. We experimentally proved the existence of varying NCTs between different groups, hoping that our findings could provide useful implications for the precise prevention and control of the disease.

2 Method

2.1 Cohort Selection

This retrospective cohort study was conducted on 471 children aged between 1 and 12 years infected with SARS-CoV-2 Omicron (BA.2) who have been admitted to Shenzhen Third People's Hospital, China, between February 14, 2022, and April 14, 2022, for centralized isolation and clinical treatment. Patients diagnosed with SARS-CoV-2 were based on the positive RT-PCR SARS-CoV-2 testing results from the oropharyngeal and nasal swabs test. A total number of 333 patients were selected out of the original 471 children according to certain eligibility criteria, which resulted in 192 (57.7%) symptomatic and 141 (42.3%) asymptomatic cases. This study was approved by the Institutional Review Board (IRB) of the Shenzhen Third People's Hospital, China. All participants have been informed of the potential benefits, risks, and alternatives associated with this research.

2.2 Group and Variable Definitions

The clinical characteristics and laboratory test results were collected from the record of each patient. The clinical characteristics include demographic information (sex, age), vaccination status (including doses), and clinical manifestations (including cough, fever, sore throat, runny nose, nasal congestion, weak, bellyache, and vomiting). The laboratory test results include white blood cell count (WBC), lymphocytes (LYMPH), platelets (PLT), prothrombin time (PT), albumin (ALB), Natriuretic Peptide Tests (NT-proBNP), IgM antibody (IgM) and IgG antibody values (IgG), IL6, Ct values for ORF1ab (ORF1ab_Ct) and N gene (N_Ct), etc. Empty values were imputed using the CART algorithm to ensure consistency in distribution [8]. The symptomatic group was identified according to the chief complaint upon admission to the hospital. Cases with a record of any aforementioned clinical manifestations are considered symptomatic. The discharge criteria are defined as the Ct values of both N genes and ORF1ab are higher than 35. The NCT is subsequently identified as the latter time for the satisfaction of the two Ct values. Thus, the negative conversion period is defined as the duration between admission and NCT[1]. The age was stratified into two groups, i.e. $1 \leq QUOTE \leq age \leq QUOTE \leq 6$ and $6 < age \leq 12$.

2.3 Statistical Analyses

In the univariate analysis, the continuous variables which satisfy normal distribution (according to the Shapiro-Wilk normality test) were expressed as the mean and standard deviation (SD) and others as the median and interquartile range (IQR). Categorical variables were described as numbers (percentages). Comparisons between groups (p-values) were estimated by univariate analyses, i.e. Chi-square test for categorical variables, and t-test and Wilcoxon Rank sum test for continuous variables. The risks of asymptomatic or symptomatic manifestations in regard to NCT were estimated using a Kaplan-Meier method that can be used with time-varying covariates. Propensity score matching (1:1 matching according to the clinical variables with the "nearest" matching strategy) and multivariate Cox proportional hazards regression (Hazard ratio [HR] and 95% confidence interval [CI]) were further leveraged to estimate the risk of negative conversion comparing the asymptomatic with the symptomatic group. All analyses were conducted using RStudio with R version 4.1.2. Two-sided p-values less than 0.05 were considered statistically significant.

3 Method

3.1 Cohort Characteristics

Among the 333 cases, 192 belong to the symptomatic group, and 141 belong to the asymptomatic group.

The characteristics of these patients are listed in Table 1. For the unmatched cohort, this descriptive analysis demonstrates that male (p = 0.037) and younger aged patients

---

[1] We use NCT to denote the negative conversion period for simplicity below.

Table 1. .

Features	Asymptomatic	Symptomatic	p-value	Symptomatic	p-value
		Before PSM		After 1:1 PSM	
Cases, n (%)	141 (42.3)	192 (57.7)		141	
Sex, n (%)			*0.037**		0.339
male	72 (51.1)	120 (62.5)		80 (56.7)	
female	69 (48.9)	72 (37.5)		61 (43.3)	
Age group, n (%)			*0.027**		0.074
≤ 6	65 (46.1)	112 (58.3)		80 (56.7)	
>6	76 (53.9)	80 (41.7)		61 (43.3)	
Vaccination, n (%)			0.134		0.302
unvaccinated	78 (55.3)	127 (66.1)		90 (63.8)	
vaccinated (1 dose)	34 (24.1)	35 (18.2)		25 (17.7)	
boosted (2 doses)	29 (20.6)	30 (15.6)		26 (18.4)	
vaccinated (1 dose + 2 doses)	63 (44.7)	65 (33.9)		51 (36.2)	
SNI, n (%)			0.63		0.812
No	66 (46.8)	95 (49.5)		71 (50.4)	
Yes	75 (53.2)	97 (50.5)		70 (49.6)	
Laboratory results					
WBC ($\times 10^9$/L), median (IQR)	6.6 (5.2, 8.5)	5.5 (4.6, 7.6)	*0.001***	5.6 (4.7, 7.9)	*0.029**
LYMPH ($\times 10^9$/L), median (IQR)	2.7 (1.9, 3.8)	2.4 (1.4, 3.4)	*0.02**	2.6 (1.8, 3.6)	0.321
PLT ($\times 10^9$/L), median (IQR)	286 (229, 342)	256 (212.8, 306)	*0.015**	270 (221, 323)	0.21
AST(g/L), median (IQR)	35.2 (28.9, 41.9)	37.5 (31.2, 45.4)	*0.002***	36.3 (29.7, 43)	0.25
ALB (g/L), mean (SD)	44.9 (43.1, 47.8)	45.1 (43.4, 46.9)	0.7	45.3 (43.4, 46.9)	0.856
PT(second), median (IQR)	13.5 (0.7)	13.7 (0.8)	0.132	13.6 (0.7)	0.414
NT.proBNP(pg/m), median (IQR)	34.8 (19.3, 68.1)	36.9 (18.5, 76.6)	0.621	34.8 (16.9, 72)	0.794
IgM (g/L), median (IQR)	1.1 (0.3, 3.1)	0.5 (0.2, 1.5)	*0.001***	0.6 (0.2, 2)	*0.044**

(*continued*)

Table 1. (*continued*)

Features	Asymptomatic	Symptomatic	p-value	Symptomatic	p-value
IgG (g/L), median (IQR)	44.4 (0.6, 108.3)	7.2 (0.3, 55.5)	*<0.001****	16.7 (0.4, 68.3)	*0.012**
IL6 (pg/ml), median (IQR)	6.9 (2.6, 11)	7.4 (4.1, 12.6)	0.073	7.4 (5, 12.6)	0.103
N_Ct, median (IQR)	36.6 (35.1, 37.8)	35.8 (33.4, 37.3)	*0.002***	36.4 (34.5, 37.6)	0.279
ORF1ab_Ct, median (IQR)	36.7 (31.4, 38.6)	35.3 (31.1, 37.9)	0.069	35.7 (31.2, 38.1)	0.2
NCT of N gene (day), median (IQR)	7 (1, 15)	13 (9, 17)	*<0.001****	13 (9, 17)	*<0.001****
NCT of ORF1ab (day), median (IQR)	4 (0, 12)	11 (7, 14)	*<0.001****	11 (8, 14)	*<0.001****
NCT, median (IQR)	10 (3, 16)	14 (11, 18)	*<0.001****	14 (11, 18)	*<0.001****

Significance levels: '***' 0.001 '**' 0.01 '*' 0.05.

($\leq$6) (p = 0.027) are more likely to be symptomatic. There are significant differences in several laboratory results including WBC (p = 0.001), LYMPH (p = 0.02), PLT (p = 0.015), AST (p = 0.002), IgM (p = 0.001), IgG (p < 0.001), and N_Ct (p = 0.002) between the two groups. Specifically, the NCTs of both N genes and ORF1ab in the asymptomatic group are shorter than those in the symptomatic group (p < 0.001), resulting in the overall NCT of the asymptomatic group being significantly shorter (10 [3, 16] days versus 14 days [11, 18], p < 0.001). After PSM, the remaining significant laboratory variables are WBC (p = 0.029), IgM (p = 0.044), and IgG (p = 0.012). And the NCTs still show significant differences (p < 0.001).

3.2 Negative Conversion Rate

The Kaplan-Meier curve showed the different negative conversions between the two groups, and the results are shown in Fig. 1. It is noticed that in the curves of both before (p < 0.001) and after PSM (p = 0.003), the asymptomatic group shows a remarkably faster negative conversion speed compared with the symptomatic counterpart.

3.3 Hazard Ratios of Negative Conversion

After adjusting to the considered variables, the results of Cox proportional hazard models showed the hazard ratio of each factor considering possible confounders. From Fig. 2, we notice that the "asymptomatic" condition is significantly associated with the negative status (1.51 [1.20–1.91], p < 0.001 and 1.49 [1.17–1.91], p = 0.001). In addition,

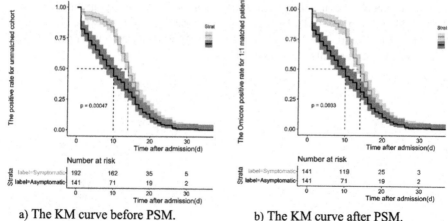

a) The KM curve before PSM.   b) The KM curve after PSM.

Fig. 1. The Kaplan-Meier curves show the different negative conversion speeds between the two exposure groups where the asymptomatic group turns negative faster.

vaccinated one dose (p = 0.017 and p = 0.036), a higher level of IgG (p = 0.049 and p = 0.036), and a lower value of the N gene Ct (p < 0.001) show increasing hazards with negative conversion, both before and after PSM.

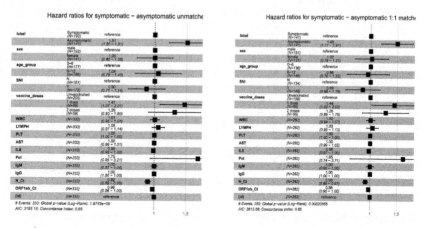

a) The cox result before PSM.   b) The cox result after PSM.

Fig. 2. The forest plot shows hazard ratios generated by the Cox model.

Sensitivity Analysis

We further split the asymptomatic patients into the two defined types (i.e. Type-I: Pre-symptomatic Infection and Type-II: Asymptomatic Infection) and see if there are specifics associated with negative conversion. Through multivariate Cox, we can still observe increasing hazards of the asymptomatic condition with negative conversion among the subcohort consisting of the symptomatic and Type-I asymptomatic patients (1.71 [1.29–2.26], p < 0.001). However, no significant associations were observed for the subcohort consisting of the symptomatic and Type-II asymptomatic patients. The KM curves and Cox results are shown in Figs. 3.

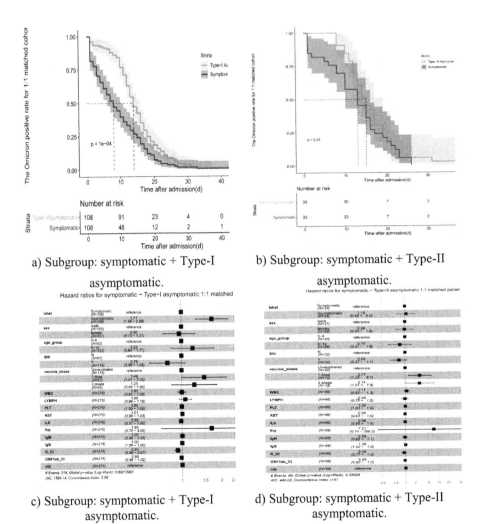

a) Subgroup: symptomatic + Type-I asymptomatic.

b) Subgroup: symptomatic + Type-II asymptomatic.

c) Subgroup: symptomatic + Type-I asymptomatic.

d) Subgroup: symptomatic + Type-II asymptomatic.

Fig. 3. KM curves and Cox results for subcohort analysis.

Since the vaccination of the second dose (the booster) is not quite prevalent among the researched cohort (only 17.7%), it is hard to determine how the vaccination of different doses functions clearly according to the small number of records. Although showing a positive hazard ratio (1.25 and 1.53 before and after PSM), the function of vaccination by two doses is not significant. Thus, we combined the patients vaccinated by one dose and two doses to form a larger group of "vaccinated patients" to verify whether vaccination is associated with faster negative conversion. The adjusted hazard ratio of vaccination generated by the Cox model (after PSM) is 1.36 (1.02–1.81) and p = 0.039, which means that vaccination accelerated the negative conversion (Fig. 4).

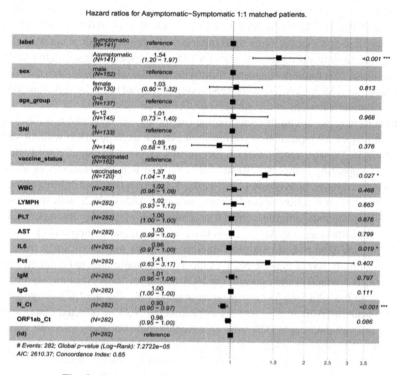

Hazard ratios for Asymptomatic–Symptomatic 1:1 matched patients.

Fig. 4. Cox results after combining the vaccination doses.

4   Discussion

The percentage of asymptomatic infections was 42.3% among pediatric patients in our study, which was higher than that of the general population reported in [9] (32.40% [25.30–39.51%]). In the pooled percentage of asymptomatic infections was 43.75% in the Omicron-positive individuals when the median age is less than 20 years, which was similar to the result in our study. The univariate analysis revealed that the WBC and lymphocytes of the asymptomatic infections are generally higher than those of the symptomatic infections (with minor exceptions). During the same period, the children infected with the Omicron variant with reduced lymphocyte proportion demonstrated a longer time of viral nucleic acid negative conversion in Shanghai [10], which was similar to those discovered in our study. This could be explained by the "cytokine storm" of symptomatic infections. The higher Th1 cytokines including IL-2, IL-8, IL-2, IL-8, IL-12p70, IFN-γ, and TNF-α, as well as Th2 cytokines including IL-10 and IL-13 lead to the depletion of WBC and lymphocytes [11].

We next compared the differences in SARS-CoV2-specific IgM and IgG antibody values and positive rates between symptomatic and asymptomatic infections (Table 1). The IgM value of the asymptomatic group was higher than that of the symptomatic group (1.1 [0.3, 3.1] vs. 0.6 [0.2, 0.2], p = 0.044, after PSM). More significantly, the IgG value of asymptomatic infected children was higher than that of the symptomatic infected children (44.4 [0.6, 108.3] vs. 16.7 [0.4, 68.3], p = 0.012, after PSM). These results may indicate that the virus in asymptomatic infected children can stimulate the immune system to produce higher levels of SARS-CoV2-specific IgM and longer-lasting IgG antibodies. Our findings suggested that asymptomatic infected children may produce higher levels of SARS-CoV2-specific IgM and IgG to avoid body damage, thus affecting the clinical manifestations and clinical type of children.

. In our study, we found that vaccination (including one dose and two doses) raises the possibility of asymptomatic manifestation (46.3% asymptomatic without vaccination versus 55.3% with vaccination), which means vaccination can effectively decrease the risk of appearing symptoms. Results also verified that vaccination was associated with a faster negative conversion (1.37, [1.04–1.80], p = 0.027). Children show some loss of cross-neutralization against all variants of SARS-CoV-2, with the most pronounced loss against Omicron, while vaccination can effectively increase high titers cross-neutralization against Alpha, Beta, Gamma, Delta, and Omicron [11].

The transmission risk of children Omicron infections may be different from that of adults. This study found that the NCT of the asymptomatic infected children averages 10 days (3, 16), which is analogous to the NCT (averages 10 days) of the asymptomatic children with the SARS-CoV-2 infection reported in [12]. But the NCT of symptomatic infected children (average 14 days) is longer than the NCT of infected Omicron adults reported in (6–9 days) [13]. The time of nasopharyngeal/pharyngeal swab viral RNA turning negative was reported as ranging from 6 to 22 days (mean 12 days) in previous research [14]. Compared with the symptomatic infected children, the NCT of asymptomatic infected children was shorter. It indicates that the risk of transmission of asymptomatic infections is lower than that of the symptomatic infections, which is similar to the result of adults in a previous study [15].

Multivariate Cox proportional hazards regression demonstrated that the NCT of asymptomatic infection was inversely correlated with the Ct thresholds of N gene (p < 0.001) and ORF1ab (mildly significant with p-value of 0.066 after PSM) in our research. It showed that even previous studies have summarized that having higher Ct values links to lower amount of viral RNA, which means cases with higher Ct values tend to being asymptomatic [15, 16].

This study has several limitations. Firstly, the study found that vaccination is more prone to asymptomatic infection with clinical features, suggesting that vaccination has a protective effect, but we did not further analyze more stratified situations. Secondly, there is a proportion of empty values in the data. In addition, symptomatic and asymptomatic children also have the risk of Long COVID disease. There is an urgent to build a follow-up survey of those children to investigate the risk of long COVID.

5 Conclusion

We conducted a systematic analysis of children infected with Omicron and found that the NCT of asymptomatic patients, is shorter than the symptomatic ones, signifying that the asymptomatic patients may be equipped with shorter periods of self- or centralized isolation, in front of determining the measures to prevent community transmission. It is also confirmed that vaccination assists in the acceleration of negative conversion. These results could provide important implications for future policy-making, e.g. informing targeted isolation periods, to lower the overall transmission risk to society.

Acknowledgment. This work is partially funded by the National Natural Science Foundation of China (Grant Number: 62106115), the Shenzhen Science and Technology Plan Project (No. JCYJ20210324132012035) and Guangdong Medical Science and Technology Research Fund (No. A2023455).

References

1. Karim, S.S.A., Karim, Q.A.: Omicron SARS-CoV-2 variant: a new chapter in the COVID-19 pandemic. Lancet **398**, 2126–2128 (2021)
2. Huang, L.: Adjusted control rate closely associated with the epidemiologic evolution of the recent COVID-19 wave in Shanghai, with 94.3% of all new cases being asymptomatic on first diagnosis. J. Infect. **85**, e89–e91 (2022)
3. Wang, L., Berger, N.A., Kaelber, D.C., et al.: Incidence rates and clinical outcomes of SARS-CoV-2 infection with the omicron and delta variants in children younger than 5 years in the US. JAMA Pediatr. **176**, 811–813 (2022)
4. Zhou, L.-K., Zhou, Z., Jiang, X.-M., et al.: Absorbed plant MIR2911 in honeysuckle decoction inhibits SARS-CoV-2 replication and accelerates the negative conversion of infected patients. Cell Discov. **6**, 54 (2020)
5. Pickering, S., Batra, R., Merrick, B., et al.: Comparative performance of SARS-CoV-2 lateral flow antigen tests and association with detection of infectious virus in clinical specimens: a single-centre laboratory evaluation study. Lancet Microbe **2**, e461–e471 (2021)
6. Chan, J.F.-W., Yip, C.C.-Y,, To, K.K.-W., et al.: Improved molecular diagnosis of COVID-19 by the novel, highly sensitive and specific COVID-19-RdRp/Hel real-time reverse transcription-PCR assay validated in vitro and with clinical specimens. J. Clin. Microbiol **58**, e00310–20 (2020)
7. To, K.K.-W., Tsang, O.T.-Y., Leung, W.-S., et al.: Temporal profiles of viral load in posterior oropharyngeal saliva samples and serum antibody responses during infection by SARS-CoV-2: an observational cohort study. Lancet Infect. Dis. **20**, 565–574 (2020)
8. Doove, L.L., Van Buuren, S., Dusseldorp, E.: Recursive partitioning for missing data imputation in the presence of interaction effects. Comput. Stat. Data Anal. **72**, 92–104 (2014)
9. Shang, W., Kang, L., Cao, G., et al.: Percentage of asymptomatic infections among SARS-CoV-2 omicron variant-positive individuals: a systematic review and meta-analysis. Vaccines **10**, 1049 (2022)
10. Yin, R., Lu, Q., Jiao, J.L., et al.: Characteristics and related factors of viral nucleic acid negative conversion in children infected with Omicron variant strain of SARS-CoV-2. Zhonghua Er Ke Za Zhi 1307–1311 (2022)

11. Tang, J., Novak, T., Hecker, J., et al.: Cross-reactive immunity against the SARS-CoV-2 Omicron variant is low in pediatric patients with prior COVID-19 or MIS-C. Nat. Commun. **13**, 2979 (2022)
12. Yin Rong, L., Quan, J.J., et al.: Characteristics and related factors of viral nucleic acid negative conversion in children infected with Omicron variant strain of SARS-CoV-2. Chin. J. Pediatr. **12**, 1307–1311 (2022)
13. Yin, Y., Lin, J., Yuan, S., et al.: The relationship between early isolation and the duration of viral shedding of mild and asymptomatic infection with SARS-CoV-2 omicron BA. 2 variant. J. Infect. **85**, e184–e186 (2022)
14. Jiehao, C., Jin, X., Daojiong, L., et al.: A case series of children with 2019 novel coronavirus infection: clinical and epidemiological features. Clin. Infect. Dis. **71**, 1547–1551 (2020)
15. Kimball, A., Hatfield, K.M., Arons, M., et al.: Asymptomatic and presymptomatic SARS-CoV-2 infections in residents of a long-term care skilled nursing facility—King County, Washington, March 2020. Morb. Mortal. Wkly Rep. **69**, 377 (2020)
16. Hall, S.M., Landaverde, L., Gill, C.J., et al.: Comparison of anterior nares CT values in asymptomatic and symptomatic individuals diagnosed with SARS-CoV-2 in a university screening program. PLoS ONE **17**, e0270694 (2022)

Author Index

H. Xu et al. (Eds.): CHIP 2023, CCIS 1993, pp. 431–432, 2024.
https://doi.org/10.1007/978-981-99-9864-7

Printed in the United States
by Baker & Taylor Publisher Services